HEADACHE AND OTHER HEAD PAIN

Wolff's
HEADACHE
and other head pain

Edited by
DONALD J. DALESSIO, M.D.
Chairman, Department of Medicine
Senior Consultant, Division of Neurology
Scripps Clinic & Research Foundation
La Jolla, California

FIFTH EDITION

New York   Oxford
OXFORD UNIVERSITY PRESS
1987

Oxford University Press

Oxford   New York   Toronto
Delhi   Bombay   Calcutta   Madras   Karachi
Petaling Jaya   Singapore   Hong Kong   Tokyo
Nairobi   Dar es Salaam   Cape Town
Melbourne   Auckland

and associated companies in
Beirut   Berlin   Ibadan   Nicosia

Published by Oxford University Press, Inc.,
200 Madison Avenue, New York, New York 10016

Oxford is a registered trademark of Oxford University Press

Library of Congress Cataloging-in-Publication Data
Wolff, Harold G. (Harold George), 1898–1962
Wolff's headache and other head pain.
Includes bibliographies and index.
1. Headache.   2. Pain.   I. Dalessio, Donald J., 1931–   .   II. Title.
III. Title: Headache and other head pain. [DNLM: 1. Headache. WL 342 W855h]
RB128.W67   1987   617′.51072   86-23669
ISBN 0-19-504356-1

1 2 3 4 5 6 7 8 9

Printed in the United States of America
on acid-free paper

To Isabel Bishop Wolff
and
Jane Dalessio

PREFACE TO THE FIFTH EDITION

Societies, species, and even diseases evolve and change with time. So it is with this book. The current edition taps the knowledge and wisdom of authors from three continents regarding head pain. We hope the book will constitute a world view of this ubiquitous complaint.

The life of this book now spans nearly forty years; the first edition was sent to press in 1948. That the volume should remain alive and useful after all this time is a source of reassurance to the current editor, who has been responsible for the last three editions.

Yet despite its age this is, in a sense, also a new book. All of the chapters have been revised, and most have been completely rewritten. We have attempted to integrate new materials with the old, and in particular to keep abreast of the changes in medical and surgical neurology resulting from the rapid advances in diagnostic technology of the last decade.

Still, the saying that today's dogma will be tomorrow's heresy is at least partly true, and much remains to be resolved. As Dr. Wolff observed in his preface to the first edition, here is the account as far as it has gone.

La Jolla
September 1986

D. J. D.

PREFACE TO THE FIRST EDITION

Since the human animal prides himself on "using his head," it is ironic and perhaps not without meaning that his head should be the source of so much discomfort. Though pain always means "something wrong," with headache it most often means "wrong direction" or "wrong pace"—a biologic reprimand rather than a threat. Thus, the vast majority of discomforts and pains of the head stem from readily reversible bodily changes, and are accompaniments of resentments and dissatisfactions. On the other hand, the headaches of brain tumor, brain abscess, fever, arteritis, meningitis, subdural and subarachnoid hemorrhage, and the pains of major neuralgias and neuritides, which call for prompt and often heroic measures, constitute only a minor proportion of the total number of pains of the head. Headache may be equally intense whether its implications are malignant or benign, and though there are few instances in human experience where so much pain may mean so little in terms of tissue injury, failure to separate the ominous from the trivial may cost life or create paralyzing fear.

Some fifteen years ago, during attempts to learn about the cerebral circulation, it was noted that the major cerebral blood vessels are covered by a network of nerve fibers having to do with pain. From these elementary observations has grown a series of investigations on headache. One part of the head after the other has been explored, and thus, piece by piece, the headache picture has been put together. Happily, in the intervening years the curiosity of bold and able workers has been aroused by the problem, and the chapters that follow are mainly the results of their efforts.

Headache as a subject for investigation has fared badly through being divided among "specialists." In an effort to unify the topic, the author and his colleagues have had the temerity to transgress divisions. By thus approaching the problem from many angles and with a variety of tools, we have tried to increase the knowledge of the natural history of headaches and other head pains, and to track down some of their mechanisms, to the end that suffering may be prevented or relieved. Doubtless there is much to correct and to clarify, but here is the account as far as it has gone.

New York Hospital   H. G. W.

CONTENTS

CONTRIBUTORS

Otto Appenzeller, M.D., Ph.D.
Professor of Neurology
University of New Mexico School of Medicine
Albuquerque, NM

Dennis E. Bullard, M.D.
Assistant Professor of Neurosurgery
Duke University Medical Center
Durham, NC

Thomas J. Carlow, M.D.
Clinical Professor of Neurology and Neuro-ophthalmology
University of New Mexico School of Medicine
Albuquerque, NM

Robert J. Coffey, M.D.
Department of Neurological Surgery
University of Florida
Gainesville, FL

Donald J. Dalessio, M.D.
Chairman, Department of Mexico
Scripps Clinic & Research Foundation
La Jolla, CA

Seymour Diamond, M.D.
Director, Diamond Headache Clinic
Adjunct Professor of Neurology
The Chicago Medical School
North Chicago, IL

Francis W. Gamache
Associate Professor of Neurosurgery
Cornell University Medical Center
New York, NY

Francis V. Howell, D.D.S.
Chairman, Department of Oral Medicine & Stomatology
Scripps Clinic & Research Foundation
La Jolla, CA

James W. Lance, M.D.
Professor of Neurology
The Prince Henry Hospital
Little Bay, New South Wales
Australia

Michael H. Lavyne
Associate Professor of Neurosurgery
Cornell University Medical Center
New York, NY

Lee Kudrow, M.D.
Director, California Medical Clinic for Headache
Encino, CA

John Stirling Meyer, M.D.
Professor of Neurology
Baylor College of Medicine
Houston, TX

Blaine S. Nashold, Jr., M.D.
Professor of Neurosurgery
Duke University School of Medicine
Durham, NC

Russell C. Packard, M.D.
Director, Headache Management and Neurology
Pensacola, FL

R. H. Patterson, Jr., M.D.
Professor of Neurosurgery
Cornell University Medical Center
New York, NY

Albert L. Rhoton, Jr., M.D.
Professor of Neurosurgery
University of Florida
Gainesville, FL

Stanley G. Seat, M.D.
Chairman, Department of Radiology
Head, Division of Diagnostic Radiology
Scripps Clinic & Research Foundation
La Jolla, CA

Ottar Sjaastad, M.D.
Professor of Neurology
Trondheim University Hospital
Trondheim
Norway

Richard A. Sternbach, Ph.D.
Director, Pain Treatment Center
Scripps Clinic & Research Foundation
La Jolla, CA

Donald D. Stevenson, M.D.
Head, Division of Allergy/Immunology
Scripps Clinic & Research Foundation
La Jolla, CA

W. E. Waters, M.D.
Professor of Community Medicine
University of Southampton Faculty of Medicine
Southampton
England

Gary W. Williams, M.D., Ph.D.
Division of Rheumatology
Scripps Clinic & Research Foundation
La Jolla, CA

Dewey K. Ziegler, M.D.
Professor of Neurology
University of Kansas Medical Center
Kansas City, KS

Jack Zyroff, M.D.
Head, Division of Neuroradiology
Scripps Clinic & Research Foundation
La Jolla, CA

HEADACHE AND OTHER HEAD PAIN

1

A Clinical Classification of Headache

DONALD J. DALESSIO

Headache has been called the most common medical complaint of civilized man; yet severe and especially chronic headache is caused only infrequently by organic disease. Hence it may be inferred that chronic headache, for the most part, represents an inability of the individual to deal in some measure with the uncertainties of life, a symptom of an underlying disorder of thought or behavior rather than structural disease of the nervous system. Nonetheless, headache may also be the presenting complaint of catastrophic illness such as brain tumor, cerebral hemorrhage, or meningitis, and to ignore the symptom in this context is to risk the life of the patient. Headache may be equally intense whether its source is benign or malignant.

What makes headaches hurt? What are the underlying mechanisms of headache? How can headaches best be classified? These questions are basic to an understanding of headache. If the clinician appreciates how and why headache generally occurs, he or she will proceed more directly to a specific diagnosis, and a decision on therapy will follow as a natural consequence.

First, one must take the time to get a reasonable history. If the physician thinks "analgesic" as soon as the patient describes headache, nothing will be accomplished. All pain is subjective; no pain can be measured effectively. All symptoms are subjective and must be described by the patient. Many patients are not good observers of their own complaints, even when those complaints are chronic. Some patients, and physicians as well, have difficulty verbalizing precisely what they are feeling. Thus, the chances are that the physician will need time to probe and find out where the patient's head pain is, what it feels like, when it occurs, how it is provoked, whether it runs in the family, and so on, before any tests are done and, most of all, before anything is prescribed.

Remember that the diagnosis of headache often depends on the patient's description of his or her symptoms. There are *no* precise clinical tests for many specific pain syndromes, including classic and common migraine, cluster headache, and the major neuralgias.

Because all physicians may be called on to treat patients with headache, it is

Table 1-1   Classification of headache

Vascular headache	Muscle contraction headache	Traction and inflammatory headache
Migraine	Cervical osteoarthritis	Mass lesions (tumors, edema, hematomas, cerebral hemorrhage)
Classic		
Common		
Hemiplegic ⎱ complicated		
Ophthalmoplegic ⎰ migraine		
Cluster (histamine)	Chronic myositis	Diseases of the eye, ear, nose, throat, teeth
Toxic vascular		Infection
Hypertensive		Arteritis, phlebitis
	Mixed headache	(Cranial neuralgias)
		Occlusive vascular disease

important to have a simple classification that will give clues to the appropriate therapy. I have divided headache into three main groups rather than a series of disparate headache syndromes, which may tax the memory. These groups are vascular, muscle contraction, and traction and inflammatory (Table 1-1).

Unfortunately, as with most classifications, patients sometimes refuse to drop neatly into separate categories. In particular, the patient with *chronic* headache will exhibit features of both vascular head pain and muscle contraction head and neck pain. For lack of a better term, these patients are characterized as having mixed headaches.

Furthermore, based on evidence continually accumulating, the established categories and descriptions of certain headaches, particularly migraine and muscle contraction headache, are being reexamined. For example, some authorities believe that the mechanisms underlying migraine are neurogenic rather than vascular, or that both systems may be involved; others have noted that there is a poor correlation between pain and muscle contraction of the head and neck in muscle contraction headache; some have suggested that there is a continuum of headache ranging from muscle contraction types to migraine. Unfortunately the matter remains to be settled. The most recent comprehensive classification of chronic pain, prepared by Merskey (1986) and his subcommittee on Taxonomy of the International Association for the Study of Pain preserves the types employed in this book; a brief description of these headache syndromes follows.

VASCULAR HEADACHE

Vascular headache includes classic and common migraine, hemiplegic migraine, ophthalmoplegic migraine, cluster (histamine) headache, and toxic vascular headache. Common to all of these is a tendency toward vascular dilatation, which represents the headache phase of the migraine attack. Vasoconstriction may also be evident and may be responsible for painless sensory phenomena prior to the onset of head pain. Hemiplegic and ophthalmoplegic migraine are considered more severe forms of classic migraine. Toxic vascular headache is evoked by a systemic vasodilatation and may be produced by fever, carbon dioxide alcohol, (CO_2) retention, agents such as nitrites, and the like.

Classic and Common Migraine

Classic and common migraine is the most troublesome form of headache; it may be viewed as a symptom complex, because migraine represents a whole spectrum of body alterations of which headache is only a single part. Classic migraine is considered to be the prototype of vascular headache. Thus, in addition to headache pain that may last from a few hours to a few days, the patient may also suffer photophobia, nausea, vomiting, constipation or diarrhea, weight gain and fluid retention followed by diuresis, scotoma or field defects, paresthesias or defects in motility, vertigo, and elevation of blood pressure. Many of these symptoms provide the basis for migraine "equivalents." These are paroxysmal, recurrent symptom complexes that occur in patients with a previous history or familial history of migraine. The headache is often replaced by this equivalent syndrome; the symptoms may be relieved with appropriate therapy, often similar to that which is used to abort the headache attack itself. Migraine equivalents may take many forms involving the abdomen, chest, pelvis, eye, cerebral cortex (hemiplegic), and perhaps other organs as well. It has been estimated that migraine equivalents occur in approximately 20% of subjects with migraine.

In classic migraine, painless sensory experiences precede the headache phase. In common migraine they do not. Most often these stimuli are expressed as scotomata or field defects. Rarely do paresthesias and defects in motility, usually unilateral, occur. These phenomena are usually attributed to intracranial vasoconstriction. It has been demonstrated that the cranial arteries of patients with migraine are especially reactive; any one of a number of stimuli may set off a migraine attack, with the vasoconstrictor phase representing the initial vector of vascular activity. In some patients, especially young women, the prodromal symptoms may be of unusual intensity and complexity. In this set of symptoms, considered by some to be related to migraine involving the basilar–vertebral arterial system, visual loss and scotomata may involve both sides of the field of vision, with associated vertigo, dysarthria, loss of consciousness, and bilateral, peripheral symptoms and signs. In at least one episode of this type, death following migraine has been described.

During the headache phase of the migraine attack the vessels involved become painful; the pain is usually described as aching and throbbing, frequently coincides with the pulse beat, and is sometimes relieved by extra-arterial pressure. After a period of vasodilatation, a sterile inflammatory reaction begins about the vessel wall, so that edema and inflammation of the affected arterial wall and the surrounding tissues may develop. By now the migraine process is in full swing. The patient is often nauseated, may vomit, and usually seeks to avoid sensory stimuli of all types, especially light. Hence, he or she retires to a dark room, goes to bed, and attempts to sleep or, at the least, to shut out the world. The pain lasts from 4 to 8 hours and sometimes longer, but eventually the patient recovers, often after a period of sleep.

Recent studies tend to confirm the longstanding hypothesis that there is a reduction of blood flow to the cerebral cortex during the preheadache phase and a substantial increase during the headache. However, these blood flow changes do not always correlate with the clinical symptoms of the attack, suggesting that the classic theory provides only a partial explanation of migraine.

Cluster Headache

There are several synonyms for cluster headache including histamine headache, Horton's headache, and migrainous neuralgia. This type of vascular headache has features that are specific enough to justify separate description, and the diagnosis can often be made on the basis of history alone. The pain occurs in attacks and is constant, of high intensity, burning, and "boring" in character. It involves the region of the eye, the temples, the neck, and often the face, and may extend into the shoulder on the involved side. It may spread to the upper teeth and occasionally to the lower teeth. Attacks often begin after middle age. Generally, the attacks last less than 1 hour, commence and often terminate suddenly, and often awaken the patient at night. The pain is so severe that the patient frequently jumps out of bed before he or she is fully awake.

The pain is associated with certain other characteristic manifestations that appear on the affected side. These are profuse watering and "congestion" of the conjunctiva, rhinorrhea and nasal obstruction, increased perspiration, and frequently evidence of vasodilatation in the skin. Swelling of the temporal vessels may be noted. During and after the attacks, marked tenderness is frequently found when pressure is applied over the branches of the external and common carotid arteries. The pain is not confined to the distribution of any cranial nerve but conforms to the ramifications of the external carotid artery.

A partial Horner's syndrome may occur in cluster headache, affecting the eye involved in the headache. Most often ptosis and meiosis are seen, related to compression of the pericarotid sympathetic fibers produced by swelling of the artery, as it passes through the skull.

Cluster headache occurs predominantly in males, with a 5:1 sex ratio. Often these are middle-aged men, commonly heavy smokers, without a family history of recurrent vascular headache. The term *cluster* is used because of the unique tempo of the recurring attacks, which vary from patient to patient but often exhibit a striking periodicity. Despite this periodicity, attempts to implicate allergen(s) in this form of headache have not been successful.

Patients with cluster headache are extremely sensitive to vasodilating agents, especially drugs such as nitroglycerin or histamine, alcohol, and the aged cheeses that contain tyramine. Sensitivity to oral nitroglycerin can be used as a provocative test if the diagnosis is suspected.

Hemiplegic Migraine

The vascular reactions of classic migraine also occur in hemiplegic migraine. Here they may be exaggerated to the point that longlasting ischemia of brain tissue occurs. This form of migraine may be familial, suggesting again that an inherited instability of vascular control is present. Whether the sequelae of this form of migraine are related to the prolongation of the vasodilator or of the vasoconstrictor phases of migraine is unknown; possibly both factors are implicated.

Ophthalmoplegic Migraine

In ophthalmoplegic migraine, ocular palsy is associated with headache. Those structures served by the third cranial nerve are most often involved. This is attributed to the pressure on the nerve exerted by the dilated and edematous wall of the internal carotid artery and its branches. Segmental narrowing of all or part of the intracranial portion of the internal carotid artery has been demonstrated by arteriography in patients during a migraine attack. It has also been suggested that brain edema produced by migraine may provoke herniation of the hippocampal gyrus sufficient to compress the third nerve, but this concept is speculative.

In patients who suffer repeated attacks, ocular palsies are usually transitory. In rare instances, however, these palsies may become persistent. It is important to differentiate between the mechanisms of ophthalmoplegic migraine and those that produce similar symptoms but are related to intracranial aneurysms, particularly of the posterior communicating artery. The sudden appearance of third-nerve signs in a patient not subject to migraine is an indication for further diagnostic study.

Toxic Vascular Headache

The category of toxic vascular headache (Table 1-2) includes all of the diseases and conditions that produce headache of a vascular nature as part of their overall symptomatology. The most common nonmigrainous vascular headache is that produced by fever. Generalized vasodilation may occur as a consequence of any significant fever, usually becoming more intense as the fever rises. Particularly intense vascular headaches may occur with pneumonia, tonsilitis, septicemia, typhoid fever, tularemia, influenza, measles, mumps, poliomyelitis, infectious mononucleosis, malaria, and trichinosis. The vasodilatation in these diseases is often intracranial as well as extracranial. Nonmigrainous headache may also occurs in a whole series of miscellaneous disorders, including such diverse entities as hangover headache and headache associated with hypoglycemia regardless of the cause. In hypoxic states headache may be a persistent complaint, especially in those in whom an increased CO_2 tension in the blood exists concurrently. Exposure to carbon monoxide may provoke a very severe form of vascular headache. Headaches may be produced by the administration of nitrates, either as medicament or unintentionally, as an industrial hazard. Many poisons may evoke headache, including lead, benzene, carbon tetrachloride, and insecticides. Treatment with monoamine oxidase inhibitors may cause a serious headache, especially when small amounts of catecholamines are ingested at the same time. The headache produced may be catastrophic, and cerebrovascular accidents as well as deaths have been reported as a result of this combination.

Withdrawal from many pharmacologic agents may provoke headache. This is especially likely after prolonged therapy with ergot derivatives but may also follow the

Table 1-2 Causes of toxic vascular headaches

Pathologic conditions		Toxic substances		Withdrawal from drugs
Febrile	Others	Nonpharmacologic	Pharmacologic	
Pneumonia	Alcohol	Carbon monoxide	Nitrates	Ergot
Tonsillitis	Hypoglycemia	Lead	Indomethacin	Caffeine
Septicemia	Hypoxia	Benzene	Oral progestational	Amphetamines
Typhoid fever	Altitude	Carbon tetrachloride	Oral vasodilators	Many phenothiazines
Tularemia	Hypercarbia	Insecticides		
Influenza	Effort	Nitrates		
Measles				
Mumps				
Poliomyelitis				
Infectious mononucleosis				
Malaria				
Trichinosis				

discontinuation of caffeine, benzedrine, and many of the phenothiazines. Treatment of arthritis with indomethacin may evoke headache, presumably by producing a chemical vasodilatation.

HEADACHE ASSOCIATED WITH ARTERIAL HYPERTENSION AND TOXEMIA OF PREGNANCY

Several kinds of headache associated with hypertension deserve discussion. A sudden rise in blood pressure during violent exercise, anger, or sexual excitement, may be associated with bilateral pounding headache, usually short-lived or transient, which is rarely of diagnostic or therapeutic importance. Effort migraine occurring in athletes after a long race, or in mountain climbers experiencing anoxia, is a related phenomenon. Such episodes do not usually require specific therapy.

Sudden and extreme elevations of the blood pressure may occur with toxemia of pregnancy, in the malignant state of essential hypertension, and with end-stage renal disease. The syndrome termed hypertensive encephalopathy consists of severe headache, nausea, vomiting, and convulsions, proceeding to confusion and coma. Papilledema is always present as a primary sign of increased intracranial pressure. The headache is more or less continuous, generalized, pounding, and difficult to relieve with simple analgesics. It is assumed that brain edema in some form produces the headache associated with hypertensive encephalopathy. The intravenous injection of osmotically active agents such as mannitol will reduce its intensity. Oral glycerol is also effective. These agents produce relative dehydration of the brain, subsequent to which traction and displacement of pain-sensitive structures are reduced.

The neurologic signs of hypertensive encephalopathy occurring in toxemia are probably related to cerebral vasospasm, thereafter producing cerebral ischemia and cerebral edema. The primary therapeutic aim in hypertensive encephalopathy is to reduce the blood pressure, which is the only effective way to relieve the symptoms.

Vascular headache may also be associated with a paroxysmal rise of blood pressure, as seen in a patient with a pheochromocytoma, but other physical findings should lead rapidly to that diagnosis.

What remains are those headaches associated with essential hypertension. With this common disease, the pain is vascular in nature and is related to the contractile state of the extracranial and intracranial arteries. Should these arteries dilate, for whatever reason, hypertensive vascular headache will occur. Usually the pain is described as dull and aching with a pounding component, often present in the morning, and improving as the patient stirs, gets up, moves about. The pain is frequently increased by effort, stooping, and by jolts to the head. Hypertensive headache is rarely present unless the diastolic blood pressure exceeds 110 mm Hg.

Patients with minimal hypertension who complain of headache need careful evaluation. Often the tendency is to blame the headache on the hypertension when this may not be the cause. As mentioned previously, unless the diastolic blood pressure exceeds 110 mm Hg, another etiology should be sought in this situation.

MUSCLE CONTRACTION HEADACHE

Perhaps the most common form of headache is that related to chronic muscular contraction occurring about the head and neck. This produces dull, bandlike, persistent pain, which may last for days or months. In treating this type of pain, a search should be made for tender and painful areas of the head and neck, as well as significant arthritis of the spine.

In chronic muscle contraction, skeletal muscle spasm is often related to local pathologic processes and their central influences and involves several reflex arcs.

MIXED HEADACHE SYNDROMES

Mixed headache has features of both vascular head pain and muscle contraction head and neck pain. Three different clinical patterns of mixed headache are recognized. The first is characterized by headache attacks with predominantly migrainous features occurring periodically over many years until the clinical expression subsides. Although a majority of the attacks are clearly migrainous (pulsatile, throbbing, unilateral with photophobia, sonophobia, and nausea and vomiting), minor, less distinct muscular elements often accompany the attack. These include dull, constant aching, pressure or tightness around the head and neck, with nonlocalizing discomfort for many days. This sometimes precedes the migrainous attack, or it may follow it. Tenderness of the scalp and neck may be present. Combing the hair may become painful.

A second clinical pattern is that of a dull, constant discomfort onto which is superimposed intermittent throbbing pain, nausea, and photophobia of a migrainous nature.

The third and probably the most common pattern is that of a transformation of

episodic migraine into a daily headache syndrome. Most of these patients start out
having typical common migraine attacks, often related to the menstrual cycle. Then,
after a number of years, a daily headache syndrome appears. The majority of these
patients wake up in the morning with head pain that might fit the description of
muscle contraction headache. They also continue to have vascular or migrainous
attacks, but less frequently, and perhaps with somewhat less intensity as years go by.

TRACTION AND INFLAMMATION HEADACHE

This category comprises headache evoked by organic disease of the skull or its components, including the brain, meninges, arteries, veins, eyes, ears, teeth, nose, and
paranasal sinuses. The term traction headache is used to describe the often nonspecific headache seen with mass lesions of the brain, such as tumors, hematomas,
abscesses, or brain edema from whatever cause. Traction headache of a particularly
intense type occurs in subarachnoid and intraventricular hemorrhage, and in cortical
venous thromboses. Traction headache is associated with inflammatory disease of the
meninges, and intracranial or extracranial arteritis or phlebitis. Inflammatory headache evoked by disease of the special sense organs and the teeth, and the major
cranial neuralgias including tic douloureux are included here.

Mass Lesions

A traction headache can be elicited by hematomas of any sort, abscesses, nonspecific
brain "edema," and lumbar puncture. It is especially a symptom of brain tumors.
Local traction on adjacent pain-sensitive structures by the tumor may occur, as well
as distant traction related indirectly to the tumor mass when internal hydrocephalus
and ventricular obstruction occur. For this reason, localization of a brain tumor by
determining the site of headache can be unreliable. It has also been possible to demonstrate localized skull tenderness at the site of meningiomas, or in the mastoid area
with a cerebellopontine angle tumor, presumably due to local involvement and extension into the skull or its structures by the tumor.

Arteritis and Infections

Headache may be produced by inflammatory processes within or outside the skull,
particularly meningitis, intracranial arteritis, phlebitis, and those inflammatory processes associated with subarachnoid hemorrhage. The pain is evoked by an inflammatory response that includes the pain-sensitive structures of the head. The head
pain, in most instances, coincides with the course of the disease, usually abating as
the disease is brought under control, and is not recurrent or paroxysmal.

Extracranial inflammation may also produce headache. The mechanism responsible
is inflammation of the extracranial arteries. The condition may be seen in a localized
form, as it occurs in cranial (temporal) arteritis, or in a more generalized disease as

part of a widespread collagen–vascular syndrome. The intracranial arteritis occurs in systemic lupus erythematosus or periarteritis nodosa and can produce excruciating headache pain of a generalized nature.

In polyarteritis nodosa multiple areas of arterial necrosis and inflammation affect many organs. The arterial lesion appears to be identical to that found in serum sickness arteritis.

A rather common form of rheumatism that affects the elderly with pains in the head, neck, back, and proximal areas of the limbs may be associated with systemic signs of disease, an elevated sedimentation rate, and a prompt therapeutic response to corticosteroids. This condition is best known as polymyalgia rheumatica. A significant number of patients with polymyalgia rheumatica will eventually develop temporal arteritis in the course of their illness, suggesting that the two diseases are in fact one and that the myalgias of polymyalgia rheumatica may represent an early stage of cranial arteritis.

In temporal arteritis the inflammatory reaction tends to be relatively limited to the cranial arteries, though it may involve other arteries as well. It is often acute and self-limited and may be associated with the development of multinucleate giant cells in the media of the blood vessels (giant-cell arteritis).

Cranial Neuritis and Neuralgias, Temporomandibular Joint (TMJ) Disease

This category includes those forms of facial pain that are mediated by the cranial nerves, including the trigeminal and glossopharyngeal neuralgias (Table 1-3). It commonly includes the atypical facial neuralgias, lower-half headache, sphenopalatine neuralgias, orofacial pains, and carotidynia. Some of these syndromes are poorly developed and may not deserve separate status. Some of them probably represent vascular pain or a form of migraine perceived in an unusual location (Table 1-3). This is particularly true of lower-half headaches, which may respond to prophylaxis with such lysergic acid derivatives as methysergide.

Categorizing Chronic Facial Pains

Perhaps the best way to categorize chronic facial pain is to separate out those specific syndromes that have a neuroanatomic basis and deal with the rest as atypical facial neuralgias. Certain discrete facial pain syndromes can be recognized by the clinician. These include especially the major neuralgias; postherpetic neuritis; cluster headache in its anatomic and verbal variations; diseases of the eyes, ears, nose, teeth, and throat; cranial arteritis; and pseudotumor of the orbit (see Tables 1-1 and 1-3).

Temporomandibular Joint (TMJ) Disease

Are there symptoms related to temporomandibular joint (TMJ) disease? The question is moot. We believe facial pain that is not neuritic in character can occur with temporomandibular joint (TMJ) disease; it is usually felt in the face adjacent to the joint,

Table 1-3 A classification of facial neuralgias

Classic neuralgia
  Trigeminal neuralgia
  Glossopharyngeal neuralgia

Other neuralgias
  Geniculate (intermedius) neuralgia of Hunt
  Postherpetic facial neuralgia
  Sphenopalatine neuralgias
    vidian neuralgia of Vail ⎫
    ciliary neuralgia (Charlin) ⎬ probably cluster
    petrosal neuralgia ⎪ headache variants
    erythroprosopalgia ⎭
  Paratrigeminal syndrome of Raeder

Facial pain related to craniofacial pathology
  Temporomandibular joint pathology (Costen's
    syndrome)
  Intracranial pathology
  Orofacial pain—burning tongue

Lower-half headache
Atypical facial pain
Carotidynia

with radiation to the jaw, the neck, and behind the ear. In our view, the syndrome consists of localized facial pain, limitation of motion of the jaw, muscle tenderness, and joint crepitus. Usually the joint itself has a normal radiologic appearance.

There is no evidence that hearing loss, damage to cranial nerves, disturbances of equilibrium, development of Meniere's syndrome, or difficulty with the eustachian tubes are in any way related to this syndrome. The current view of etiology is that occlusal disharmony and psychophysiologic factors play primary roles, with most of the dysfunction resident in the masticatory muscles rather than in the TMJ itself. Those pathologic changes that affect the joint, such as rheumatoid arthritis, may cause similar complaints, but they are, by definition, different problems, which need not be discussed here. The syndromes delineated as trigeminal neuralgia (tic douloureux) and glossopharyngeal neuralgia are better characterized.

Trigeminal Neuralgia (Tic Douloureux)

In tic douloureux, pain is experienced chiefly in areas of the face supplied by the second and, to a lesser extent, the third and first divisions of the fifth cranial nerve. It may be felt in any part of the face, but never below the ramus of the jaw or in back of the ear, and rarely in the entire distribution of the fifth nerve at any one time. The pain has an aching and burning quality and may occur spontaneously, but it is more often initiated by cold air or a light touch on the skin of the cheek, or by the motion of biting, chewing, laughing, swallowing, talking, yawning, sneezing, or similar movements. The pain is usually described as a high-intensity "jab" of 20 to

30 seconds duration, followed by a period of abatement lasting from a few seconds to a minute, and then followed by another jab of high-intensity pain. The spasms do not last longer than a minute. The entire attack or series of such brief pains usually lasts one or more hours.

A familiar characteristic of trigeminal neuralgia is the patient's ability to point out trigger zones. These zones are 2 to 4 mm in diameter and are hyperexcitable areas of skin or mucous membrane that, when given a minimal stimulus, are capable of producing paroxysmal pain in one or more divisions of the trigeminal nerve. These zones are clustered around the mouth and nares.

Glossopharyngeal Neuralgia

Glossopharyngeal tic is a related phenomenon. Severe pain similar to that described for tic douloureux is experienced in the tonsillar area and ear. It is often initiated by eating, yawning, or swallowing. Syncope may occur during the painful episode, presumably resulting from cardiac asystole.

REFERENCE

Merskey, H. (1986) Classification of Chronic Pain. *Pain Suppl. 3*:S71-S79.

2

Modern Concepts of Pain

RICHARD A. STERNBACH

An understanding of the evolving concepts of pain and analgesic mechanisms is obviously fundamental to a specialized interest in face and head pain. In the following discussion, neurophysiologic and psychological processes in pain and analgesia will be described, irrespective of body locus. The head participates with the rest of the body in spinal and supraspinal mechanisms, sharing in the spinal events by virtue of the innervation from the first and second cervical roots. In addition, as is well known, there is innervation by the three branches of the trigeminal (fifth cranial) nerve. Despite the transmission of pain along these fibers, in other respects the following information regarding receptors, fibers, descending inhibitory mechanisms, and so on is applicable to pains of the head and face as well as to pains in other parts of the body. Dubner et al. (1978) give specific details of oral and face pain mechanisms.

In this area of rapidly changing information about pain and analgesic mechanisms,it is obviously difficult to be exhaustive or even thorough in a single chapter. Furthermore, when psychological factors as well are considered, the task becomes nearly impossible. The following gives only brief highlights of relevant topics and information. Readers interested in a more comprehensive review may consult Yaksh and Hammond (1982).

NEUROPHYSIOLOGIC MECHANISMS: PAIN RECEPTORS AND FIBERS

Recent developments in dissection and recording techniques have made it possible to show that there are three general classes of nociceptors (pain receptors): high-threshold mechanoreceptors, heat nociceptors, and "polymodal" nociceptors responsive to both noxious mechanical and noxious thermal stimuli (Bessou & Perl, 1969). Polymodal and heat nociceptors can be sensitized after repeated or prolonged stimulation, or during regeneration following section of nerve, so that their thresholds for activation can be lowered to levels of stimulus intensity that are ordinarily innocuous. This may account for the pain states following burns or nerve injury.

Perl and his colleagues (Bessou & Perl, 1969; Burgess & Perl, 1967; Perl, 1968;

Perl, 1971) found that a large proportion of both A-delta and C fibers in cat and monkey cutaneous nerve were specifically responsive to tissue damage. That is, these fibers responded only to intensities of peripheral stimulation that were at or near levels sufficient to produce injury. See the reviews by Burgess and Perl (1973) and Lynn (1984).

Several investigators have used microelectrode recording techniques in normal human subjects, and have recorded from single cutaneous C fibers (Torebjork & Hallin, 1973, 1974a; Van Hees & Gybels, 1972). These reports, along with the work of Price (1972, 1976), suggest that the activation of A-delta fibers is associated with the experience of "first" pain: fast, sharp, and well localized. Activation of C fibers is associated with the experience of "second" pain: slow, aching, burning, longlasting, and poorly localized.

From these studies it appears that pain is a specific sensory event (Perl, 1971), and not merely excessive stimulation of other sensory modalities, as was formerly supposed (Keele, 1957). There would seem to be specialized nociceptors whose information is transmitted to the spinal cord over specific A-delta and C fibers.

SPINAL MECHANISMS

In the past decade important advances have been made in our understanding of the course and termination of primary afferent fibers. This has been due to the development and use of autoradiography and horseradish peroxidase labeling, and the use of immunocytochemistry to map the distribution of peptides in central terminal fields (Fitzgerald, 1984).

There appear to be two types of pain-related sensory neurons in the dorsal horn of the spinal cord. Christensen and Perl (1970) described a Class 1 nociceptive cell, located in the marginal zone or most superficial layer of the dorsal horn (lamina 1). Class 1 cells are specifically responsive to injurious or near-injurious levels of stimulation.

Class 2 nociceptive cells are located primarily in lamina 5, and respond to low-intensity stimulation, but as the intensity of stimulation is increased to noxious levels these cells follow with more vigorous and sustained discharge (Hillman & Wall, 1969; Price & Browe, 1973; Willis et al., 1974).

Class 2 cells are impinged on by inputs from both visceral and somatic sources; they may thus be involved in visceral referred pain (Pomeranz et al., 1968). They show "windup" or temporal summation with repetitive C-fiber activation (Price & Wagman, 1970), and they also show prolonged afterdischarges to noxious heat stimuli (Handwerker et al., 1975).

The axons of many Class 1 and Class 2 cells project directly to the brain; others ascend multisynaptically or contribute to reflex paths (Kerr, 1975). A large proportion of both types of cells ascend in the contralateral anterolateral quadrant and terminate in the thalamus. Mayer et al. (1975) studied the effects of direct stimulation of the anterolateral columns in conscious patients undergoing cordotomy for relief of pain. These results were compared with similar data on Class 1 and Class 2 cells projecting to the anterolateral columns in monkeys (Price & Mayer, 1975). Refractory periods and electrical thresholds for Class 2 cells in the monkey were more similar to the periods and thresholds that caused sensations of pain in humans. These authors suggest that although Class 1 cells may be involved in pain perception, activation of Class 2 cells alone may be a sufficient condition for some kinds of human pain.

GATE CONTROL THEORY

The gate control theory of pain proposed by Melzack and Wall (1965) suggests a dynamic interaction among large and small afferent fibers, mediated through the small cells of the substantia gelatinosa (laminas 2 and 3 in the dorsal horn of the spinal cord). Substantia gelatinosa cells are proposed to exert presynaptic inhibition on both large and small fiber terminals as they synapse on dorsal horn transmission cells whose axons project to the brain. Large fibers excite the substantia gelatinosa, thus increasing presynaptic inhibition (closing the gate) to noxious impulses incoming through small fibers. Small fibers inhibit the substantia gelatinosa, thus decreasing presynaptic inhibition (opening the gate). Pain is perceived when a threshold level of firing is attained by the central transmission cells. The gating mechanism could be influenced also by higher centers through descending fibers projecting to spinal cord cells.

The gate theory has been modified and expanded to encompass recent developments in neurophysiology, including evidence that postsynaptic is more important than presynaptic inhibition (Melzack, 1973). The theory has been criticized from an anatomic point of view (Kerr, 1975), as well as conceptually (Perl, 1971), but many clinical observations, as well as experimental studies, are compatible with it. The gating mechanism, susceptible to influence from centrifugal as well as centripetal sources, appears to be a useful concept. Wall (1984) now considers that a gate control establishes the short-term effects of stimulation, and a connectivity control, acting more slowly, influences which afferents fire which cells.

Transmission Pathways

The injury signals that relay in the dorsal horns of the spinal cord and the trigeminal nuclei are then transmitted to appropriate nuclei in the brain stem and thalamus. Several different pathways are involved, including the spinothalamic, spinoreticular, spinomesencephalic, spinocervical, and second-order dorsal column tracts. Of these, the anterolateral spinothalamic tracts are probably the most important in humans (Willis, 1984).

The anterolateral columns project to a number of discrete regions of the brain. The one most thoroughly studied is the nucleus gigantocellularis (NGC) of the bulbar reticular formation. Casey and his colleagues have found that many cells of this nucleus respond maximally to activation of A-delta and C fibers or to intense natural stimuli of the skin (Casey, 1971a,b,c; Morrow & Casey, 1976). There do not appear to be any significant number of nociceptive cells in the NGC. Rather, the great majority appear to have properties like those of Class 2 and not of Class 1 dorsal horn cells in that they respond maximally but not uniquely to noxious stimuli. Also like Class 2 cells, the NGC cells have large, peripheral receptive fields, and thus are not likely to have a significant sensory discriminative role in nociception. The NGC cells may be part of an affective component of pain.

Most studies of more rostral brain regions have used anesthetized animals and may be misleading with respect to nociception. For example, Poggio and Mountcastle (1960) found that 60% of the units studied in the posterior nuclear region of the thalamus responded specifically to noxious stimuli. But Casey (1966), using an una-nesthetized animal, found that none of these cells was specifically nociceptive during waking. He also found that many cells throughout the diencephalon and rostral mid-brain responded differentially to noxious and nonnoxious stimuli, and most of these had wide peripheral receptive fields.

Attempts have been made to postulate brain mechanisms based on studies of the effects of lesions designed to relieve pain in chronic pain states. These studies are fraught with difficulties. Changes in emotionality typically follow limbic system le-sions, and these alterations in the affective component of pain make an assessment of its severity difficult. Furthermore, such lesions seldom occur in those with a long life expectancy; thus, long-term follow-up is rare. Even highly successful anterola-teral cordotomies frequently fail after 12 to 18 months in chronic pain states. Casey and Melzack (1967) note that the progressive divergence of the pain signals at higher levels makes it unlikely that focal lesions will significantly or permanently interrupt the sensory-discriminative aspects of nociception.

Central Peptides and Amines

Substance P, present in peripheral afferents and the dorsal horns, seems to be a neuropeptide whose role may be that of a neurotransmitter in the nociceptive path-ways. It can also coexist in serotonin-containing neurons in the raphe system (Ter-enius, 1984).

The opioid peptides are widely distributed in the limbic system, periaqueductal gray, brain stem, and frontal cortex. A number of such peptides are now known to exist, with varying degrees of analgesic potential and binding to several opiate recep-tors. The enkephalins have a high affinity for delta and mu receptors and may have the most important role in analgesia. However, alpha-neoendorphin and dynorphin, with affinity for the kappa receptors, have analgesic effects as well, and metke-phamid, a delta-receptor agonist, is also analgesic (Terenius, 1984).

The role of these endogenous opioids is not yet clear. When binding to opiate receptors, they usually inhibit the central nervous system (CNS) neurons, and thus may trigger descending inhibitory systems by inhibiting inhibitory neurons—a disin-hibition process. In any event they seem to be involved in a bulbospinal analgesic system that has both serotonergic and noradrenergic components. This system in-cludes connections from the midbrain periaqueductal gray to the raphe nuclei and, through the dorsolateral funiculus, descends to the dorsal horn where, apparently, inhibitory interneurons are stimulated to modulate second-order nociceptive neurons (Fields & Basbaum, 1984). Depleting brain serotonin by inhibiting its synthesis or by lesioning the raphe nuclei will block the analgesic effect of systemic opiates.

A number of pain-related behaviors are also serotonergically mediated; sleep is one of these (Jouvet, 1969). Sleep disturbance is one of the symptoms patients with chronic pain most frequently complain of (Sternbach, 1974a). It is now reported that patients with painful fibromyositis syndrome have abnormal stage 4 sleep patterns (Moldofsky et al., 1975). Normal subjects whose stage 4 sleep pattern is experimentally interrupted develop painful fibrositis symptoms (Moldofsky & Scarisbrick, 1975).

Patients with chronic pain typically develop depressive reactions (Sternbach, 1974a,b). There is some evidence suggesting that there may be two kinds of depression associated with underactivity of brain norepinephrine or of brain serotonin (Maas, 1975; Asberg et al., 1976); pain patients seem to have the serotonin-type of depression. Akil and Liebeskind (1975) showed that brain norepinephrine tends to antagonize the analgesic-promoting effects of brain serotonin. We showed that administration of chlorimipramine, a tricyclic antidepressant that acts primarily to block reuptake of brain serotonin, reduces pain in chronic pain patients more than amitriptyline, which did no better than placebo; chlorimipramine exerted its effect by increasing pain tolerance (Sternbach et al., 1976b).

ANALGESIC STIMULATION

Central

Liebeskind et al. (1974) have shown that electrical stimulation of mesencephalic periaqueductal gray matter, in the region of the dorsal raphe nucleus, produces a very significant analgesia. This stimulation-produced analgesia (SPA) has been obtained using many different pain tests in many species, including humans (Adams, 1976; Giesler & Liebeskind, 1976; Goodman & Holcombe, 1976; Hosobuchi et al., 1977; Mayer & Liebeskind, 1974; Melzack & Melinkoff, 1974; Richardson & Akil, 1977a,b; Soper, 1976). After only a few seconds of stimulation, the analgesia may last as long as several hours. The analgesia may be subtotal, so that the animal completely ignores a strong pinch to one limb but responds normally to a pinch to another limb. The analgesia can be equivalent to large doses of morphine (Mayer & Liebeskind, 1974), but the animals are normally reactive to other stimuli and can engage in normal behaviors (Mayer et al., 1971).

SPA appears to result from stimulation of medial structures from the nucleus raphe magnus in the rostral medulla, through midbrain central gray, to the caudal diencephalon. It can completely inhibit the pain-evoked discharges of Class 2 dorsal horn cells, without affecting their responsiveness to nonpainful stimuli (Oliveras et al., 1974). Akil has shown that this is a serotonergic system (Akil & Mayer, 1972; Akil & Liebeskind, 1975). Either chemical or dietary depletion of brain serotonin levels increases sensitivity to pain, which can be restored to normal levels by administration of the precursors tryptophan or 5-hydroxytryptophan. SPA can be blocked by selective destruction of the spinal cord dorsolateral funiculus in which the serotonin-containing fibers descend from the nucleus raphe magnus (Basbaum et al., 1976).

The sites where microinjections of morphine are effective in producing analgesia are virtually identical to the effective sites of SPA (Mayer & Murfin, 1976), and cross-tolerance develops between morphine- and stimulation-induced analgesia (Mayer & Hayes, 1975). Alteration of brain monoamine levels alter SPA and morphine analgesia similarly (Akil & Liebeskind, 1975). The morphine antagonist, naloxone, reverses SPA (Adams, 1976; Akil et al., 1976; Hosobuchi et al., 1977; Oliveras et al., 1975). These reports suggest that SPA responds to pharmacologic manipulations as does morphine.

There are also anatomic and electrophysiologic studies to suggest that the opiate system is involved in a pain-inhibiting mechanism. Microinjection of morphine in the central gray results in a greater analgesia than injection in the ventricles or elsewhere (Jacquet & Lajtha, 1974; Pert & Yaksh, 1974), and stereospecific binding sites for opiates have been found in central gray (Kuhar et al., 1973). Both morphine and SPA selectively suppress nociceptive responding units in the dorsal horn (Kitahata et al, 1974) and in the brain stem (Oleson & Liebeskind, 1976).

Mayer and Price (1976) have reviewed the literature on central mechanisms of analgesia, and have proposed a model involving both a serotonergic and an enkephalinlike neurotransmitter system. Both ascending and descending serotonin pathways are involved with periaqueductal–periventricular structures of the brain stem, especially the nucleus raphe magnus, being critical loci or funnels in this system. In series or in parallel with this system is an enkephalin system. Electrical or chemical stimulation of either produces analgesia, whereas chemical or surgical blockade of either prevents analgesia. This powerful descending pain-inhibitory mechanism is still being unraveled.

Peripheral

Acupuncture analgesia has a long history in the United States as well as in Asia, for Osler (1912) cites it (and electrical stimulation) as a treatment for neuralgias. Travell and Rinzler (1952) long ago reported the special effect of dry needling of certain trigger points for myofascial syndromes, and Melzack et al. (1977) have shown the similarity of traditional acupuncture points and trigger points for referred pain sites.

Well-controlled studies of the efficacy of acupuncture are few, and their outcomes are frequently contradictory. Some studies report a strong analgesic effect (Gaw et al., 1975; Mann et al, 1973), others only a weak effect (Day et al., 1975; Li et al., 1975). The mechanism of action is unclear, but the typical 20 minute delay of analgesia suggests a humoral process. This is supported by the finding that naloxone reverses acupuncture analgesia but not hypnotic analgesia, suggesting a chemical rather than a psychological mechanism (Goldstein & Hilgard, 1975; Mayer et al., 1976).

Transcutaneous electrical neurostimulation (TENS) may involve a mechanism similar to that of acupuncture. Melzack and Wall's (1965) gate control theory of pain predicted that activation of large fibers by somatosensory stimulation would "close the gate'' to noxious input along small fibers. Wall and Sweet (1967) confirmed that direct electrical stimulation of peripheral fibers relieved pain due to peripheral neuropathy for many minutes or hours after the brief stimulation.

The mechanism of this analgesic effect may, indeed, involve a central closing of a gate; this is supported by the finding that TENS can relieve the pain of postherpetic neuralgia, which involves pathologic lesions of dorsal root ganglia and dorsal columns (Nathan & Wall, 1974). However, studies by Taub and Campbell (1974), Torebjork and Hallin (1974b), and Ignelzi and Nyquist (1976) also suggest a direct ''fatiguing'' effect on small peripheral fibers, in evoked potential studies. Somatosensory changes in patients using TENS successfully for pain relief also suggest that the effect is primarily peripheral (Ignelzi et al., 1976). The notion that suggestion, or a placebo effect, is not important is shown in follow-up studies, which show continued increased activity levels after 1 year of regular daily use (Sternbach et al., 1976a). There is no clear habituation effect with TENS as with narcotic analgesia, and there may even be increasing sensitivity to electrical analgesia (Melzack, 1975).

PSYCHOLOGICAL MECHANISMS

One of the compelling arguments for a gating model of pain is the lack of a 1:1 relationship between stimulus intensity and the subjective experience of stimulus magnitude. Pain does not involve a straight-through transmission system, but is subject to ascending and descending modulating processes (Melzack, 1973). Some of these processes show consistent patterns, or ''lawfulness,'' and we will consider those that have been best documented.

Perceptual Parameters

Pain Threshold

The pain threshold is the lowest intensity of stimulation at which pain is perceived or the least intensity of stimulation that can be called painful. It is the ''absolute threshold'' for pain in the same sense that the term is used for vision and hearing. In operational psychophysical terms, it is the point of stimulus intensity at which pain is reported 50% of the time in a series of ascending and descending (!) stimulus presentations.

Unlike the other modalities, in which a judgment of ''present'' or ''not present'' is made, the decision of ''painful'' versus ''not painful'' usually involves comparing the quality of two stimuli, rather than detecting the presence of one stimulus. That is, determining the point at which a warm stimulus becomes a pricking pain or a cold one becomes an ache or a pressure becomes painful is rather different from noting whether or not a flash or a tone appears. The nature of the comparative judgment depends on what form of painful stimulation is used. With any noninvasive technique, it is arguable whether or not ''pure'' pain can occur: sensations of heat, cold, or pressure are also usually involved, taking on the added quality of pain.

Using the radiant heat technique, Hardy et al. (1952) found that psychological factors such as the site of the stimulation, the skin temperature, the blackness or wetness of the site, the presence of injury, and repetition and duration of the administered heat were important determinants of threshold, whereas the race, sex, age, fatigue, and emotional state of the individual seemed not to be marked influences. Similar findings have been obtained with electrical shock techniques. Although thresholds can be modified somewhat by acquired attitudes toward pain (Sternbach & Tursky, 1965), they are relatively stable and apparently a function of physiologic parameters (Tursky, 1974).

Attempts have been made to measure deep somatic pain as well as superficial cutaneous pain. Wolff and Jarvik (1965), using hypertonic saline injections in the gluteus medius muscle, found that age increases the pain threshold, particularly for men; and women have a slightly (not significantly) lower threshold than men. The authors also compared radiant heat, ice water, and hypotonic as well as hypertonic saline, and obtained some significance in correlations of thresholds that ranged from 0.42 to −0.53. They concluded that different stimuli applied to different body loci can elicit correlated pain thresholds under certain conditions.

Pain Tolerance

Pain tolerance is the maximum pain level, the point at which the subject no longer voluntarily accepts pain; it is thus the upper threshold for pain. In several respects the pain tolerance level may be a more useful concept for clinical applications than the pain threshold, although it is more difficult to measure. One of the technical difficulties is that humanitarian and ethical considerations make it necessary to employ only an ascending series of stimuli and preclude use of a descending series. This introduces a measurement error that is avoided by using both series in determining the lower pain threshold.

Hardy et al. (1952) admitted to difficulties with assessing pain tolerance to radiant heat because of resultant tissue damage and an inability to obtain repeated measures within a reasonable period of time. In studies with electric shock, pain tolerance was found to be easily influences by coaxing subjects and was more susceptible to attitudes associated with ethnic membership than was pain threshold (Sternbach & Tursky, 1965). In a very large sample of more than 40,000 subjects subjected to pressure on the Achilles tendon delivered by a calibrated motor-driven device, it was found that pain tolerance decreases with age, more so for men than women; pain tolerance at every age is greater for men than for women; and whites tolerate more pain than blacks, who tolerate more pain than orientals (Woodrow et al., 1972).

Several authors using different techniques have noted significant correlations between pain thresholds and pain tolerances. Wolff and Jarvik (1963), using radiant heat, obtained a correlation of 0.91 between the two levels. Merskey and Spear (1964), using the pressure algometer, obtained correlations in three groups of subjects of 0.70, 0.82, and 0.84. Tursky and O'Connell (1972), using electric shock, obtained within-day correlations of 0.97 to 0.99, and day-to-day correlations ranging from 0.73 to 0.85.

Clearly there is a significant association between pain threshold and pain tolerance. One reason the correlations are not better, however, is that the latter is more readily influenced by subjects' sets (attitudes). Among the factors that have been shown to influence pain tolerance are suggestion, distraction, manipulation of anxiety, and motivation (Sternbach, 1968). Recently, social modeling has also been shown to alter tolerance; that is, if a model appears to endure more or less pain, this influences the subject's tolerance in the same direction (Craig et al., 1975). In general, when studies have examined the effects of experimental variables on both pain threshold and pain tolerance, the effects on tolerance have been more marked.

Pain Sensitivity Range

The pain sensitivity range is the difference between the pain threshold and pain tolerance. Other terms have been used, such as "pain interval" and "pain duration," but they imply a time scale. Wolff's (1971) suggestion of the term *pain sensitivity range* (PSR) is becoming more widespread. Wolff and Jarvik (1963) noted that the PSR correlated more highly with pain tolerance than with pain threshold, and Merskey and Spear (1964) did also.

Wolff (1971) performed a factor analysis on data he obtained from 60 chronic arthritis patients, using several different experimental pain techniques: cold pressor, radiant heat, cutaneous shock, deep muscle shock, and hypertonic saline. For each stimulation method, the pain threshold, pain tolerance, and the PSR were calculated.

The factors obtained in analysis constituted a "cutaneous sensitivity" factor, which contained all the cutaneous parameters except the PSR responses, and two "gluteal (deep) sensitivity" factors. However, a separate PSR factor emerged, representing the PSR measures independent of type or depth of pain or body locus. Wolff (1971) termed this the *pain endurance factor*. This factor had a small but significant positive correlation with successful postoperative painful rehabilitation in the patients. Thus, the PSR is an experimental factor with clinical relevance.

In an application of this concept, ischemic pain has been used to match the intensity of clinical pain experienced by patients and is expressed as a percentage of the patient's ischemic pain tolerance. In a factor analysis of pain and personality measures, the matched level and maximum tolerance level emerged as separate factors, confirming the concept of pain endurance as a specific pain factor related to clinical pain experience (Timmermans & Sternbach, 1974). A canonical correlation analysis of patients' ischemic pain scores, their numerical estimates of clinical pain severity, and personality measures, showed that patients' pain estimates were associated with the impact of pain on daily activities but that ischemic pain scores were associated with the level of depression (Timmermans & Sternbach, 1976). However, technical problems continue to impede the clinical application of the tourniquet pain test (Sternbach, 1983).

Just Noticeable Difference

The just noticeable difference (JND) measure represents the traditional psychophysical difference limen which is the smallest interval that can be discriminated between levels of pain intensity. Hardy et al. (1952), using the radiant heat method, found 21 JNDs from pain threshold to pain tolerance. From this they created a dol scale, in which one dol represented two JNDs, so that there were 10½ clearly discriminable dols from threshold to tolerance. Using the Weber ratio $\Delta I/I$ in which $I =$ stimulus intensity, they found that it did not remain constant, as expected, but increased from 0.03 at threshold to 0.29 at tolerance; they concluded that the Weber law was not obeyed for pricking pain.

Interest in psychophysics shifted from JNDs to the power function. Stevens et al. (1958), using electric shock and a magnitude estimation technique, obtained a slope whose exponent was 3.5. Sternbach and Tursky (1964) obtained exponents of 1.8 to 1.9 in four different magnitude estimation studies, much closer to the slopes for other sensory modalities, and a range of slopes of 1.25 to 2.68, depending on the psychophysical technique used.

Craig et al. (1975) found that social modeling can influence the psychophysical relationship. This is impressive because previously cited studies have shown that the pain threshold can be influenced only slightly by psychological factors, and pain tolerance is easily influenced by these factors, but there had been no suggestion that social context can influence the psychophysical exponent. In fact, Sternbach and Tursky (1964, 1965) failed to find significant differences among ethnic groups in their magnitude estimation exponents. But Craig et al. (1975) found that their pain tolerant model had the effect of significantly reducing the size of the exponent in certain groups compared with control groups with pain intolerant models.

Signal Detection

One of the difficulties with traditional psychophysical analyses is that error variances cannot be parceled out into those due to errors of sensory discrimination and those due to other biasing factors. This difficulty has been overcome by the relative operating characteristic (ROC) technique that emerged from statistical decision theory and electronic signal detection theory (Swets, 1973). The approach has important implications for experimental pain research, because it provides a measure of "sensory discriminability," and a measure of affective and motivational factors reflecting "response bias" (Clark, 1974). Analgesic effects of placebo and suggestion result only from a change in response bias (Clark, 1969, 1974; Feather et al., 1972), whereas nitrous oxide alters both bias and discriminability (Chapman et al., 1973). Recent studies of the effectiveness of acupuncture analgesia have also shown changes in bias and discriminability (Chapman et al., 1977), although there is some dispute about whether or not pain can be assessed by this technique (Rollman, 1977).

PERSONALITY PARAMETERS

Anxiety

There are now many experimental and clinical studies to show that anxiety enhances sensitivity to pain, or increases pain responsiveness (Sternbach, 1968). This is one of the major aspects of the "reaction component" of pain described by Beecher (1959). He showed that the significance of the injury suffered (anxiety) determined the degree of pain more than the extent of tissue injury.

When studies are made of those whose anxiety is very great—psychiatric patients—it is found that complaints of pain occur most frequently in those diagnosed as having anxiety neurosis or anxiety hysteria. And medical patients with complaints of pain are more likely to be diagnosed as anxious than medical patients without pain symptoms (Merksey & Spear, 1967). Furthermore, the severity of postoperative pain and complications in surgical patients are in large measure a function of neurotic anxiety (Parbrook et al., 1973a,b).

Although anxiety is highly associated with the occurrence and severity of pain, it should be noted that in both the experimental and clinical situations it is acute pain that is correlated with anxiety; chronic pain is associated with depression, as described later (Sternbach, 1978).

Expressiveness

Clinicians have long held that the patient who complains about pain more than the average has a "low pain threshold." This is an error. The readiness to communicate the experience of pain is a function of expressiveness, and this in turn is associated with degree of extroversion and also with group membership.

In experimental studies, Lynn and Eysenck (1961) found that the pain tolerance of college students to radiant heat was negatively correlated with neuroticism and positively correlated with extroversion. Eysenck (1961) found that among 100 married and 100 unmarried women having their first babies, extroversion correlated significantly with experienced pain; the more extroverted the woman, the more she recalled her labor as having been painful. Neuroticism was not related to the pain ratings.

In several studies of groups of patients with advanced cancer, Bond and his colleagues (Bond & Pilowsky, 1966; Bond & Pearson, 1969; Pilowsky & Bond, 1969; Bond, 1971, 1973) have shown rather convincingly that the experimental findings on extroversion apply as well to the clinical situation. To summarize the conclusions of these studies, it appears that the degree of *pain experienced* is positively correlated with the degree of neuroticism, but the *complaint* of pain (and the receipt of analgesics) is associated with the degree of extroversion. Of those with the greatest amount of pain (by rating), the amount of pain expression seemed to be a function of extroversion, so that neurotic introverts might suffer silently, with little relationship between pain severity and pain complaint, but those with high extroversion scores had little difficulty communicating.

Social learning influences expressiveness as well, including that related to pain communication. Craig (1984) has shown that learned expressions of pain (which can be evaluated by observers) begin in the second year of infancy. Zborowski (1969) interviewed "Old American," Irish, Italian, and Jewish veterans who were surgical patients in pain, and their families, to determine their attitudes toward pain and pain expression. He found that Old Americans have a phlegmatic, matter-of-fact, doctor-helping orientation associated with their not complaining. The Irish, who also do not complain much, have a fearful, lonesome attitude with a great concern not to appear weak. The Italians and Jews are not inhibited in their expression of pain. The Italians express a desire for immediate pain relief. The Jews express a concern for the meaning of pain as a symptom and the future implications of the pain.

Sternbach and Tursky (1965) interviewed and tested Yankee, Irish, Italian, and Jewish housewives, and corroborated the differences in attitudes toward pain and its expression. The Yankees felt one simply "took it in stride." The Irish were similarly undemonstrative, but anxious, and felt it important to "keep a stiff upper lip" and to not "be a baby." The Italians felt pain was an accident of fate and not to be endured, and expression of their pain helped to rally support and obtain relief. The Jews were similarly demonstrative, in part because of a belief in the cathartic value of "getting it out of your system," and because of a concern to direct attention to the underlying disease the pain represented. These various attitudes were associated with differences in laboratory findings. Italian women had significantly lower pain tolerance to electric shocks, and the Yankees demonstrated a more rapid and complete adaptation of diphasic palmar skin potentials to repeated strong shocks. In addition, there were significant group differences in a number of autonomically innervated variables (Tursky & Sternbach, 1967).

These findings indicate that culturally acquired attitudes toward pain and its expression can modulate the physiological responses to pain. There are many anecdotal reports which suggest even greater differences among various cultures in defining what constitutes pain (Melzack, 1973). However, almost all such observations lack any semblance of methodological rigor (Wolff & Langley, 1968).

Depression

There is a clear difference between the physiologic and psychological reactions in chronic pain, compared with acute pain (Sternbach, 1981, 1984). Anxiety is associated with acute pain, but depression is associated with chronic pain.

In clinical situations, anxiety is associated with the *anticipation* of pain (body harm), or of loss (separation). Depression is associated with the *consequence* of these, in the form of intropunitive anger or of mourning. In view of this relationship, it might be expected that anxiety will be found in acute pain states, as noted above, and depression in chronic pain states. Sternbach et al. (1973) found that patients with low back pain of less than 6 months' duration obtained MMPI profiles within normal limits, whereas those with low back pain of longer duration had markedly elevated scores for depression, hypochondriasis, and hysteria.

Merksey and Spear (1967) found that in 200 consecutive admissions to a psychiatric clinic, pain was a symptom in 53%. Depression was the most common diagnosis, and pain occurred in 56% of the 85 depressives. Pilling et al. (1967) reported on 562 patients seen in psychiatric consultation at the Mayo Clinic; 32% had a pain as a presenting symptom. In both men and women, about 64% of those with pain were thought to have depressive symptoms. This supports the inference from Kenyon's (1964) study of hypochondriasis that pain can "stand for" and affective disorder, as in "masked" depressions.

Bradley (1963) studied the response to antidepressant treatment of 35 patients with pain and depression. In 16 whose pain preceded the depression, depression alone responded to treatment, but there was an increased tolerance of the pain. In the 19 whose pain and depression occurred together, both were relieved by treatment of the depression. Others have also reported on the effects of antidepressants in relieving chronic pain, sometimes in combination with other psychotropic agents (Merskey & Hester, 1972; Taub & Collins, 1974).

Hypochondriasis

A frequent accompaniment of the depression is hypochondriasis, which often "masks" the depression so that the patient and observer are unaware of the depressed affect but focus instead on physical symptoms. Hypochondriasis is the "fascinated absorption by the experience of a physical or mental impairment" (Ladee, 1966).

Pilowsky (1967) found three factors basic to the concept of hypochondriasis: bodily preoccupation, disease phobia, and conviction of the presence of disease with nonresponse to reassurance. Any one or combination of these factors may be present in a pain patient.

Kenyon (1964) examined the records of all patients seen at Bethlem Royal and Maudsley Hospitals in the 10-year period from 1951 to 1960, and chose those receiving an only or primary diagnosis of hypochondriasis (N = 301) to compare with those diagnosed as hypochondriacal secondary to some other diagnosis (N = 211). The symptom most often presented was pain, occurring in 75% of the primary group and in 62% of the secondary group. Affective symptoms of anxiety and depression were the next most frequent, occurring in about 40% of the primary group and in 60% of the secondary group. Of those receiving a secondary diagnosis of hypochondriasis, 82% received a primary diagnosis of an affective disorder.

Pilowsky (1968) found that anxiety and depression were correlated with a good outcome in hypochondriacal patients; treatment of the associated affective disorder diminished the hypochondriasis. Poor treatment outcome was associated with the presence of organic pathology, among other variables. Pilowsky also found that older males and younger females did less well in treatment.

SUMMARY

Pain is a specific sensory event normally initiated by tissue damage or impending tissue damage. Specialized nociceptors transmit information to the spinal cord over specific A-delta and C fibers. Class 1 nociceptive cells, located in lamina 1 of the dorsal horn, respond specifically to injurious stimuli; Class 2 cells in lamina 5 respond to the full range from low intensity to noxious levels of stimulation. The gate control theory predicts that such responses can be inhibited both by large-fiber input and by centrifugal mechanisms. Peripheral analgesic stimulation, whether from acupuncture, transcutaneous neurostimulation, or other mechanisms, seems to involve both a direct effect on peripheral fibers and a central inhibitory mechanism that depends partly on a serotonin system in the periaqueductal gray and periventricular areas and partly on an enkephalin system in overlapping areas, which also involves other structures of the limbic system. Direct stimulation of these areas produces analgesia, which is reversible by naloxone. Other forms of central analgesia, such as motivation, attention, and hypnosis, are not reversible by naloxone.

Pain threshold and pain tolerance can be determined fairly accurately by several experimental techniques, and they show high reliability. Age, sex, race, ethnic group, and other factors can influence both, but pain tolerance is especially susceptible to these. Men have a higher tolerance than women; with aging there is a slight increase in the pain threshold and a marked decrease in pain tolerance, especially for men, which thus narrows the pain sensitivity range with age. This pain sensitivity range has been shown to be a significant pain endurance factor of relevance to clinical pain, and a version of it has been used to measure the severity of clinical pain. The slope of the psychophysical relationship (stimulus intensity versus perceived sensation) depends on the technique used to assess it but seems to have a slightly larger exponent in pain than in most of the other perceptual modalities; it is also susceptible to such influences as the social context of the experimental situation. Signal detection techniques are useful in separating pain sensitivity from biasing factors such as placebo effects.

In both laboratory and clinical situations, the intensity of the subjective pain experience is almost directly proportional to the individual's degree of neuroticism. The neuroticism consists chiefly of anxiety in the acute pain situation and of depression in the chronic situation. Experimentally, extroversion and the presence of a model who is pain tolerant may make the pain experience less intense. Clinically, the pain experience may be potentiated by hypochondriasis. In both the laboratory and clinical situations the readiness to describe the pain experience appears to depend on both the degree of extroversion and ethnic or cultural group membership. Certain groups encourage the expression of pain, albeit for different reasons, and others inhibit such expression, also for different reasons. The clinical pain complaint appears to be an endpoint of both the pain experience and pain expression. As such, it seems to be a function of neuroticism, extroversion, and social learning. In cases of "psychogenic" pain, these seem to be adequate causes. In cases of "somatogenic" pain, these seem to be the factors that make the pain intractable and the patient demanding and manipulative (Sternbach, 1978).

REFERENCES

Adams, J.E. (1976). Naloxone reversal of analgesia produced by brain stimulation in the human. *Pain 2*:161–166.

Akil, H., and J.C. Liebeskind (1975). Monoaminergic mechanisms of stimulation-produced analgesia. *Brain Res. 94*:279–296.

Akil, H., and D.J. Mayer (1972). Antagonism of stimulation-produced analgesia by p-CPA, a serotonin synthesis inhibitor. *Brain Res. 44*:692–697.

Akil, H., D.J. Mayer, and J.C. Liebeskind (1976). Antagonism of stimulation-produced analgesia by naloxone, a narcotic antagonist. *Science 191*:961–962.

Asberg, M., P. Thoren, L. Traskman et al. (1976). "Serotonin depression"—A biochemical subgroup within the affective disorders? *Science 191*:478–480.

Basbaum, A.I., N. Marley, and J. O'Keefe (1976). Spinal cord pathways involved in the production of analgesia by brain stimulation. In *Advances in Pain Research and Therapy, Vol. 1, Proceedings of the First World Congress on Pain* (J.J. Bonica and D. Albe-Fessard, eds.), pp. 511–515. Raven Press, New York.

Beecher, H.K. (1959). *Measurement of Subjective Responses: Quantitative Effects of Drugs.* Oxford University Press, New York.

Bessou, P., and E.R. Perl (1969). Response of cutaneous sensory units with unmyelinated fibers to noxious stimuli. *J. Neurophysiol. 32:*1025–1043.

Bond, M.R. (1971). The relation of pain to the Eysenck Personality Inventory, Cornell Medical Index and Whiteley Index of Hypochondriasis. *Br. J. Psychiatry 119:*671–678.

Bond, M.R. (1973). Personality studies in patients with pain secondary to organic disease. *J. Psychosom. Res. 17:*257–263.

Bond, M.R. and I.B. Pearson (1969). Psychological aspects of pain in women with advanced cancer of the cervix. *J. Psychosom. Res. 13:*13–19.

Bond, M.R. and I. Pilowsky (1966). Subjective assessment of pain and its relationship to the administration of analgesics in patients with advanced cancer. *J. Psychosom. Res. 10:*203–208.

Bradley, J.J. (1963). Severe localized pain associated with the depressive syndrome. *Br. J. Psychiatry 109:*741–745.

Burgess, P.R. and E.R. Perl (1967). Myelinated afferent fibres responding specifically to noxious stimulation of the skin. *J. Physiol. (Lond.) 190:*541–562.

Burgess, P.R. and E.R. Perl (1973). Cutaneous mechanoreceptors and nociceptors. In *Handbook of Sensory Physiology, Vol. 2* (A. Iggo, ed.), pp. 29–78. Springer-Verlag, Berlin.

Casey, K.L. (1966). Unit analysis of nociceptive mechanisms in the thalamus of the awake squirrel monkey. *J. Neurophysiol. 29,*727–750.

Casey, K.L. (1971a). Responses of bulboreticular units to somatic stimuli eliciting escape behavior in the cat. *Int. J. Neurosci. 2:*15–28.

Casey, K.L. (1971b). Escape elicited by bulboreticular stimulation in the cat. *Int. J. Neurosci. 2:*29–34.

Casey, K.L. (1971c). Somatosensory responses of bulboreticular units in awake cat: Relation to escape-producing stimuli. *Science 173:*77–80.

Casey, K.L. and R. Melzack (1967). Neural mechanisms of pain: A conceptual model. In *New Concepts in Pain and Its Clinical Management* (E.L. Way, ed.), pp. 13–31. F.A. Davis, Philadelphia.

Chapman, C.R., A.C. Chen, and J.J. Bonica (1977). Effects of intrasegmental electrical acupuncture on dental pain: Evaluation by threshold estimation and sensory decision theory. *Pain 3:*213–227.

Chapman, C.R., T.M. Murphy, and S.H. Butler (1973). Analgesic strength of 33 percent nitrous oxide: A signal detection theory evaluation. *Science 179:*1246–1248.

Christensen, B.N. and E.R. Perl (1970). Spinal neurons specifically excited by noxious or thermal stimuli: Marginal zone of the dorsal horn. *J. Neurohysiol. 33:*293–307.

Clark, W.C. (1969). Sensory decision theory analysis of the placebo effect on the criterion for pain and thermal sensitivity (d'). *J. Abnorm. Psychol. 74:*363–371.

Clark, W.C. (1974). Pain sensitivity and the report of pain: An introduction to sensory decision theory. *Anesthesiology 40:*272–287.

Craig, K.D. (1984). Emotional aspects of pain. In *Textbook of Pain* (P.D. Wall and R. Melzack, eds.), pp. 153–161. Churchill-Livingstone, Edinburgh.

Craig, K.D., H. Best, and L.M. Ward (1975). Social modelling influences on psychophysical judgments of electrical stimulation. *J. Abnorm. Psychol. 84:*366–373.

Day, R.L., L.M. Kitahata, F.F. Kao et al. (1975). Evaluation of acupuncture anesthesia: A psychophysical study. *Anesthesiology 43:*507–517.

Dubner, R., B.J. Sessle, and A.T. Storey (1978). *The Neural Basis of Oral and Facial Function*. Plenum Press, New York.

Eysenck, S.B.G. (1961). Personality and pain assessment of childbirth of married and unmarried mothers. *J. Ment. Sci. 107:*417–430.

Feather, B.W., C.R. Chapman, and S.B. Fisher (1972). The effect of a placebo on the perception of painful radiant heat stimuli. *Psychosom. Med. 34:*290–294.

Fields, H.L. and A.I. Basbaum (1984). Endogenous pain control mechanisms. In *Textbook of Pain* (P.D. Wall and R. Melzack, eds.), pp. 142–152. Churchill-Livingstone, Edinburgh.

Fitzgerald, M. (1984). The course and termination of primary afferent fibres. In *Textbook of Pain* (P.D. Wall and R. Melzack, eds.), pp. 34–48. Churchill-Livingstone, Edinburgh.

Gaw, A.C., L.W. Chang, and L.-C. Shaw (1975). Efficacy of acupuncture on osteoarthritic pain. *N. Engl. J. Med. 293:*375–378.

Giesler, G.J. Jr., and J.C. Liebeskind (1976). Inhibition of visceral pain by electrical stimulation of the periaqueductal gray matter. *Pain 2:*43–48.

Goldstein, A., and E.R. Hilgard (1975). Lack of influence of the morphine antagonist naloxone on hypnotic analgesia. *Proc. Natl. Acad. Sci. 72:*2041–2043.

Goodman, S.J. and V. Holcombe (1976). Selective and prolonged analgesia in monkey resulting from brain stimulation. In *Advances in Pain Research and Therapy, Vol. 1, Proceedings of the First World Congress on Pain* (J.J. Bonica and D. Albe-Fessard, eds.), pp. 495–502. Raven Press, New York.

Handwerker, H.O., A. Iggo, and M. Zimmerman (1975). Segmental and supraspinal actions on dorsal horn neurons responding to noxious and non-noxious skin stimuli. *Pain 1:*147–165.

Hardy, J.D., H.G. Wolff, and H. Goodell (1952). *Pain Sensations and Reactions*. Williams & Wilkins, Baltimore.

Hillman, P., and P.D. Wall (1969). Inhibitory and excitatory factors influencing the receptive fields of lamina 5 spinal cord cells. *Exp. Brain Res. 9:*284–306.

Hosobuchi, Y., J.E. Adams, and R. Linchitz (1977). Pain relief by electrical stimulation of the central gray matter in humans and its reversal by naloxone. *Science 197:*183–186.

Ignelzi, R.J. and J.K. Nyquist (1976). Direct effect of electrical stimulation on peripheral nerve evoked activity: Implications in pain relief. *J. Neurosurg. 45:*159–165.

Ignelzi, R.J., R.A. Sternbach, and M. Callaghan (1976). Somatosensory changes during transcutaneous electrical analgesia. In *Advances in Pain Research and Therapy, Vol. 1, Proceedings of the First World Congress on Pain* (J.J. Bonica and D. Albe-Fessard, eds.), pp. 421–425. Raven Press, New York.

Jacquet, Y.F. and A. Lajtha (1974). Paradoxical effects after microinjection of morphine in the periaqueductal gray matter in the rat. *Science 185:*1055–1057.

Jouvet, M. (1969). Biogenic amines and the states of sleep. *Science 163:*32–41.

Keele, K.D. (1957). *Anatomies of Pain*. Blackwell, Oxford.

Kenyon, F.E. (1964). Hypochondriasis: A clinical study. *Br. J. Psychiatry 110:*478–488.

Kerr, F.W.L. (1975). Neuroanatomical substrates of nociception in the spinal cord. *Pain 1:*325–356.

Kitahata, L.M., Y. Kosaka, A. Taub, et al. (1974). Lamina-specific suppression of dorsal-horn unit activity by morphine sulfate. *Anesthesiology 41:*39–48.

Kuhar, M.J., C.B. Pert, and S.H. Snyder (1973). Regional distribution of opiate receptor binding in monkey and human brain. *Nature 245:*447–450.

Ladee, G.A. (1966). *Hypochondriacal Syndromes*. Elsevier, Amsterdam.

Li, C.L., D. Ahlberg, H. Lansdell, et al. (1975). Acupuncture and hypnosis: Effects on induced pain. *Exp. Neurol. 49:*272–280.

Liebeskind, J.C., D.J. Mayer, and H. Akil (1974). Central mechanisms of pain inhibition: Studies of analgesia from focal brain stimulation. In *Advances in Neurology*, Vol. 4 (J.J. Bonica, ed.), pp. 261–268. Raven Press, New York.

Lynn, B. (1984). The detection of injury and tissue damage. In *Textbook of Pain* (P.D. Wall and R. Melzack, eds.) pp. 19–33. Churchill-Livingstone, Edinburgh.

Lynn, R. and H.J. Eysenck (1961). Tolerance for pain, extraversion and neuroticism. *Percept. Mot. Skills 12:*161–162.

Maas, J.W. (1975). Biogenic amines and depression: Biochemical and pharmacological separation of two types of depression. *Arch. Gen. Psychiatry 32:*1357–1361.

Mann, F., D. Bowsher, J. Mumford et al. (1973). Treatment of intractable pain by acupuncture. *Lancet 2:*57–60.

Mayer, D.J. and R. Hayes (1975). Stimulation-produced analgesia: Development of tolerance and cross-tolerance to morphine. *Science 188:*941–943.

Mayer D.J. and J.C. Liebeskind (1974). Pain reduction by focal electrical stimulation of the brain: An anatomical and behavioral analysis. *Brain Res. 68:*73–93.

Mayer, D.J. and R. Murfin (1976). Stimulation-produced analgesia (SPA) and morphine analgesia (MA): Cross-tolerance from application at the same brain site. *Fed. Proc. 35:*385.

Mayer, D.J. and D.D. Price (1976). Central nervous system mechanisms of analgesia. *Pain 2:*379–404.

Mayer, D.J., D.D. Price, J. Barber, and A. Rafii (1976). Acupuncture analgesia: Evidence for activation of a pain inhibitory system as a mechanism of action. In *Advances in Pain Research and Therapy, Vol. 1, Proceedings of the First World Congress on Pain* (J.J. Bonica and D. Albe-Fessard, eds.), pp. 751–754. Raven Press, New York.

Mayer, D.J., D.D. Price, and D.P. Becker (1975). Neurophysiological characterization of the anterolateral spinal cord neurons contributing to pain perception in man. *Pain 1:*51–58.

Mayer, D.J., T.L. Wolffe, H. Akil et al. (1971). Analgesia from electrical stimulation in the brainstem of the rat. *Science 174:*1351–1354.

Melzack, R. (1973). *The Puzzle of Pain*. Basic Books, New York.

Melzack, R. (1975). Prolonged relief of pain by brief, intense transcutaneous somatic stimulation. *Pain:* 357–373.

Melzack, R., and D.F. Melinkoff (1974). Analgesia produced by brain stimulation: Evidence of a prolonged onset period. *Exp. Neurol. 43:*369–374.

Melzack, R. and P.D. Wall (1965). Pain mechanisms: A new theory. *Science 150:*971–979.

Melzack, R., D.M. Stillwell, and E.J. Fox (1977). Trigger points and acupuncture points for pain: Correlations and implications. *Pain 3:*3–23.

Merskey, H. and R.N. Hester (1972). The treatment of chronic pain with psychotropic drugs. *Postgrad. Med. J. 48:*594–598.

Merskey, H. and F.G. Spear (1964). The reliability of the presure algometer. *Br. J. Soc. Clin. Psychol. 3:*130–136.

Merskey, H. and F.G. Spear (1967). *Pain: Psychological and Psychiatric Aspects*. Bailliere, Tindall, and Cassell, London.

Moldofsky, H. and P. Scarisbrick (1975). Induction of neurasthenic musculoskeletal pain syndrome by selective sleep stage deprivation. *Psychosom. Med. 38:*35–44.

Moldofsky, H., P. Scarisbrick, R. England, and H. Smythe (1975). Musculoskeletal symptoms and non-REM sleep disturbance in patients with "fibrositis syndrome" and healthy subjects. *Psychosom. Med. 37:*341–351.

Morrow, T.J. and K.L. Casey (1976). Analgesia produced by mesencephalic stimulation: Effect on bulboreticular neurons. In *Advances in Pain Research and Therapy, Vol. 1, Proceedings of the First World Congress on Pain* (J.J. Bonica and D. Albe-Fessard, eds.), pp. 503–510. Raven Press, New York.

Nathan, P.W. and P.D. Wall (1974). Treatment of post-herpetic neuralgia by prolonged electric stimulation. *Br. Med. J. 3*:645–647.

Oleson, T.D. and J.C. Liebeskind (1976). Modification of midbrain and thalamic evoked responses by analgesic brain stimulation in the rat. In *Advances in Pain Research and Therapy, Vol. 1, Proceedings of the First World Congress on Pain.* (J.J. Bonica and D. Albe-Fessard, eds.), pp. 487–494. Raven Press, New York.

Oliveras, J.L., J.M. Besson, G. Guilbaud, and J.C. Liebeskind (1974). Behavioral and electrophysiological evidence of pain inhibition from midbrain stimulation in the cat. *Exp. Brain Res. 20*:32–44.

Oliveras, J.L., F. Redjemi, G. Guilbaud, and J.M. Besson (1975). Analgesia induced by electrical stimulation of the inferior centralis nucleus of the raphe in the cat. *Pain 1*:139–145.

Osler, W. (1912). *The Principles and Practice of Medicine,* 8th ed. pp. 1092–1093. Appleton, New York.

Parbrook, G.D., D.G. Dalrymple, and D.F. Steel (1973a). Personality assessment and post-operative pain and complications. *J. Psychosom. Res. 17*:277–285.

Parbrook, G.D., D.F. Steel, and D.G. Dalrymple (1973b). Factors predisposing to postoperative pain and pulmonary complications. *Br. J. Anaesthesia 45*:21–33.

Perl, E.R. (1968). Myelinated afferent fibres innervating the primate skin and their response to noxious stimuli. *J. Physiol (Lond.) 197*:593–615.

Perl, E.R. (1971). Is pain a specific sensation? *J. Psychiatr. Res. 8*:273–287.

Pert, A. and T. Yaksh (1974). Sites of morphine induced analgesia in the primate brain: Relation to pain pathways. *Brain Res. 80*:135–140.

Pilling, L.F., T.L. Brannick, and W.M. Swenson (1967). Psychologic characteristics of psychiatric patients having pain as a presenting symptom. *Can. Med. Assoc. J. 97*:387–394.

Pilowsky, I. (1967). Dimensions of hypochondriasis. *Br. J. Psychiatry 113*:89–93.

Pilowsky, I. (1968). The response to treatment in hypochondriacal disorders. *Aust. N. Z. J. Psychiatry 2*:88–94.

Pilowsky, I. and M.R. Bond (1969). Pain and its management in malignant disease: Elucidation of staff-patient transactions. *Psychosom. Med. 31*:400–404.

Poggio. G.F. and V.B. Mountcastle (1960). A study of the functional contributions of the lemniscal and spinothalamic systems to somatic sensibility. *Bull. Johns Hopkins Hosp. 106*:266–316.

Pomeranz, B., P.D. Wall, and W.V. Weber (1968). Cord cells responding to fine myelinated afferents from viscera, muscle and skin. *J. Physiol. (Lond.) 199*:511–532.

Price, D.D. (1972). Characteristics of second pain and flexion reflexes indicative of prolonged central summation. *Exp. Neurol. 37*:371–387.

Price, D.D. (1976). Modulation of first and second pain by peripheral stimulation and by psychological set. In *Advances in Pain Research and Therapy, Vol. 1, Proceedings of the First World Congress on Pain* (J.J. Bonica and D. Albe-Fessard, eds.), pp. 427–431. Raven Press, New York.

Price, D.D. and A.C. Browe (1973). Responses of spinal cord neurons to graded noxious and non-noxious stimuli. *Brain Res. 64*:425–429.

Price, D.D. and D.J. Mayer (1975). Neurophysiological characterization of the anterolateral quadrant neurons subserving pain in *Macaca mulatta. Pain 1*:59–72.

Price, D.D. and I.H. Wagman (1970). Physiological roles of A and C fiber inputs to the spinal dorsal horn of *Macaca mulatta. Exp. Neurol. 29*:383–399.

Richardson, D.E. and H. Akil (1977a). Pain reduction by electrical brain stimulation in man. I. Acute administration in periaqueductal and periventricular sites. *J. Neurosurg. 47*:178–183.

Richardson, D.E. and H. Akil (1977b). Pain reduction by electrical brain stimulation in man. II. Chronic self-administration in the periventricular gray matter. *J. Neurosurg. 47*:184–194.

Rollman, G.B. (1977). Signal detection theory measurement of pain: A review and critique. *Pain 3*:187–211.

Soper, W.Y. (1976). Effects of analgesic midbrain stimulation on reflex withdrawal and thermal escape in the rat. *J. Comp. Physiol. Psychol. 90*:91–101.

Sternbach, R.A. (1968). *Pain: A Psychophysiological Analysis.* Academic Press, New York.

Sternbach, R.A. (1974a). Pain and depression. In *Somatic Manifestations of Depressive Disorders* (A. Kiev, ed.), pp. 107–119. Excerpta Medica, Princeton, N.J.

Sternbach, R.A. (1974b). *Pain Patients: Traits and Treatment.* Academic Press, New York.

Sternbach, R.A. (ed.) (1978). *The Psychology of Pain.* Raven Press, New York.

Sternbach, R.A. (1981). Chronic pain as a disease entity. *Triangle 20*:27–32.

Sternbach, R.A. (1983). The tourniquet pain test. In *Pain Measurement and Assessemnt* (R. Melzack, ed.), pp. 27–31. Raven Press, New York.

Sternbach, R.A. (1984). Acute versus chronic pain. In *Textbook of Pain* (P.D. Wall and R. Melzack, eds.), pp. 173–177. Churchill-Livingstone, Edinburgh.

Sternbach, R.A. and B. Tursky (1964). On the psychophysical power function in electric shock. *Psychonom. Sci. 1*, 217–218.

Sternbach, R.A. and B. Tursky (1965). Ethnic differences in psychophysical and skin potential responses to electric shock. *Psychophysiology 1*:241–246.

Sternbach, R.A., R.J. Ignelzi, L.M. Deems, and G. Timmermans (1976a). Transcutaneous electrical analgesia: A follow-up analysis. *Pain 2*:35–41.

Sternbach, R.A., D.S. Janowsky, L.Y. Huey, and D.S. Segal (1976b). Effects of altering brain serotonin activity on human chronic pain. In *Advances in Pain Research and Therapy, Vol. 1, Proceedings of the First World Congress on Pain* (J.J. Bonica and D. Albe-Fessard, eds.), pp. 601–606. Raven Press, New York.

Sternbach, R.A., S.R. Wolf, R.W. Murphy, and W.H. Akeson (1973). Traits of pain patients: The low-back "loser." *Psychosomatics 14*:226–229.

Stevens, S.S., A.S. Carton, and G.M. Shickman (1958). A scale of apparent intensity of electric shock. *J. Exp. Psychol. 56:* 328–334.

Swets, J.A. (1973). The relative operating characteristic in psychology. *Science 182*:990–1000.

Taub, A. and J.N. Campbell (1974). Percutaneous local electrical analgesia: Peripheral mechanisms. In *Advances in Neurology, Vol. 4* (J.J. Bonica, ed.), pp. 727–732. Raven Press, New York.

Taub, A. and W.F. Collins, Jr. (1974). Observations on the treatment of denervation dysesthesia with psychotropic agents: Postherpetic neuralgia, anesthesia dolorosa, peripheral neuropathy. In *Advances in Neurology,* Vol. 4 (J.J. Bonica, ed.), pp. 727–732. Raven Press, New York.

Terenius, L. (1984). The endogenous opioids and other central peptides. In *Textbook of Pain* (P.D. Wall and R. Melzack, eds.), pp. 133–141. Churchill-Livingstone, Edinburgh.

Timmermans, G. and R.A. Sternbach (1974). Factors of human chronic pain: An analysis of pain and personality measures. *Science 184*:806–807.

Timmermans, G. and R.A. Sternbach (1976). Human chronic pain and personality: A canonical correlation analysis. In *Advances in Pain Research and Therapy, Vol. 1, Proceedings of the First World Congress on Pain* (J.J. Bonica and D. Albe-Fessard, eds.), pp. 307–310. Raven Press, New York.

Torebjork, H.E. and R.G. Hallin (1973). Perceptual changes accompanying controlled preferential blocking of A and C fibre responses in intact human skin nerves. *Exp. Brain Res. 16*:321–332.

Torebjork, H.E. and R.G. Hallin (1974a). Identification of afferent C units in intact human skin nerves. *Brain Res. 67*:387–403.

Torebjork, H.E. and R.G. Hallin (1974b). Excitation failure in thin nerve fiber structures and accompanying hypalgesia during repetitive electric skin stimulation. In *Advances in Neurology, Vol. 4* (J.J. Bonica, ed.), pp. 733–736. Raven Press, New York.

Travell, J. and S.H. Rinzler (1952). The myofascial genesis of pain. *Postgrad. Med. 11*:425–434.

Tursky, B. (1974). Physical, physiological, and psychological factors that affect pain reaction to electric shock. *Psychophysiology 11*:95–112.

Tursky, B. and D. O'Connell (1972). Reliability and interjudgment predictability of subjective judgments of electrocutaneous stimulation. *Psychophysiology 9*:290–295.

Tursky, B. and R.A. Sternbach (1967). Further physiological correlates of ethnic differences in responses to shock. *Psychophysiology 4*:67–74.

Van Hees, J. and J.M. Gybels (1972). Pain related to single afferent C fibers from human skin. *Brain Res. 48*:397–400.

Wall, P.D. (1984). The dorsal horn. In *Textbook of Pain* (P.D. Wall and R. Melzack, eds.), pp. 80–87. Churchill-Livingstone, Edinburgh.

Wall, P.D. and W.H. Sweet (1967). Temporary abolition of pain in man. *Science 155*:108–109.

Willis, W.D. (1984). The origin and destination of pathways involved in pain transmission. In *Textbook of Pain* (P.D. Wall and R. Melzack, eds.), pp. 88–99. Churchill-Livingstone, Edinburgh.

Willis, W.D., D.L. Trevino, J.D. Coulter, and R.A. Maunz (1974). Responses of primate spinothalamic tract neurons to natural stimulation of the hindlimb. *J. Neurophysiol. 37*:358–372.

Wolff, B.B. (1971). Factor analysis of human pain responses: Pain endurance as a specific pain factor. *J. Abnorm. Psychol. 78*:292–298.

Wolff, B.B. and M.E. Jarvik (1963). Variations in cutaneous and deep somatic pain sensitivity. *Can. J. Psychol. 17*:37–44.

Wolff, B.B. and M.E. Jarvik (1965). Quantitative measures of deep somatic pain: Further studies with hypertonic saline. *Clin. Sci. 28*:43–56.

Wolff, B.B. and S. Langley (1968). Cultural factors and the response to pain: A review. *Am. Anthropologist 70*:494–501.

Woodrow, K.M., G.D. Friedman, A.B. Siegelaub, and M.F. Collen (1972). Pain tolerance: Differences according to age, sex and race. *Psychosom. Med. 34*:548–556.

Yaksh, T.L. and D.L. Hammond (1982). Peripheral and central substrates involved in the rostrad transmission of nociceptive information. *Pain 13*:1–85.

Zborowski, M. (1969). *People in Pain*. Jossey-Bass, San Francisco.

3

Pain-Sensitive Cranial Structures

ROBERT J. COFFEY
ALBERT L. RHOTON, JR.

The foundation for any study of the causes and treatments of headache is knowledge of the pain-sensitive structures and pain-conducting pathways within the cranium. Anatomic studies of postmortem human and animal material form the cornerstone on which further knowledge is built. The recent use of histochemical tracer techniques adds another dimension to the anatomic evidence regarding intracranial sensory innervation. Brain surgery performed under local anesthesia on awake patients has also contributed significant data regarding the pain sensitivity of intracranial structures to direct stimulation. The most well known of these studies is the landmark paper of Ray and Wolff (1940) on which this chapter was based in earlier editions. Experimental stimulation during intracranial surgery on anesthetized lower animals provides corroborative, although less direct information. Finally, the examination of patients after the ablation of cranial sensory pathways by deliberate surgical interventions or destructive pathologic processes serves to correlate clinical observations with anatomic data.

The present chapter reviews the anatomic, physiologic, and clinical evidence contributing to our current knowledge of the pain-sensitive intracranial structures. Pathways involved in the pains of superficial scalp origin, cranial neuralgias, cervical spondylosis, and ocular, paranasal sinus, or dental disease are discussed in separate chapters devoted to those entities. The cranial bone itself, and its endosteal venous channels, are insensitive to pain.

The following discussion considers first the anatomic evidence and intraoperative data regarding structures within the supratentorial compartment and then a similar examination of the posterior fossa contents. The results of animal and human experimentation and observation are presented to correlate anatomic principles with cranial pain syndromes.

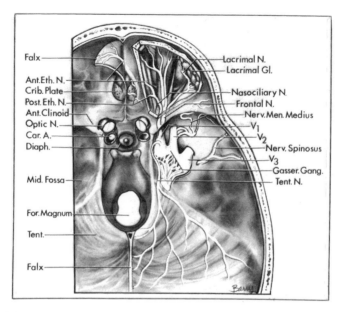

Figure 3-1. View of the anterior skull base showing the trigeminal sensory innervation of the supratentorial dura, dural sinuses, and meningeal arteries. The tentorial nerve (Tent. N.) arises from the ophthalmic division (V1) just proximal to the superior orbital fissure. Anterior and posterior ethmoidal nerves (Ant. Eth. N., Post. Eth. N.) arise from the nasociliary branch (Nasociliary N.) of the ophthalmic division within the orbit. The nervus meningeus medius (Nerv. Men. Medius) branches from the maxillary division (V2) proximal to the cavernous sinus. The nervus spinosus (Nerv. Spinosus) arises from the mandibular division (V3) outside the foramen ovale and reenters the skull through the foramen spinosum with the middle meningeal artery. Abbreviations: anterior clinoid (Ant. Clinoid), carotid artery (Car. A.), cribriform plate (Crib. Plate), diaphragm sellae (Diaph.), foramen magnum (For. Magnum), frontal nerve (Frontal N.), gasserian ganglion (Gasser. Gang.), lacrimal gland (Lacrimal Gl.), lacrimal nerve (Lacrimal N.), middle fossa (Mid. Fossa), optic nerve (Optic N.), tentorium (Tent.)

SUPRATENTORIAL DURA, DURAL SINUSES, AND MENINGEAL ARTERIES

Anatomic Data

The ophthalmic division of the trigeminal nerve (Figure 3-1) is a major source of pain-sensitive afferents for large areas the supratentorial dura and associated venous structures. (Figure 3-2). The tentorial nerve of Arnold arises as a group of branches from the superior margin of the proximal ophthalmic division within the lateral wall of the cavernous sinus just before that division enters the superior orbital fissure (Arnold, 1851). It immediately turns posteriorly within the most anterior portion of the free tentorial edge and courses close to the trochlear nerve with which it was originally confused by Arnold (Penfield & McNaughton, 1940). As the tentorium fans out in a triangular fashion, the fibers of the tentorial nerve spread out within its leaves. Here, the nerve bears no constant relation to the tentorial artery. Upon reaching the posterior tentorial margin at the transverse sinus, terminal branches of the tentorial nerve turn upwards within the dura of the parieto-occipital convexity. The more medial branches within the tentorium reach the straight sinus at the junction of

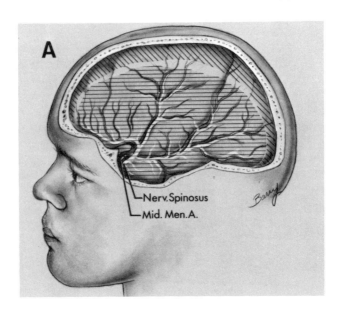

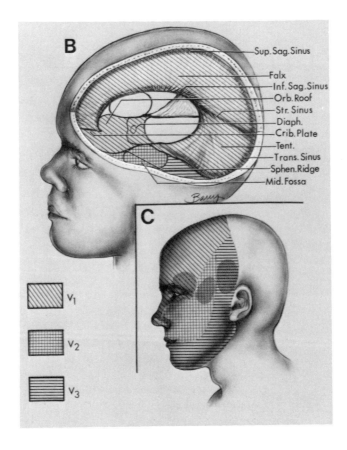

the tentorium and falx cerebri. Here, branches turn forward to distribute themselves along the posterior two thirds of the falx for its entire width from convexity to free margin. In this fashion the tentorial nerves supply the tentorium, the superior surface of the transverse and straight sinuses, and the caudal two thirds of the falx, including the superior and inferior sagittal sinuses (Feindel et al., 1960; Kimmel, 1961b; Lance, 1982; McNaughton, 1938; McNaughton & Feindel, 1977; Netter & Mitchell, 1983; Penfield & McNaughton, 1940). Evidence gathered during awake brain surgery suggests that major surface tributary veins of the previously named sinuses also receive ophthalmic division innervation by means of the tentorial nerve (see below).

The dura of the diaphragma sellae is also supplied by the ophthalmic division through a small branch that arises variably from the first division or its tentorial or frontal branches. According to Kimmel (1961b) this branch reaches the superior hypophyseal artery, (branch of supraclinoid internal carotid artery), accompanies it for a short distance, and then joins the dura forming the intercavernous venous sinuses. It divides into anterior and posterior dural branches, which enter the diaphragm sellae.

Upon entering the orbit, the ophthalmic division divides into the frontal, nasociliary, and lacrimal nerves. The nasociliary nerve traverses the common annular tendon and gives off an inconstant posterior ethmoidal nerve as well as a more constant anterior ethmoidal nerve. Other branches of the nasociliary nerve include the infratrochlear and long ciliary nerves as well as the sensory root of the ciliary ganglion, neither of which is concerned with intracranial sensation. The posterior and anterior ethmoidal nerves, in addition to innervating mucous membranes of the ethmoidal sinuses and nasal cavity, contribute twigs to the anterior meningeal nerves. These are formed by variable contributions from all three trigeminal divisions and provide innervation to the dura over the cribriform plate of the ethmoid bone, the medial orbital roof, the crista galli, and the rostral one third of the falx including the superior and inferior sagittal sinuses (Feindel et al, 1960; Kimmel, 1961b; Lance, 1982; McNaughton; 1938; McNaughton & Feindel, 1977; Netter & Mitchell, 1983; Penfield & McNaughton, 1940).

The maxillary division of the trigeminal nerve gives off a dural branch, the nervus meningeus medius of Arnold (1860), before it enters the cavernous sinus. It courses laterally and anteriorly within the dura of the middle fossa floor to join the middle meningeal artery, most often the anterior branch, but occasionally the main trunk or

Figure 3-2. The supratentorial dural structures with their contained sinuses and meningeal arteries, shown according to their predominant sensory supply from the three divisions of the trigeminal nerve, as shown by the accompanying key. *(A)* Lateral view of the dura covering the cerebral hemisphere, showing the nervus spinosus branch of the mandibular division (Nerv. Spinosus) closely following the ramifications of the middle meningeal artery (Mid. Men. A.). The narrow band of dura on either side of the superior sagittal sinus receives its innervation from the ophthalmic division through the ethmoidal and tentorial nerves (see Figures 3-1, 3-2B, and the text). *(B)* Schematic view of the tentorium (Tent.), falx, and anterior and middle fossa dural structures after removal of the convexity dura. *(C)* The dermatomal distribution of the trigeminal divisions is shown on the face. Within each dermatome is a smaller, shaded area, which represents the most common sites of referred pain from stimulation during intracranial surgery on awake patients of dural or vascular structures innervated by each division. Abbreviations: cribriform plate (Crib. Plate), diaphragm sellae (Diaph.), inferior sagittal sinus (Inf. Sagg. Sinus), middle fossa (Mid. Fossa), orbital roof (Orb. Roof), sphenoid ridge (Sphen. Ridge), straight sinus (Str. Sinus), superior sagittal sinus (Sup. Sagg. Sinus), tentorium (Tent.), transverse sinus (Trans. Sinus).

posterior branch. Closely applied to the artery and its branches, it supplies the dura of the anterior floor of the middle fossa along with a variable contribution from branches of the mandibular division. Branches of the nervus meningeus medius, along with the middle meningeal artery, cross the sphenoidal ridge to innervate the dural covering of the orbital roof, especially its lateral portion (Feindel et al., 1960; Kimmel, 1961b; Lance, 1982; McNaughton, 1938; McNaughton & Feindel, 1977; Netter & Mitchell, 1983; Penfield & McNaughton, 1940).

The mandibular division of the trigeminal nerve consists of a large preganglionic sensory root and the smaller motor/proprioceptive root (portio minor), which unite immediately upon leaving the foramen ovale. The nerve then lies between the lateral pterygoid and tensor veli palatini muscles just anterior to the extracranial portion of the middle meningeal artery. Here, the otic ganglion is suspended from the medial surface of the nerve by its preganglionic root. The nervus spinosus of Luschka (1850) leaves the mandibular nerve posteriorly at this level to join the middle meningeal artery and reenter the cranial cavity with that vessel through the foramen spinosum. According to Penfield and McNaughton (1940), the nervus spinosus sometimes passes directly from the third division to the artery without first leaving the skull. In all cases the nerve closely follows the middle meningeal artery and its ramifications to supply the dura over the lateral floor of the middle fossa and most of the convexity of the cranium. Upon reaching the vertex between the anterior and middle thirds of the superior sagittal sinus, branches of the nervus spinosus extend onto that structure and the adjacent falx. Thus, the third trigeminal division through the nervus spinosus provides innervation to the "sensory watershed" region of the falx between the portions supplied by the first division through the tentorial and anterior meningeal nerves (Feindel et al., 1960; Kimmel, 1961b; McNaughton, 1938; McNaughton & Feindel, 1977; Netter & Mitchell, 1983; Penfield & McNaughton, 1940).

Cadaver dissection reveals fibers originating in all divisions of the trigeminal nerve supplying the supratentorial dura in an orderly and generally constant fashion. The first division fibers through the tentorial nerve are largely distributed along venous structures, the major supratentorial dural sinuses, while second- and third-division fibers of the nervus meningeus medius and nervus spinosus closely follow arterial structures, the middle meningeal artery, and its branches.

The data gathered by investigators using the technique of retrograde axonal transport of horseradish peroxidase (HRP) agree in most respects with earlier studies based on dissection of anatomic specimens. Steiger et al. (1982) applied HRP to various regions of supratentorial dura in the cat. When HRP was applied to the "medial aspect of the anterior cranial fossa," labeled cell bodies were found in the ophthalmic division of the trigeminal ganglion. When applied more laterally to the orbital roof dura, HRP label appeared predominantly in the maxillary division of the ganglion. Application to the tentorial dura led to labeling of first-division neurons (tentorial nerve), whereas HRP placed centrally along the middle fossa floor appeared in third-division neurons. Most labeled neurons in all divisions were small, supporting the notions that they subserve pain and that dural sensitivity is limited to that modality. In other recent studies, also in cats (Mayberg at al., 1984; Moskowitz, 1984), HRP applied directly to the middle meningeal artery appeared in trigeminal ganglion cells of all divisions, predominantly the ophthalmic. Likewise, tracer applied to either the anterior or the posterior third of the sagittal sinus appeared in first-division neurons.

Sinus ligation and falcine transection, either rostral or caudal with respect to the HRP application site, prevented label from appearing in ganglion cells.

Despite some differences between these studies, the data are remarkably consistent with those of earlier morphologic investigations and support the notion that the trigeminal system is the sole source of sensory innervation to the supratentorial dura, venous sinuses, and meningeal arteries.

Stimulation Studies

Beginning with Cushing (1904), neurosurgeons have taken the opportunity to study and record the reactions of awake patients to stimulation of the various tissues exposed during intracranial operations. Both faradic and mechanical stimulation were commonly used. The observations of most investigators are in accord with those presented by Ray and Wolff (1940) in their landmark study (Cushing, 1909; Fay, 1931, 1937, 1939; Feindel et al., 1960; Kerr, 1961; McNaughton & Feindel, 1977; Penfield, 1935; Penfield & Norcross, 1936; Ray & Wolff, 1940; Tasker et al., 1982; Wirth & Van Buren, 1971; Wolff, 1938, 1955).

The dura over the cerebral convexity and middle fossa floor is itself insensitive to all modalities of stimulation except immediately along or within 2 mm of the meningeal arteries or dural sinuses. In contrast, the dura of the anterior fossa floor is sensitive over its entire surface. Pain arising there is referred to the ipsilateral eye and forehead. It is most intense with stimulation medially at the olfactory groove and diminishes progressively as the stimulus moves anteriorly toward the frontal convexity or laterally toward the sphenoid ridge. In those regions pain sensitivity along branches of the anterior meningeal artery is maintained and referred to the forehead or back of the eye. Stimulation of the middle meningeal artery or its small branches well out onto the convexity yields pain roughly localized to the area of stimulation.

The superior surface of the tentorium, torcular, transverse, and straight sinuses as well as the posterior portion of the superior and inferior sagittal sinuses all refer pain to the ipsilateral forehead and eye when stimulated. The anatomic basis of this phenomenon is the distribution of the tentorial nerves discussed earlier. Major surface venous tributaries of the superior sagittal, sphenoparietal, and transverse sinuses also refer pain to the cutaneous field of the ipsilateral ophthalmic division. Only one study found random pain referral phenomena, including a number of cases with bilateral or contralateral pain (Wirth & Van Buren, 1971). In general, the patterns of localized and referred pain elicited during awake intracranial surgery correspond to the distribution of trigeminal fibers found in anatomic studies.

It has been the experience of most investigators that the pial surface remote from large basal vessels is insensitive to painful stimulation. However, during functional stereotactic operations on awake patients, Tasker (Tasker et al., 1982) obtained painful responses to the mechanical passage of a probe or electrical stimulation through the probe in the region of the dorsal midbrain pia. The majority of these responses consisted of pain referred within the ipsilateral trigeminal ophthalmic division. Probe location was predicted from a computerized correlation of ventriculographic and stereotactic brain atlas data. Whether these responses truly represent ophthalmic division innervation of the midbrain pia or reflect incidental stimulation of the tentorium or nearby vascular structures known to have trigeminal innervation remains to be shown conclusively. The application of advanced imaging techniques such as computed tomography and magnetic resonance imaging to probe localization during stereotactic surgery may ultimately settle the question.

SUPRATENTORIAL CEREBRAL ARTERIES

Anatomic Data

The details of innervation of the vessels of the circle of Willis and their penetrating cerebral branches (Figure 3-3) has remained an area of active investigation and controversy since the turn of the century (Gulland, 1898; Hassin, 1929; Huber, 1899). All modern studies have demonstrated a rich nerve plexus, probably of mixed sensory and vasomotor function, on the main arterial trunks at the base of the brain and their proximal pial surface branches (Lance, 1982).

Despite a few reports of vascular nerves accompanying penetrating intracerebral vessels (Chorobski & Penfield, 1932; Penfield, 1932a; Clark, 1934; Mcnaughton, 1938; Stohr, 1932), a recent electron micrographic study failed to disclose any nerve supply to those deep vessels (Dahl, 1976). The bulk of evidence suggests that the source of afferent sensory fibers on supratentorial arterial trunks is the ophthalmic division of the trigeminal nerve. However, no direct connection between the trigeminal nerve and the circle of Willis has yet been conclusively demonstrated. Thus, aside from showing a network of nerve fibers investing the major basal and surface arteries, classic anatomic techniques have done little to elucidate the source of afferent vascular nerves.

In 1981, Mayberg et al. first reported the results of applying HRP to the proximal middle cerebral artery (MCA) in the cat. They found labeled cells in the ipsilateral trigeminal ganglion, predominantly the ophthalmic division, and in the ipsilateral superior cervical sympathetic ganglion (SCG). Subsequent studies employing HRP and wheat germ agglutinin (WGA) confirmed these findings (Liu-Chen et al, 1983c; Mayberg et al, 1984; Moskowitz, 1984). The authors microscopically examined the ganglia of the trigeminal, facial, glossopharyngeal, and vagus nerves as well as the superior cervical ganglion bilaterally. Tracer application to distal MCA branches yielded fewer labeled cells in the trigeminal ganglion than proximal application, suggesting a more sparse innervation distally on the vessel. Ligation and transection of the proximal MCA prevented any retrograde transport of tracer, and no labeled cells were found. Thus, even though the neural pathway between the trigeminal nerve and the circle of Willis has not been found, it is clear that the supratentorial vascular sensory nerves have their first-order neuron in the ophthalmic division of the trigeminal ganglion.

The second-order neuron mediating somesthetic function from dural, venous, and arterial trigeminal afferents lies within the descending (spinal) trigeminal nucleus, which itself merges with the substantia gelatinosa (lamina II of Rexed) of the upper cervical cord. Projections from the spinal nucleus of V travel in the crossed and uncrossed ventral trigeminothalamic tracts (trigeminal lemniscus) to reach the ventral posteromedial thalamic nuclei as well as the intralaminar nuclei bilaterally. General

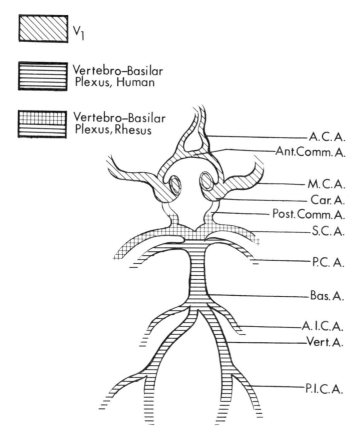

Figure 3-3. The major arterial trunks at the base of the brain are illustrated according to the source of their sensory nerve supply. The ophthalmic division of the trigeminal nerve (V1) provides the general somatic sensory supply to the intracranial carotid (Car. A.), middle cerebral (M.C.A.), anterior cerebral (A.C.A.), anterior communicating (Ant. Comm. A.), and possibly the proximal posterior communicating arteries (Post. Comm. A.). The vertebrobasilar plexus provides a mixed sensory–autonomic nerve supply to the vertebral (Vert. A.), basilar (Bas. A), posterior inferior cerebellar (P.I.C.A.), anterior inferior cerebellar (A.I.C.A.), and superior cerebellar arteries (S.C.A.) in the human. This plexus extends more rostrally in the rhesus monkey to supply the posterior cerebral arteries (P.C.A.) as well. The precise origin of the vertebrobasilar plexus remains unsettled (see text).

somatic afferent (GSA) impulses originating in the trigeminal, vagal, and upper cervical nerves converge on the second-order neuron pool within the descending nucleus of V at the cervicomedullary junction. This may represent the anatomic basis of pain referral phenomena seen in the pathologic conditions affecting the foramen magnum region (see below) (Kerr, 1961, 1962, 1967).

Stimulation Studies

The small cortical surface vessels over the convexity are insensitive to all forms of stimulation. In contrast, stimulation of the supraclinoid internal carotid artery, the proximal middle cerebral artery, and the anterior cerebral artery (pre- and postcommunicating segments) elicits pain referred to the ipsilateral eye and forehead or pterion. The large superficial middle cerebral vein and its bridging segment refer pain in the same distribution.

In summary, the trigeminal system, in addition to being the sole source of supratentorial dural and meningeal vessel sensory afferents, is also, through the ophthalmic division, the source of sensory fibers to the vessels of the anterior circulation.

INFRATENTORIAL DURA, DURAL SINUSES AND MENINGEAL ARTERIES

Anatomic Studies

The interpretation of data from cadaver dissection studies of the posterior fossa dural nerves (Figure 3-4) has generated a controversy for more than one and a quarter centuries, which is only now being sorted out. Various authors have implicated the facial, glossopharyngeal, vagal, spinal accessory, sympathetic, and upper three cervical nerves either alone or in various combinations as supplying painful sensation to the posterior fossa dura and associated vascular structures (Keller et al., 1985b; Kerr, 1961, 1962; Kimmel, 1961a, 1961b; Lance, 1982; Netter & Mitchell, 1983; Pearson, 1939).

Kimmel, in 1961 (Kimmel, 1961a,b), studied the posterior fossa nerves in serially sectioned human embryos. He rejected the notion of a cranial nerve source for any of the infratentorial general somatic afferents and advanced the theory that cells in the upper three cervical dorsal root ganglia sent fibers through the foramen magnum, hypoglossal canal, and jugular foramen in company with the respective cranial nerves. More recent studies have shown Kimmel's theory to be at least partly true. General somatic afferent fibers with cell bodies in the superior vagal ganglion form a recurrent meningeal branch, which travels back through the jugular foramen. The cells of the upper two or three cervical spinal ganglia probably contribute to the recurrent meningeal branch of the vagus through interconnections at the level of the superior vagal ganglion. The superior cervical sympathetic ganglion also contributes fibers, probably with vasomotor function, to the meningeal branch at this level. Once inside the cranium, branches of the nerve travel superiorly and anteriorly along the walls of the sigmoid sinus to innervate dura over the petrous surface of the temporal bone. Other fibers turn posteriorly at the level of the inferior wall of the transverse sinus to reach the falx cerebelli, occipital sinus, and dura covering the suboccipital cerebellar surface. The central processes of vagal GSA cells synapse on second-order neurons in the ipsilateral spinal trigeminal nucleus.

Sensory fibers entering the posterior fossa through the hypoglossal canal all originate in cells of the upper two cervical spinal ganglia. They travel with the hypoglossal nerve and meningeal branch of the ascending pharyngeal artery, form a plexus within the hypoglossal canal, and emerge onto the posterior fossa floor as two branches. One extends anteriorly and laterally to innervate dura to the level of the inferior petrosal sinus. The posterior branch travels along the posterolateral margin of the foramen magnum to supply the dura of the medial posterior fossa floor.

The dura lining the anterior floor of the posterior fossa, clivus, and ventral cran-

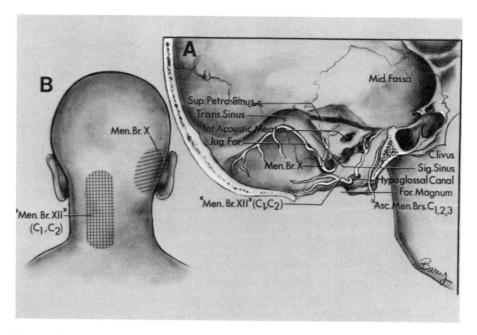

Figure 3-4. *(A)* The dura, dural sinuses, and meningeal arteries of the posterior fossa with their accompanying sensory nerve supply. The recurrent meningeal branch of the vagus nerve (Men. Br. X) enters the jugular foramen (Jug. For.) to innervate the dura covering the petrous surface of the temporal bone as well as the suboccipital cerebellar convexity and adjacent sinuses: sigmoid sinus (Sig. Sinus), superior petrosal sinus (Sup. Petro. Sinus), and transverse sinus (Trans. Sinus). The meningeal branch of the hypoglossal nerve (Men. Br. XII) enters the hypoglossal canal with the posterior meningeal branch of the ascending pharyngeal artery. The fibers actually arise in the upper two cervical dorsal root ganglia and provide innervation to the lateral margin of the foramen magnum (For. Magnum) and lateral posterior fossa floor. Ascending branches of meningeal rami from the upper three cervical nerves (ASC. Men. Brs. C1, 2, 3) traverse the dura along the anterior craniospinal junction to supply the clivus. These reach almost to the level of the posterior clinoid processes. Abbreviations: internal acoustic meatus (Int. Acoustic Meatus), middle fossa (Mid. Fossa). *(B)* Stimulation of structures innervated by the recurrent meningeal branch of the vagus nerve elicits referred pain behind the ipsilateral ear in the distribution of the auricular (cutaneous) branch of the vagus. Sensations evoked by stimulation of the dural structures innervated by upper cervical fibers forming the meningeal branch of the hypoglossal nerve are referred to the ipsilateral occipitonuchal region within the highest cervical dermatomes. Stimulation of the ventral posterior fossa dura innervated by the ascending meningeal branches of C1, C2, and C3 (Asc. Men. Brs. C1, 2, 3) in the awake patient has not been reported.

iospinal junction is supplied by ascending branches of meningeal rami from the upper three cervical nerves. The majority of fibers originate at the second cervical level. Within the ventral dura near the midline, interconnections between branches from opposite sides of the body occur. The rostral extent of these branches is almost to the level of the posterior clinoid processes (Kimmel, 1961a, 1961b).

Studies of posterior fossa dural innervation using current neuroanatomic tracer techniques have only recently been reported (Keller et al., 1985b). In the cat, application of HRP to the dura of the inferior leaf of the tentorium, the suboccipital cerebellar surface, and the clivus leads to bilateral tracer uptake in the upper three cervical dorsal root ganglia. Tracer applied to tentorial dura appears in the ophthalmic division of the trigeminal ganglion as well. Application to the suboccipital dura leads to labeling of cells in the superior vagal ganglion, presumably through the recurrent meningeal branch. No pathway to explain the appearance of HRP-labeled cells in the mandibular division of the trigeminal ganglion after application to suboccipital dura has yet been found. HRP placed on dura covering the clivus labels cells in the superior vagal ganglion as well as the cervical dorsal root ganglia. The finding of bilateral labeling in many cases is likely due to the intermingling of fibers from both sides of the body mentioned earlier.

Significantly, no tracer appears in the geniculate, inferior vagal (nodose), or the superior or inferior glossopharyngeal ganglia. These findings are in general agreement with current concepts of posterior fossa innervation based on anatomic dissection. Interspecies variation, which is most significant in the context of the trigeminal system's contribution to posterior fossa innervation, must be kept in mind.

Stimulation Studies

The patterns of referred pain elicited during the stimulation of posterior fossa dura and associated vascular channels during awake brain surgery confirm the anatomic data presented earlier (Dalessio, 1980a; Kerr, 1967; Penfield & McNaughton, 1940; Pickering, 1955). As in the supratentorial compartment, the dura itself over the suboccipital cerebellar convexity is for the most part, insensitive to all forms of stimulation (Ray & Wolff, 1940).

The dura covering the medial petrous surface and lateral posterior fossa floor, including the sigmoid sinus, is sensitive to stimulation, having pain referred to an area behind the ipsilateral ear. Stimulation along the lower margin of the transverse sinus and adjacent superior portion of the occipital sinus yields pain referred to the same area. All of the previously named dural structures are innervated by the recurrent meningeal branch of the vagus nerve. The area of pain referral corresponds to the cutaneous distribution of the auricular branch of the vagus, which arises from the superior ganglion at the same level as the meningeal branch. Furthermore, intracranial section of the vagus nerve abolishes pain sensitivity in these dural structures.

The mesial posterior fossa floor surrounding the foramen magnum, the dorsal suboccipitocervical junction, and the lower portion of the occipital sinus are all sensitive to stimulation, having pain referred to the low occipital and upper cervical regions. Stimulation of branches of the posterior meningeal artery along the floor of the posterior fossa also yields low occipital–upper cervical pain. This corresponds to the dural and cutaneous fields of the upper cervical roots, the pain being abolished by intradural section of the upper three cervical dorsal roots. The ventral margin of the foramen magnum, posterior fossa floor, and clivus, also receiving upper cervical sensory fibers, have not been exposed and stimulated in awake patients.

Kerr found a unique role for the first cervical dorsal root, which he exposed in awake surgical patients (Kerr, 1961, 1962, 1967). Electrical stimulation of Cl intradural fibers caused frontal headache in the distribution of the ipsilateral trigeminal ophthalmic division. Central processes from pseudounipolar cells in the first cervical spinal ganglion synapse with their second-order neuron within the spinal trigeminal nuclear complex at the cervicomedullary junction. Kerr proposed central processing at this level as a mechanism to explain the phenomenon of fronto-orbital headache due to tonsillar herniation or a foramen magnum lesion compressing and irritating the first cervical root.

INFRATENTORIAL CEREBRAL ARTERIES

Anatomic Studies

Aside from revealing the presence of a perivascular nerve plexus on the surface of the vertebrobasilar vessels and their branches, studies of stained cadaver material have contributed little to uncovering the origin of such nerves (see Figure 3-3). A sympathetic contribution through the perivertebral plexus exists, but its relevance to sensory innervation is doubtful.

Cadaver dissections have shown that the rostral extent of the vertebrobasilar nerve plexus varies among species. In the human, it includes the superior cerebellar arteries whereas in the rhesus monkey the vertebrobasilar plexus extends onto the posterior cerebral arteries (McNaughton, 1938). Thus, the application of data from anatomic tracer studies or physiologic experimentation performed on lower animals to explain headache phenomena observed in humans must be viewed with caution. This applies especially to the posterior cerebral and posterior communicating arteries, which may represent a sensory watershed between the trigeminal and vagocervical innervation territories.

Keller and others (Keller et al., 1985a) examined the ganglia of the trigeminal, facial, glossopharyngeal, and vagal nerves as well as dorsal root ganglia of the upper three cervical nerves, and the superior cervical, stellate, and sphenopalatine ganglia in a series of cats after application of HRP or WGA–HRP to the caudal basilar artery. They found positive label uptake in cells of the superior cervical, stellate, sphenopalatine, trigeminal, and superior vagal ganglia (although the label in the latter was felt to be spurious). Of these ganglia, only the trigeminal mediates general somatic (pain) sensation. The few intraoperative observations of basilar artery branch stimulation in humans suggests a nontrigeminal source for sensory nerves to that vessel (see below). Thus, the issue of the precise origins and pathways mediating painful sensation from posterior fossa arterial structures remains unsettled (Lance, 1982).

Stimulation Studies

Ray and Wolff (1940) stimulated a circumferential pontine perforating branch of the basilar artery and the internal auditory artery. Both caused pain referred behind the ipsilateral ear, suggesting sensory innervation by the vagus nerve.

Stimulation of the intradural segment of the vertebral artery or its branch, the posterior inferior cerebellar artery, causes diffuse pain referred to the occiput or to the upper cervical dermatomes. Thus, the pain-referral patterns observed during the stimulation of posterior fossa structures in awake surgical patients correspond to the distribution of general somatic afferent fibers revealed by some anatomic studies, but questioned by others.

CLINICAL OBSERVATIONS

Since Cushing reported the loss of middle fossa dural sensitivity following removal of the trigeminal ganglion (Cushing, 1904), clinical observation of a large number of patients after surgical, pharmacologic, or pathologic interruption of intracranial pain pathways has contributed to an understanding of the anatomic principles underlying headache mechanisms.

The trigeminal and vagus nerves along with the dorsal roots of the upper three cervical spinal nerves are the only structures whose destruction has consistently abolished pain sensitivity in the appropriate distributions, as outlined previously in this chapter. Ganglionectomy, rhizotomy, chemical gangliolysis, brain stem injury, or syringomyelia with accompanying anesthesia in intracranial regions appropriate to the locale of the lesion abolish the headache due to histamine injection, direct dural or vascular stimulation, pneumography, or migraine in the anesthetic zone (Carmichael & Woollard, 1933; Cushing, 1904; Graham & Wolff, 1937; Northfield, 1938; Penfield, 1935; Pickering, 1939; Pickering, 1955; Schumacher et al., 1940; Sutherland & Wolff, 1938; Von Storch et al., 1940; Wolff, 1938).

Among the structures that clinical observation has shown are not important in the generation or conduction of head pain are the facial, glossopharyngeal, and sympathetic nerves. Destruction of these nerves has no effect on dural pain sensitivity, histamine headache, or migraine. A detailed discussion of operations performed specifically for the relief of headache is the subject of a later chapter. It is appropriate to mention here, however, that procedures not based on sound anatomic principles have not withstood the test of time.

Thus, operations such as superficial temporal or middle meningeal artery ligation (Craig, 1933), cervical or periarterial sympathectomy (Dandy, 1931; Penfield, 1932b), petrosal neurectomy (Gardner et al., 1947), and therapeutic pneumography or lysis of subdural adhesions (Penfield & Norcross, 1936; Penfield & McNaughton, 1940) as treatments for headache are now rarely if ever performed. Most of Penfield's patients were relieved of their headaches only after a denervation procedure, which included the ophthalmic division of the trigeminal nerve. The effects of trigeminal lesions on the pressor response elicited by painful stimulation of intracranial structures in anesthetized animals lends further support for the exclusive role of the fifth nerve in mediating supratentorial pain sensations (Leake et al., 1927; Levine & Wolff, 1932; Wall & Pribram, 1950).

More recently, the effects of lesions of the trigeminal ganglion, cervical dorsal roots, and cervical sympathetic ganglia on the levels of substance P (SP) and other pain-associated peptides in the pial vessels of various species have been studied. Depletion of SP in the anterior circle of Willis after trigeminal ganglionectomy again underscores the key role of the trigeminal system in mediating head pain from supratentorial structures. Evidence regarding the source of SP in the vertebrobasilar circulation is much less conclusive (Liu-Chen et al., 1983a, 1983b, 1983c; Moskowitz, 1984; Moskowitz et al., 1983; Norregaard et al., 1983).

So far, the mechanisms and pathways involved in the transmission of pain due to pathologic processes within the cerebral parenchyma or ventricular system have not been addressed. The cerebral substance itself and the ventricular ependyma are insensitive to all forms of stimulation. Thus, pain associated with intracerebral lesions or hydrocephalus arises as a consequence of effects on the pain-sensitive structures discussed in the previous sections of this chapter.

Depending on the size, location, and mass effect of a particular lesion, the affected pain-sensitive structures may be located either nearby, at a distance, or both. A more detailed discussion of headache and brain tumor follows in a later chapter; however, the anatomic principles of pain sensitivity associated with intracranial mass lesions bear mentioning here. According to Ray and Wolff (1940) and Kunkle, Ray, and Wolff (1942), the mechanisms include the following: (1) traction on venous sinuses or their tributaries; (2) traction on meningeal arteries; (3) traction on the large arteries at the base of the brain; (4) direct pressure on cranial or cervical pain-sensitive nerves; (5) dilatation of intracranial arteries; and (6) inflammation of any pain-sensitive structure.

Processes that affect local pain-sensitive structures reproduce the various pain syndromes elicited during awake brain surgery stimulation studies described in this chapter. However, those that produce displacements or herniation syndromes at a distance will elicit pain of a generalized or falsely localizing nature. One special instance is the phenomenon of displacement of the underlying large vessels of the circle of Willis by distension of the third ventricle in cases of hydrocephalus or tumor. This produces severe generalized headache. Another is the production of frontal headache by tonsillar herniation or mass lesions of the foramen magnum associated with upper cervical root traction. Central processing of afferent signals at the level of the spinal trigeminal nucleus has been discussed earlier as a possible mechanism in such cases.

In summary, all available evidence supports an orderly somatotopic representation of the supratentorial pain-sensitive meningeal and vascular structures within the trigeminal system. Pain sensation from posterior fossa structures is carried centrally by the vagus nerve, the upper three cervical nerves, and possibly by trigeminal afferents as well. The patterns of pain referral from experimental or pathologic stimulation of sensitive structures generally follow the dermatomal distribution of the structures' nerve supply. The convergence of trigeminal, vagal, and cervical afferents on second-order neurons in the spinal trigeminal nucleus and dorsal horn at the cervicomedullary junction unites pain impulses encoded from all portions of the cranium centrally.

The anatomic principles outlined in this chapter are fundamental to an understanding of the mechanisms and rational treatment of head pain.

REFERENCES

Arnold, F. (1851). *Handbuch der Anatomie des Menschen*. A. Emmerling and Herder, Freiberg, Germany. (Quoted by Penfield and McNaughton, 1940).

Arnold, F. (1860). *Icones Nervorum Capitis*. J.C.B. Mohr, Heidelberg, Germany.

Carmichael, E.A. and H.H. Woollard (1933). Some observations on the fifth and seventh cranial nerves. *Brain 56*:109.

Chorobski, J. and W. Penfield (1932). Cerebral vasodilator nerves and their pathway from the medulla oblongata, with observations on the pial and intracerebral vascular plexus. *Arch. Neurol. Psychiatry 28*:1257.

Clark, S.L. (1934). Innervation of the choroid plexuses and the blood vessels within the central nervous system. *J. Comp. Neurol. 60*:21.

Craig, W.M. (1933). Localized headache associated with lesion of meningeal vessels. *JAMA 100*:816.

Cushing, H. (1904). The sensory distribution of the fifth cranial nerve. *Bull. Johns Hopkins Hosp. 15*:213.

Cushing, H. (1909). A note upon the faradic stimulation of the postcentral gyrus in conscious patients. *Brain 32*:44.

Dahl, E. (1976). Microscopic observations on cerebral arteries. In *The Cerebral Vessel Wall* (J. Cervos-Navarro et al., ed.), Raven Press, New York.

Dalessio, D.J. (1980a). Pain sensitive structures within the cranium. In *Wolff's Headache and Other Head Pain* (D.J. Dalessio, ed.), Chapter 3. Oxford, New York.

Dalessio, D.J. (1980b). Clinical observations on headache. In *Wolff's Headache and Other Head Pain* (D.J. Dalessio, ed.), Chapter 25. Oxford, New York.

Dandy, W.E. (1931). Treatment of hemicrania (migraine) by removal of the inferior cervical and first thoracic sympathetic ganglion. *Bull. Johns Hopkins Hosp. 48*:357.

Fay, T. (1931). Certain fundamental cerebral signs and symptoms and their response to dehydration. *Arch. Neurol. Psychiatry 26*:452.

Fay, T. (1937). Mechanism of headache. *Arch. Neurol. Psychiatry 37*:471.

Fay, T. (1939). Problems of pain reference to the extremities, their diagnosis and treatment. *Am. J. Surg. 44*:52.

Feindel, W., W. Penfield, and F. McNaughton (1960). The tenotorial nerve and localization of intracranial pain in man. *Neurology 10*:555.

Gardner, W.S., A. Stowell, and R. Dutlinger (1947). Resection of the greater superficial petrosal nerve in the treatment of unilateral headache. *J. Neurosurg. 4*:105.

Graham, J.R., and H.G. Wolff (1937). Mechanism of migraine headache and action of ergotamine tartarate. *Assoc. Res. Nerv. Dis. Proc. 18*:638.

Gulland, L. (1898). The occurrence of nerves on intracranial blood vessels. *Br. Med. J. 2*:781.

Hassin, G.B. (1929). The nerve supply of the cerebral blood vessels, a histologic study. *Arch. Neurol. Psychiatry 22*:375.

Huber, C.G. (1899). Observations on the innervation of the intracranial vessels. *J. Comp. Neurol. 9*:1.

Keller, J.T., A. Beduck, M.C. Saunders (1985a). Origin of fibers innervating the basilar artery of the cat. *Neuroscience Letters 58*:263.

Keller, J.T., M.C. Saunders, A. Beduk, J.G. Jollis (1985b). Innervation of the posterior fossa dura of the cat. *Brain Res. Bull. 14*:97.

Kerr, F.W.L. (1961). A mechanism to account for frontal headache in cases of posterior fossa tumors. *J. Neurosurg. 18*:605.

Kerr, F.W.L. (1962). Facial, vagal and glossopharyngeal nerves in the cat: Afferent connections. *Neurology 6*:264.

Kerr, F.W.L. (1967). Evidence for a peripheral etiology of trigeminal neuralgia. *J. Neurosurg. 26* (Suppl.):168.

Kimmel, D.L. (1961a). Innervation of spinal dura mater and dura mater of the posterior cranial fossa. *Neurology 11*:800.

Kimmel, D.L. (1961b). The nerves of the cranial dura mater and their significance in dural headache and referred pain. *Chicago Med. School Q. 22*:16.

Kunkle, E.C., B.S. Ray, and H.G. Wolff (1942). Studies on headache: The mechanisms and significance of the headache associated with brain tumor. *Bull. N.Y. Acad. Med. 18:*400.

Lance, J. (1982). Causes of headache. In *Mechanism and Management of Headache.* 4th ed., Chapter 5. Butterworths, London.

Leake, C.D., A.S. Loevenhart, and C.W. Muehlberger (1927). Dilatation of cerebral blood vessels as a factor in headache. *JAMA 88:*1076.

Levine, M. and H.G. Wolff (1932). Cerebral circulation: Afferent impulses from the blood vessels of the pia. *Arch. Neurol. Psychiatry 28:*140.

Liu-Chen, L.Y., P.H. Han, and M.A. Moskowitz (1983a). Pia arachnoid contains substance P originating from trigeminal neurons. *Neuroscience 9:*803.

Liu-Chen, L.Y., M.R. Mayberg, and M.A. Moskowitz (1983b). Immunohistochemical evidence for a substance p-containing trigeminovascular pathway to pial arteries in cats. *Brain Res. 268:*162.

Liu-Chen, L.Y., T. Liszcak, S.A. Gillespie et al. (1983c). Substance p-containing fibers in middle cerebral arteries—origin and ultrastructure. *Neurosci. Soc. 13:*294.

Luschka, H. (1850). *Die Nerven in der harten Hirnhaut.* H. Laupp, Tubingen, Germany. (Quoted by Penfield and McNaughton, 1940; Kimmel, 1961b).

Mayberg, M., R.S. Langer, N.T. Zervas, and M.A. Moskowitz (1981). Perivascular meningeal projections from cat trigeminal ganglia: Possible pathways for vascular headaches in man. *Science 213:*228.

Mayberg, M.R., N.T. Zervas, and M.A. Moskowitz (1984). Trigeminal projections to supratentorial pial and dural blood vessels in cats demonstrated by horseradish peroxidase histochemistry. *J. Comp. Neurol. 223:*46.

McNaughton, F.L. (1938). The innervation of the intracranial blood vessels and dural sinuses. *Assoc. Res. Nerv. Dis. Proc. 18:*178.

McNaughton, F.L. and W.H. Feindel (1977). Innervation of intracranial structures: A reappraisal. In *Physiological Aspects of Clinical Neurology* (F.C. Rose, ed.), Chapter 19. Blackwell, Oxford.

Moskowitz, M.A. (1984). The neurobiology of vascular head pain. *Ann. Neurol. 16:*157.

Moskowitz, M.A., T.V. Norregaard, L.Y. Liu-Chen et al. (1983). VIP, CCK, and met-enkephalin in pia arachnoid and cerebral arteries after unilateral lesions of the cat trigeminal ganglia. *Neurosci. Soc. 13:*576.

Netter, F.H. and G.A.G. Mitchell (1983). Cranial nerves. In *The CIBA Collection of Medical Illustrations,* Vol. 1, Part I, Sect. 5 (prepared by F.H. Netter). CIBA, West Caldwell, N.J.

Norregaard, T.V., R.C. Weatherwax, and M.A. Moskowitz (1983). The effects of lesioning the trigeminal, superior cervical sympathetic, C2 and C3 ganglia on substance-p in cat cerebral arteries. *Neurosci. Soc. 13:*455.

Northfield, D.W.C. (1938). Some observations on headache. *Brain 61:*133.

Pearson, A.A. (1939). The hypoglossal nerve in human embryos. *J. Comp. Neurol. 71:*21.

Penfield, W. (1932a). Intracerebral vascular nerves. *Arch. Neurol. Psychiatry 27:*30.

Penfield, W. (1932b). Operative treatment of migraine and observations on the mechanism of vascular pain. *Trans. Am. Acad. Ophthalmol. 37:*50.

Penfield, W. (1935). A contribution to the mechanism of intracranial pain. *Assoc. Res. Nerv. Dis. Proc. 15:*399.

Penfield, W. and N.C. Norcross (1936). Subdural traction and posttraumatic headache, study of pathology and therapeusis. *Arch. Neurol. Psychiatry 36:*75.

Penfield, W. and F. McNaughton (1940). Dural headache and innervation of the dura mater. Arch. Neurol. Psychiatry 44, 43.

Pickering, G.W. (1939). Experimental observations on headache. *Br. Med. J. 1:*4087.

Pickering G.W. (1955). Experimental observations on headache. *Int. Arch. Allergy 7:*1955.

Ray, B.S. and H.G. Wolff (1940). Experimental studies on headache pain-sensitive structures of the head and their significance in headache. *Arch. Surg. 41:*813.

Schumacher, G.A., B.S. Ray, and H.G. Wolff (1940). Experimental studies on headache. Further analysis of histamine headache and its pain pathways. *Arch. Neurol. Psychiatry 44:*701.

Steiger, H.J., J.M. Tew Jr., and J.J. Keller (1982). The sensory representation of the dura mater in the trigeminal ganglion of the cat. *Neurosci. Lett. 31:*231.

Stohr, P.J. (1932). Nerves of the blood vessels, heart, meninges, digestive tract and urinary bladder. In *Cytology and Cellular Pathology of the Nervous System*, Vol. 1, Sect. 8 (W. Penfield, ed.), p. 383. Hoeber, New York.

Sutherland, A.M. and H.G. Wolff (1938). Experimental studies on headache. Observations on the mechanism of headache in migraine, hypertension and fever therapy. *Trans. Am. Neurol. Assoc. 64:*103.

Tasker, R.R., L. Organ, and P.A. Hawrylyshyn (1982). Pial Responses. In *The Thalamus and Midbrain of Man*, Chapter 12. Charles C Thomas, Springfield, Ill.

Von Storch, J.J.C., L. Secunda, and C.M. Krinsky (1940). Production and localization of headache with subarachnoid and ventricular air. *Arch. Neurol. Psychiatry 43:*326.

Wall, P.D. and K.H. Pribram (1950). Trigeminal neurotomy and blood pressure response from stimulation of lateral cerebral cortex of macaca mulatta. *J. Neurophysiol. 13:*409.

Wirth, F.P., Jr. and J.M. Van Buren (1971). Referral of pain from dural stimulation in man. *J. Neurosurg. 34:*630.

Wolff, H.G. (1938). Headache and cranial arteries. *Trans. Assoc. Am. Phys. 53:*193.

Wolff, H.G. (1955). Headache mechanisms. *Int. Arch. Allergy 7:*210.

4

Inheritance and Epidemiology of Headache

W. E. WATERS

Headache is one of the most common of all symptoms. It is sometimes of almost trivial impact and, partly because of this, its inheritance and epidemiology have received surprisingly little detailed study until recent years. Many clinicians through the centuries, however, have made epidemiologic observations based on the experience of their patients. These should no longer be accepted at face value as we know that clinical impressions, and even detailed statistical data based on consecutive series of patients, may not be confirmed when a rigorous epidemiologic study is carried out. At least with the more common forms of headache, evidence now exists that those individuals who consult a medical practitioner are often different from those who do not. Of course, it is to be expected that those who go to a doctor with headache may have more severe pain, more prolonged headaches, or more frequent headaches than others who do not seek medical attention. This has proved to be the case, but in addition those seeking medical attention for migraine, for example, are likely to differ in other respects, such as intelligence and social class (see below). These findings make any review of the inheritance and epidemiology of headache difficult because most of the reports in the medical literature are based on selected series of patients (in that any series of patients may be selected because many sufferers of headache and migraine do not seek medical attention).

The other important difficulty in reviewing the inheritance and epidemiology of headache is the problem of definitions. Most headaches have no known morbid anatomy and no biochemical, physiologic, or other test is useful for diagnosis in epidemiologic research. Even the presence or absence of headache may not always be easy to determine in epidemiologic surveys because some headaches are so mild they may not be reported by individuals either on direct questioning by doctors or on administered or self-administered questionnaires. Even published information derived from population-based studies is sometimes difficult to assess because such studies have widely different response rates and those who do not cooperate in such surveys may be different from those who do. The various epidemiologic studies have often used different definitions of, for example, migraine. The studies may also have been conducted in different ways, which may make direct comparisons inappropriate. These and other epidemiologic problems have recently been considered in more detail (Linet & Stewart, 1984; Waters, 1986). This chapter emphasizes those findings that are based on representative populations; the methods used will be mentioned because this information will determine how confident one can be about the accuracy and comparability of the results.

The problem of defining various types of headache in a way that is suitable for epidemiologic study is perhaps even greater than that of providing a general definition. Definitions such as those given by the World Federation of Neurology (1970), which include the characteristic features of the condition, are not precise enough for use in epidemiologic studies. Indeed, epidemiologic studies have questioned whether migraine is a separate entity, distinct from other headaches, or simply a spectrum of varying degrees of severity (Waters, 1973; Ziegler, 1976).

INHERITANCE

Many studies of headache acknowledge, and some stress, that migraine is inherited. It is difficult to determine from most collections of data if this is true inheritance or if the condition simply runs in families. Because families tend to share the same living conditions, headache that runs in families may be environmentally or genetically determined. Many reports in the literature are surprisingly vague and nonspecific. They may, for example, simply mention a "positive family history," and often do not define what "positive" or "family" means. Some authors, and the World Federation of Neurology (1970) itself, even include the familial element of migraine in their definition. However, in any study of inheritance or clustering in families, it is essential that this aspect be excluded from the definition and the identification of cases since its inclusion would lead to bias.

Patients with headache and migraine frequently report similar attacks in other members of their families. As shown below, migraine is very prevalent in the general population, so the important point is whether or not migraine is more prevalent in the relatives of those with migraine than it is in the relatives of those who do not have migraine.

Although the literature is almost unanimous in stating that migraine is inherited, there is no consensus on the type of inheritance. Dominant inheritance (Allan, 1928), dominant with greater penetration in females (Barolin, 1970), recessive with incomplete penetrance (Goodell et al., 1954), and multifactorial inheritance related to several genes (Dalsgaard-Nielsen & Ulrich, 1973) have all been proposed.

Epidemiologic Evidence

In a study using random samples of subjects with no headache, headache, and migraine, all selected from an epidemiologic study, first-degree relatives of all the groups living in a defined area were visited at home and asked questions about their headaches in the previous year by a trained interviewer (Waters, 1971). The response rate

Table 4-1 Details of three twin studies of inheritance of headache

Country	Sample	Findings	Reference
Denmark	Danish twin study —1900 unselected twins	Migraine found in only 84 subjects (2.2%). There were 6 concordant pairs of monozygotic twins among 18 with migraine in at least one, and 3 concordant pairs of dizygotic twins among 57 with migraine in at least one.	Harvald and Hauge (1956)
United States	Wide advertisements yielded 106 twins	Of 41 pairs of monozygotic twins, 11 had at least one individual and 2 had both affected by severe headaches. Of 65 pairs of dizygotic twins, 16 had at least one individual and 2 had both affected by severe headaches.	Ziegler, Hassanein, Harris, and Stewart (1975)
England	1300 twins on London Institute of Psychiatry's twin register	Concordance rates for migraine were 26% in monozygotic twins and 13% in dizygotic twins.	Lucas (1977)

was over 99% of the 524 first-degree relatives: a prevalence of migraine (strictly defined) of 10% was found in the relatives of the probands with migraine compared with only 5 or 6% in the relatives of the other groups. These differences are less than expected from the literature and were in fact not statistically significant. But the findings came from interviews of first-degree relatives of migraine sufferers and suitable controls, all identified from a community study. Dalsgaard-Nielsen et al. (1970) found that headache reports from patients were often inaccurate, thus, studies of family pedigree based on secondhand histories may be unreliable.

Twin Studies

A standard method of looking at the genetic aspects of the more common diseases involves the comparison of the prevalences in monozygotic and dizygotic twins because such studies have "built-in" controls (Lucas, 1977). Members of a twin pair are concordant when they are affected similarly and discordant when only one is affected. Many twin studies on migraine have been based on small numbers and some others have lacked detailed information on zygosity. Table 4-1 shows the three most important studies of headache in twins.

Although these findings do give some evidence of inheritance, for both migraine and severe headache, it is much less convincing than might have been suspected from the numerous uncontrolled clinical studies. The evidence is actually rather weaker than that shown in the table because migraine is more common in women than in

Table 4-2 Prevalence of headache in the previous year
(percentages)

	Age groups (years)			
	21–34	35–54	55–74	75 and over
Men	74.0	69.0	53.3	21.7
Women	92.3	82.6	66.2	55.2

(*Source:* Pontypridd survey, Waters, 1986.)

men, and therefore one would expect some degree of concordance when the data are presented as in the table. In fact, when Lucas (1977) analyzed the dizygotic twins of the same sex, the concordance rate was similar to that in monozygotic twins. Care was taken in these studies to reduce errors, however, the possibility of some bias exists in studies of this sort. Lucas (1977) concluded that there is "a much lower genetic factor in migraine than previously thought."

PREVALENCE OF HEADACHE AND MIGRAINE

Adults

The most appropriate measure of headache is a *period prevalence,* which determines the proportion of the population having at least one attack in a defined period of time. Many studies have used the year immediately preceding the survey, and data obtained by postal questionnaires sent to a sample of the general population are presented in Table 4-2. It can be seen that headache is more common in women than in men; in both sexes, the prevalence declines with age.

As discussed earlier there are no agreed-upon definitions of migraine suitable for epidemiologic studies. Some of the characteristic features of migraine are surprisingly common in those with headache in the general population. For example, of all women with a headache in the previous year, 48% had a unilateral distribution, 48% had nausea with the headache, and 28% had a warning that the attack was coming, all sometime in the previous year (Waters, 1986). Migraine is usually a clinical diagnosis, therefore, comparison between a neurologist's clinical diagnosis and the data obtained from questionnaires is an appropriate method of determining the prevalence of migraine (Waters & O'Connor, 1975). Data from such a study are shown in Table 4-3, which gives much higher prevalences of migraine than most previous studies. The prevalence of migraine in other studies has varied greatly from less than 1% to more than a quarter of the total population (Waters, 1986).

The variety of definitions of migraine almost certainly contribute greatly to this variation, but it should be pointed out that many earlier studies were based on patients consulting a doctor. Nearly half the patients clinically diagnosed as having migraine in the clinical validation of the questionnaire had never consulted a doctor because of their headaches and only 23% had done so in the previous year (Waters & O'Connor, 1971). Studies based on patients seeking medical help will, therefore,

Table 4-3 Prevalence of migraine (based on clinical validation of a questionnaire) in the previous year (percentages)

	Age groups (years)			
	21–34	35–54	55–74	75 and over
Men	16.8	16.4	12.6	4.9
Women	30.1	26.0	16.6	10.3

(*Source:* Pontypridd survey, Waters and O'Connor, 1975.)

considerably underestimate the true prevalence of migraine. Whatever the view of the actual prevalences shown in Table 4-3—and this depends on definitions and diagnosis—the table does present data in different age groups and in men and women separately, and all these figures were obtained in a similar way. With this "internal consistency," it is evident that migraine, like all headache, is more prevalent in women than in men and that its prevalence declines with age in both sexes.

Children

Pioneering studies of migraine in children were conducted in Sweden especially by Bille (1962). Although the definition of migraine used by Bille has not been followed in all subsequent studies, he showed that the prevalence of migraine was similar in boys and girls aged 7 to 10 years but higher in girls in older age groups. Other studies have confirmed that headaches are prevalent in children: at ages 13 to 15 years about 85% of boys and 95% of girls have had a headache in the previous year (Waters, 1986). The symptoms that are characteristic of migraine are also common in children, as assessed by self-administered questionnaires, but there has been no satisfactory clinical validation of such questions in children.

Cluster Headache

Most studies reporting on the frequency of cluster headache are based on the "relative incidence" of such attacks compared with cases of migraine. The figures have varied between 1:5.6 and 1:47.1. There was, however, one study of its prevalence in some 10,000 18-year-old men being considered for national service in Sweden. A questionnaire was followed by a clinical examination when a prevalence of 0.09% was reported (Ekbom et al., 1978).

CHARACTERISTICS OF SUBJECTS WITH HEADACHE AND MIGRAINE

Many characteristics have been recorded in the literature as being more, or less, frequent in subjects with headache and migraine. Any such associations should, however, be based on epidemiologic surveys and not simply on patients attending a doctor, because these may be selected in various ways. Thus, the clinical impression that migraine sufferers were more intelligent and of a higher social class has often been reported. Bille (1962) found that this was not the case in school children: he used various school classes as a 'measure' of intelligence. Later, epidemiologic studies in adults used occupation as a measure of social class and used intelligence testing on representative groups; no evidence of any association of either social class or intelligence with migraine was found (Waters, 1971). However, there was some evidence that, among those with migraine, those who had attended a medical practitioner were more likely to be of a higher social class and to be, on the average, more intelligent. This was evidence of *selection*—those who sought medical attention were biased toward higher social class and intelligence than other migraine sufferers who did not consult a doctor. A number of other hypotheses about possible causal factors such as visual acuity, ocular muscle imbalance, and blood pressure have been similarly tested in representative groups of subjects with no-headache, headache, and migraine, however, little convincing evidence that these are actually associated with migraine has emerged (Waters, 1986). The only statistically significant result from the eye-testing was that a higher proportion of the group with migraine had hyperphoria with near vision, and this may well be a true association. In conducting such studies for example, of visual acuity, manifest, and latent squints, it is important whenever possible to make the assessments "blindly"—that is, with the observer being unaware of the symptoms of the subjects when these tests are being performed—so as to reduce the danger of bias. These studies have demonstrated that defects of visual acuity, ocular muscle imbalance, and blood pressure are unlikely to be frequent etiologic factors, or statistical associations, in headache or migraine. They cannot show that in a few cases the headache or migraine may not be relevant to these conditions but simply that in the general population these defects, or abnormalities, are roughly equally common in those with migraine, those with headache, and those with neither. In view of the fact that these defects, or abnormalities, vary with age, all comparisons between the headache, migraine, and no-headache groups must be standardized for age and usually also for sex.

A few studies have looked at personality and headache. Migraine, muscle tension, and mixed cases of headache selected from a community sample were studied by Philips (1976). These groups were indistinguishable from each other on any of the four personality dimensions measured by the personality questionnaire, but differences were found in those taking certain treatments. Using a random sample of civil servants with migraine, nonmigrainous headaches, and no-headache, Henryk-Gutt and Rees (1973) obtained details of personal, medical, and family histories by interview. This study did give evidence that migraine was associated with increased N scores of the Eysenck Personality Inventory, increased anxiety and somatization scores on the Minnesota Multiphasic Personality Inventory (women only), and also increased hostility scores on the Buss Scale. Although these differences were statistically significant, it should be pointed out that in the initial study only 54% of questionnaires were returned correctly completed and it is possible that this may have introduced bias, as the response rate varied between 31 and 77% in various groups (Henryk-Gutt & Rees, 1973). Recently a study in schoolchildren in Holland failed to find many of the recorded differences between those with migraine, headache, and no-headache but it did find that sufferers from migraine and tension headache were characterized by the following personality traits: achievement motivation, rigidity, fear of failure, and low impulsiveness (Passchier, 1985).

REFERENCES

Allan, W. (1928). The inheritance of migraine. *Arch. Intern. Med. 42*:590–599.

Barolin, G.S. (1970). Migraine families and their EEGs. In *Background to Migraine: Third Migraine Symposium*, pp. 28–36. Heinemann, London.

Bille, B. (1962). Migraine in school children. *Acta Paediatrica (Suppl. 136)51*:1–151.

Dalsgaard-Nielsen, T., H. Engberg-Pedersen, and H.E. Holm (1970). Clinical and statistical investigations of the epidemiology of migraine; an investigation of the onset age and its relation to sex, adrenarche, menarche and the menstrual cycle in migraine patients, and of the menarche age, sex, distribution and frequency of migraine. *Dan. Med. Bull. 17*:138–148.

Dalsgaard-Nielsen, T. and M.D. Ulrich (1973). Prevalence and heredity of migraine and migrainoid headaches among 461 Danish doctors. *Headache 12*:168–172.

Ekbom, K., B. Ahlborg, and R. Schele (1978). Prevalence of migraine and cluster headache in Swedish men of 18. *Headache 18*:9–19.

Goodell, H., R. Lewontin, and H.G. Wolff (1954). Familial occurrence of migraine headache. *Arch. Neurol. Psychiatry 72*:325–334.

Harvald, B. and M. Hauge (1956). A catamnestic investigation of Danish twins. *Dan. Med. Bull. 3*:150–158.

Henryk-Gutt, R. and W.L. Rees (1973). Psychological aspects of migraine. *J. Psychosom. Res. 17*:141–153.

Linet, M.S. and W.F. Stewart (1984). Migraine headache: Epidemiologic perspectives. *Epidemiol. Rev. 6*:107–139.

Lucas, R.N. (1977). Migraine in twins. *J. Psychosom. Res. 21*:147–156.

Passchier, J. (1985). *Headache and Stress.* VU Uitgeverij, Amsterdam.

Philips, C. (1976). Headache and personality. *J. Psychosom. Res. 20*:535–542.

Waters, W.E. (1971). Migraine: Intelligence, social class, and familial prevalence. *Br. Med. J. 2*:77–81.

Waters, W.E. (1973). The epidemiological enigma of migraine. *Int. J. Epidemiol. 2*:189–194.

Waters, W.E. (1986). *Headache,* pp. 1–156. Croom Helm, London.

Waters, W.E. and P.J. O'Connor (1971). Epidemiology of headache and migraine in women. *J. Neurol. Neurosurg. Psychiatry 34*:148–153.

Waters, W.E. and P.J. O'Connor (1975). Prevalence of migraine. *J. Neurol. Neurosurg. Psychiatry 38*:613–616.

World Federation of Neurology (1970). Definition of migraine. In *Background to Migraine: Third Migraine Symposium*, pp. 181–182. Heinemann, London.

Ziegler, D.K. (1976). Epidemiology and genetics of migraine. In *Pathogenesis and Treatment of Headache*, pp. 19–29. Spectrum, New York.

Ziegler, D.K., R.S. Hassanein, D. Harris, and R. Stewart (1975). Headache in a non-clinic twin population. *Headache 14*:213–218.

5

The Pathophysiology of Migraine

JAMES W. LANCE

In *Dr. Willis' Practice of Physicke,* published in 1684, nine years after the death of Thomas Willis, headache is ascribed to increased blood flow to the head, which "distends the vessels, greatly blows up the membranes, and pulls the nervous fibres one from another, and so brings to them painful corrugations or wrinklings" (Knapp, 1963). Vascular distension as the primary cause of headache was questioned by Liveing (1873), who subtitled his classic monograph *A Contribution to the Pathology of Nerve-Storms.* Gowers (1893) wrote: "We must not ascribe too much significance to throbbing, or to the increase in the pain by the causes of vascular distension; these may be due merely to the over-sensitiveness of the central structures."

While the studies of Wolff and his colleagues concentrated on the reactions of extracranial vessels during migraine, Wolff (1963) left open the possibility that vascular changes were secondary to a central neural discharge.

> According to the neurogenic concept of vascular headache of the migraine type, any noxious factor within the brain that threatens survival of the cerebrum may induce cerebral vasodilatation. If this be sufficiently great, the cranial arteries on the outside of the head dilate. With the liberation of chemical factors such as proteases and polypeptides, edema and a lowering of the pain threshold are engendered. Tenderness and headache ensue. . . . It is conceivable that the initial event within the head is vasoconstriction, resulting in ischemia.

Whether the symptoms of migraine are determined by changes in the cerebral, meningeal, and extracranial circulations and humoral agents that react with them or the primary event is a neural discharge remains controversial to the present day. These hypotheses are not mutually exclusive and may well prove to be complementary. Certain groups of symptoms can be recognized within the conceptual framework of migraine that may recur in a specific phase of each attack, may be present in some episodes but not in others, and probably employ diverse neurovascular mechanisms.

SYMPTOMS COMPLEXES IN MIGRAINE

Any attempt to explain the pathophysiology of migraine has to account for the following components of the attack:

Premonitory symptoms. Mood changes (commonly a sense of elation associated with hyperactivity), increased appetite (particularly for sweet foods), and excessive yawning may precede migraine by as long as 24 hours on a least some occasions in about one third of migrainous patients (Blau, 1980; Drummond & Lance, 1984). These symptoms are presumably of hypothalamic origin.

Focal neurologic symptoms. These may arise from the cerebral cortex, brain stem, or cerebellum and may anticipate the onset of headache as in the prodromal phase of classic migraine or may appear during the headache phase. In either case, the neurologic symptoms may progress as a ''slow march,'' for example, spreading fortification spectra or paresthesias that indicate sequential involvement of areas of cerebral cortex, or as a patchy impairment of neurologic function that suggests a diffuse but unevenly distributed process affecting cortical function.

Headache. Headache is unilateral in two thirds of patients and commonly starts as a dull ache at the occipitonuchal junction, or in one temple, which then spreads over that side of the head or the whole head or may remain localized as a ''bar of pain'' extending from the eye to the occiput. The pain is usually constant and unremitting but assumes a pulsatile or throbbing quality when severe. It may consistently affect the same side of the head or may move from side to side, even in the one migrainous episode. Pain may radiate down the neck to the shoulder or, in some cases, to the arm and even the leg on the same side of the body, suggesting that the spinothalamic tract has collaborated with trigeminal pathways in the production of pain.

Prominent scalp vessels. The frontal branches of the superficial temporal artery become distended in about one third of patients, venous engorgement may be seen, and heat loss increases from the affected area while pressure over the prominent vessels eases the headache to some extent (Drummond & Lance, 1983). Most patients appear pale and ''dark under the eyes'' as the headache worsens, although exceptional patients flush before or during the attack.

Sensory hyperacuity. Light may be perceived as dazzling or may provoke pain, sounds may appear unnaturally loud, and smells may be more intense during (or even before) the headache phase. Sensitivity of the scalp to touch and muscular hyperalgesia may develop during, and outlast, the headache phase.

Gastrointestinal symptoms. Nausea sometimes precedes the onset of headache but commonly evolves as the attack progresses and may culminate in vomiting. Diarrhea is associated in about 20% of patients (Lance & Anthony, 1966).

THE ORIGIN OF MIGRAINE HEADACHE

Brain substance is insensitive to pain. The studies of Ray and Wolff (1940) showed that pain may be referred to the frontotemporal area from the dura, the intracranial segment of the internal carotid artery, the proximal few centimeters of the anterior and middle cerebral arteries, a portion of the cerebral veins and venous sinuses, the middle meningeal artery, and the superficial temporal artery. Afferent nerves from these blood vessels contain substance P, and have their cell bodies in the part of the

Gasserian ganglion corresponding to the ophthalmic division of the trigeminal nerve (Moskowitz, 1984). Stimulation of structures in the posterior fossa causes pain in the occipital region and upper neck (Ray & Wolff, 1940) while stimulation of the upper three cervical posterior roots refers pain to the vertex as well as the back of the head and neck. Kerr (1961a) reported that stimulation of the first cervical root in humans consistently caused frontal and orbital pain. He also demonstrated that afferent fibers from the first and second cervical roots converged with fibers in the spinal tract of the trigeminal nerve on second-order neurons in the posterior horn of the spinal cord (Kerr, 1961b). This convergence provides a pathway for referral of pain from the neck to the front of the head and vice versa.

Graham and Wolff (1938) observed that the severity of migraine headache lessened after the injection of ergotamine tartrate as the amplitude of temporal artery pulsation declined. This, together with the old observation that compression of the common carotid or temporal arteries often alleviated the pain, suggested that arterial distension was an important factor in producing migraine headache. From studies of more than 5000 records of temporal artery pulsations in 75 patients, Tunis and Wolff (1953) selected 10 migrainous patients for special analysis. They found that temporal artery pulse amplitudes became more variable and larger for up to 3 days before the onset of headache and that the mean amplitude during headache was greater than in headache-free periods. Blau and Dexter (1981) assessed the contribution of extra-cranial arteries to migraine headache by inflating a sphygmomanometer cuff around the patient's head. Of 47 patients, only 21 experienced relief from headache after inflation of the pericranial cuff whereas the majority complained that their headaches were aggravated by coughing, jolting, or holding their breath, indicating an intra-cranial component to head pain. Drummond and Lance (1983) compared the pulse amplitude of the superficial temporal artery and its main frontotemporal branch with the intensity of pain felt in the temple while the ipsilateral common carotid and temporal arteries were compressed alternately. Of 62 patients, selected only by the presence of a unilateral migrainous headache, the pain appeared to be of extracranial vascular origin in about one third, was of mainly intracranial (or meningeal) vascular origin in one third, and had no detectable vascular component in the remaining one third. In the subgroup with increased arterial pulsation in the frontotemporal region, thermography demonstrated increased heat loss from this area, and temporal artery compression eased the headache.

Headache does not depend on increased cerebral perfusion since common migraine is not usually associated with alteration of cerebral blood flow (Olesen et al., 1981b) and the headache of classic migraine may start while blood flow is still reduced (Lauritzen et al., 1983a). On the other hand, migrainous headache may be relieved by ergotamine (Norris et al., 1975) or codeine (Sakai & Meyer, 1978) although cerebral perfusion remains increased. In any event, vascular dilatation by itself would not cause headache. In periarterial fluid sampled during migraine headache Chapman et al. (1960) found a polypeptide similar to the polypeptide found in blister fluid that they named "neurokinin." This bradykininlike substance was postulated to set up a sterile inflammatory response in the vessel, which thus became pain-sensitive. Serotonin may also be implicated because it is known to be released from platelets during migraine headache (Anthony et al., 1967) and potentiates the pain-producing effect of bradykinin when injected into a human arm vein (Sicuteri, 1967).

Pain from muscle contraction may add a nonvascular component to migraine headache. Excessive contraction of the temporal, masseter, and neck muscles is common in migrainous patients (Lous & Olesen, 1982), more so than in patients with "tension headache," and becomes evident just before the headache reaches its maximum (Bakke et al., 1982). Tfelt-Hansen et al.(1981) found that infiltration of tender muscle areas with local anesthetic or normal saline relieved migraine headache within 70 minutes in 28 of 48 patients. Serotonin and bradykinin potentiated the pain-producing effects of one another when injected into the temporal muscle of normal volunteers but did not evoke headache (Jensen et al., 1985). The sites of muscle contraction in migraine correlate with the spatial distribution of pain and tenderness, suggesting that it is a secondary phenomenon but one that nonetheless contributes to headache. The possibility of a reduction in activity of the endogenous pain control system or of a primary discharge in central trigeminal pain pathways initiating migraine headache, with the vascular changes being secondary, will be considered later in this chapter.

In summary, the headache of migraine is not necessarily associated with dilatation of extracranial arteries or increased cerebral perfusion, although it is aggravated by vascular pulsation. It appears to be of intracranial origin at least as often as extracranial origin, and it may be related to increased sensitivity of vessels or perivascular structures. Whether or not central trigeminal pathways are also hyperexcitable, and whether or not their spontaneous discharge may initiate migraine headache, remains uncertain.

VASCULAR CHANGES

Vascular Reactivity Between Headaches

Pulsation of the superficial temporal artery in migrainous patients does not differ from that of normal controls at rest, nor does it differ on changing posture from sitting to standing, but it does increase more during exercise on the side habitually affected by migraine headache (Drummond & Lance, 1981). A similar increase was noted in migrainous patients during a stressful mental arithmetic test (Drummond, 1982) or when subjects viewed slides of fatal traffic accidents (Pratt, 1985). However, Goudswaard et al. (1985) found that, during the sustained stress of a student examination, temporal pulse amplitude did not increase in migrainous patients as much as it did in control subjects. Physiologic reactions in a target organ participating in the production of symptoms is known as "symptom specificity" and could indicate that some neurovascular reflexes are hyperactive in migrainous patients even between attacks.

Reactivity of intracranial vessels is also asymmetrical in the resting state. The vasodilator response to carbon dioxide is greater in migrainous patients than in normal subjects, more so on the side affected most recently by headache (Sakai & Meyer, 1979). Moreover, blockade of alpha-adrenergic receptors or stimulation of beta receptors was shown to increase cerebral blood flow more on the side of headache or the side recently affected by headache (Yamamoto & Meyer, 1980). Conversely,

Table 5-1   Cerebral and extracranial blood flow in migraine

Reference	No. of patients	Change during prodrome (%)	Change during headache (%)	Change after headache (%)
O'Brien, 1971	18	↓ 23	↑ 8	
Skinhøj, 1973	10	↓ 50	↑ 0–90	
Simard and Paulson, 1973	1	↓ 50	↑ –	
Hachinski et al., 1978	5	↓ 0–40	↑ 0–30	↑ 20
Henry et al., 1978	12	–	↑ 0–40	
Sakai and Meyer, 1978	43	↓ 20 (general)	↑ 35 (i.c.)	↑ 20
		↓ 35 (focal)	↑ 50 (e.c.)	
Olesen, Larsen, and Lauritzen, 1981	8	↓ 20 (general)	–	
		↓ 36 (focal)	–	

Key to symbols and abbreviations: Arrows indicate the mean increase or decrease in blood flow for the group; i.c. = intracranial circulation; e.c. = extracranial circulation.

(Reproduced from Lance, J.W. (1982). The Mechanism and Management of Headache, 4th ed. Butterworths, London.)

alpha stimulation diminished cerebral perfusion more on the affected side. Yamamoto and Meyer explained these findings by sympathetic denervation hypersensitivity.

Observations on Cerebral Blood Flow

Since the introduction of radioactive xenon measurement techniques, cerebral blood flow has been shown to diminish by about 20% during the prodromal phase of classic migraine (Table 5-1). Studies undertaken in Copenhagen over the last few years to measure the regional cerebral blood flow (rCBF) from one hemisphere by 254 detectors after intracarotid injection of xenon-133 (^{133}Xe) (which precipitates classic migraine in some patients) have given a more precise picture of the sequence of events. In some patients with classic migraine, patchy areas of increased blood flow were seen before the cerebral blood flow diminished. Diminution of the flow started in the occipital region and extended forward as a "spreading oligemia" (Olesen et al., 1981a). The wave of oligemia progressed over the cortex at 2.2 mm per minute, irrespective of arterial territories, stopping short at the central and lateral sulci, although the frontal lobes also become oligemic independently in some patients (Lauritzen et al., 1983a). Spreading oligemia typically began before the patient noticed focal neurologic symptoms, reached the sensorimotor area only after the appropriate symptoms had started, and outlasted these symptoms. The headache usually started while cerebral blood flow was still diminished. From this study, the authors concluded that cortical oligemia was a reflection of the "spreading depression of Lāeo" responsible for the slow march of fortification spectra and other neurologic symptoms previously calculated to traverse the cortex at about 3 mm per minute. Lauritzen and his colleagues (1982) showed that induced spreading depression in the rat was accompanied by a transient hyperemia for some 3 minutes, followed by a 20 to 25% depression of cerebral blood flow for 60 minutes or more. Spreading depression has been observed in human patients undergoing specific neurosurgical procedures (Sramka et al., 1977–78).

Reevaluation of cerebral blood flow studies to allow for the influence of scattered radiation on the recording from areas of low flow has shown that flow dropped to 16 to 23 ml/100 g/minute, below the critical level for cortical function, in the most underperfused areas in the majority of patients (Skyhøj-Olsen et al., 1984). This degree of ischemia is sufficient to explain transient and possibly persistent neurologic deficits.

During classic migraine attacks, the increase in rCBF usually seen with physiologic activation of the cortex was found to be impaired in underperfused areas although autoregulation was retained (Lauritzen et al., 1983b). Between migraine attacks, all aspects of cerebral circulation were regulated normally. In contrast to the findings in classic migraine, no changes in rCBF took place during four attacks of common migraine precipitated by drinking red wine (Olesen et al., 1981b).

More recently, rCBF has been studied during *spontaneous* attacks of migraine after the inhalation of ^{133}Xe by single photon emission computerized tomography (Lauritzen & Olesen, 1984). Of 11 patients examined during attacks of classic migraine in the headache phase, areas of cortical hypoperfusion were found on the appropriate side in 8, posteriorly in 7, and anteriorly in 1. The mean decrease in rCBF was $17 \pm 7\%$, (rCBF 41—66 ml/100 g/minute), which persisted for about 4 to 6 hours. Three patients did not exhibit any flow changes when studied $\frac{1}{2}$ to 3 hours after the onset of the attack. In no patient was rCBF increased, although patients were examined during severe headache. Twelve patients with common migraine showed no alteration in rCBF when estimations were made 3 to 20 hours after the onset of headache.

It therefore appears that the focal neurologic symptoms of classic migraine, whether arising as a prodrome or developing during the headache phase, are accompanied by diminished cortical perfusion of the appropriate part of the opposite cerebral hemisphere. On some occasions a wave of hypoperfusion may advance slowly over the cortex in association with a slow march of visual or other neurologic symptoms whereas on other occasions it may persist as a local or diffuse cortical oligemia. It is not possible to deduce with certainty from current techniques whether constriction of the cortical microcirculation precedes or follows diminution in cortical neuronal activity.

It is clear that the presence or absence of headache does not depend on changes in cerebral blood flow.

Observations on Extracranial Blood Flow

Extracranial blood flow generally increases during migraine headache (Sakai & Meyer, 1978), although thermographic studies have demonstrated increased heat loss from the frontotemporal region of the affected side in only one third of patients (Drummond & Lance, 1983). Dilatation of scalp arteries in this area contributes to the intensity of headache in this subgroup because compression of the temporal artery eases the pain. The nerve supply to human temporal arteries contains substance P, which could be implicated in transmission of pain impulses, and vasoactive intestinal polypeptide (VIP) (Edvinsson et al., 1984). The increase in extracranial blood flow that results from stimulation of brain-stem nuclei such as locus ceruleus in experimental animals, mediated by the greater superficial petrosal nerve and sphenopalatine ganglion, depends on the release of VIP (Goadsby & Macdonald, 1985). Blegvad et al. (1985) reported that plasma VIP increased from a mean of 6.8 pmol/liter in headache-free periods to 9.7 pmol/liter during attacks, although this change did not reach statistical significance in the 20 patients studied. It is therefore possible that the dilatation of frontotemporal vessels observed in some migrainous patients is mediated by the release of VIP.

BLOOD PLATELETS, VASOACTIVE AGENTS, AND BIOCHEMICAL CHANGES

Blood Platelets

Do platelets aggregate more easily in migrainous patients, particularly during a headache? Kalendovsky and Austin (1975) demonstrated that platelets from migrainous patients aggregated more readily than controls, a difference most marked in those patients with complicated migraine, of whom 4 out of 7 also showed increased coagulability of the blood. Hyperaggregability of blood platelets in migrainous patients was confirmed by Couch and Hassanein (1977) and Deshmukh and Meyer (1977), who found that platelet aggregation increased during the prodromal phase but diminished during headache. Kruglak et al. (1984), however, could find no significant difference between the platelets of migrainous patients and those of controls in headache-free periods and only a small *increase* in aggregability during headache, which was of statistical but questionable clinical significance. A recent study by Hanin et al. (1985) could not demonstrate any variation from normal controls of platelets from blood taken during the migraine attack or in headache-free periods.

How can this conflicting evidence be reconciled? Perhaps platelet aggregation takes place in subgroups of migrainous patients or is demonstrable only by certain techniques. Certainly the changes are not so constant as to influence views on the pathogenesis of migraine, although they may be a factor in the vascular thrombosis of "complicated migraine."

Irrespective of the degree of platelet aggregation, there is evidence for a platelet release reaction in migraine, as judged by the increase in beta thromboglobulin, a measure of total platelet activation, during headache (Gawel et al., 1979). This has relevance to the changes in plasma serotonin levels in migraine, discussed below. The monoamine oxidase content of platelets (MAO B), which assists the metabolism of phenylethylamine (not serotonin), has been reported to be low in migrainous patients, but Glover et al. (1981) found that this was true only for male patients. With the possible exception of MAO content, blood platelets in migrainous patients seems to be remarkably normal and their role in migraine is probably limited to aggregation in some instances and to serotonin release in the majority (Fozard, 1982).

Serotonin

Platelet serotonin content increases before migraine attacks and falls during the headache phase in most migraine patients (Anthony et al., 1967, 1969). Anthony et al.

first reported that a serotonin-releasing factor was present in the blood during migraine headache, an observation since confirmed by Dvilansky et al. (1976) and Mück-Šeler et al. (1979). The agent concerned is of less than 50,000 molecular weight (Anthony & Lance, 1975) and has not been identified although adrenaline, noradrenaline, free fatty acids, and immune complexes are possible contenders. The main metabolite of serotonin, 5-hydroxyindoleacetic acid, is excreted in excess in the urine of some patients during migraine attacks (Sicuteri et al., 1961; Curran et al., 1965). The intramuscular injection of reserpine lowers plasma serotonin and evokes a typical headache in those susceptible to migraine, which is relieved by the intravenous injection of serotonin (Kimball et al., 1960; Anthony et al., 1967). Normal subjects experience only a dull, nonspecific headache after reserpine.

Free serotonin, after release from platelets, could possibly exert vasomotor effects before it is adsorbed to vessel walls or metabolized because it is a potent constrictor of extracranial arteries in the monkey (Spira et al., 1976) and in humans (Lance et al., 1967; Carroll et al., 1974). The isolated human basilar artery constricts more readily to serotonin than to noradrenaline (Carroll et al., 1974), but the infusion of serotonin into the monkey vertebral artery does not produce any significant change (Lambert et al., 1984b), presumably because of autoregulation in the intact circulation. It seems unlikely that the amount of serotonin released from platelets during migraine headache would be sufficient to cause any vascular constriction, at least in the anesthetized monkey (Spira et al., 1976), but it may possibly combine with bradykinin to render the arterial wall sensitive to painful dilatation.

Changes in plasma serotonin may be an index of changes of serotonergic transmission within the central nervous system. Serotonin is implicated in two important pathways of potential application to migraine: a direct projection from the raphe nuclei of the brain stem to the cerebral cortex and the inhibitory system descending from nucleus raphe magnus that operates the enkephalinergic pain control system.

Serotonin receptors have not yet been classified definitively. There appear to be two specific binding sites in the brain, one, termed the $5HT_1$ receptor, at which serotonin (5-hydroxytryptamine [5HT]) has a high affinity and one, termed $5HT_2$, at which spiperone and ketanserin have a high affinity. $5HT_2$ receptors also exist in the periphery and mediate smooth muscle contraction, similar to D receptors in the original classification by Gaddum and Picarelli (1957). Another peripheral receptor mediates neuronal depolarization, for example, when serotonin evokes pain from blood vessels, and is blocked by cocaine and new preparations code-named MDL72222 and ICS205-930. These are similar but not identical to Gaddum and Picarelli's M receptor. There are probably two other peripheral receptors, one prejunctional, which inhibits the release of noradrenaline, and one that mediates vasodilator effects of 5HT (Humphrey, 1984).

Catecholamines

In contrast with studies of serotonin levels in migraine that are reasonably consistent between different laboratories, the reports for noradrenaline differ widely. Hsu et al. (1978) found that noradrenaline levels were higher in the 3 hours preceding headache, whereas Fog-Møller et al. (1978) reported a progressive decline during the headache phase that reached statistical significance 1 to 2 hours before headache reached its peak. Anthony (1981) followed 10 patients through a migraine attack, observing that noradrenaline levels rose by 30% in the headache phase (P < 0.05). Gotoh et al. (1984) reported that levels in migrainous patients between headaches were significantly lower than those of nonheadache controls. On the other hand, Schoenen et al. (1985) found that noradrenaline levels were significantly higher in headache-free migraineurs than in patients with tension headache. No comparisons are available between tension headache patients and normal controls. Such an investigation may be of importance because platelet serotonin is lower in tension headache patients than in control subjects (Rolf et al, 1981) and even lower than in migrainous patients during headache (Anthony & Lance, 1986). It is possible that noradrenaline levels may be lower in tension headache patients than in migraineurs, who in turn have lower levels than control subjects. In this case, the level may rise before migraine attacks and be sustained at the onset of headache, progressively decreasing as the headache intensifies. This hypothesis would unify the present observations but obviously requires experimental verification.

The final enzyme in the synthesis of noradrenaline is dopamine beta hydroxylase (DBH), so that serum levels reflect the amount of sympathetic activity. Serum DBH activity in migrainous patients without headache is almost double that of patients with tension headache and normal controls (Gotoh et al., 1976) and was shown in increase in 19 out of 20 patients at some stage during migraine headache. The high level of DBH in migraine has been confirmed by Anthony (1981). One of the main catabolites of catecholamines, vanillylmandelic acid (VMA), also known as p-hydroxy-m-methoxymandelic acid (HMMA), is excreted in excessive amounts by some, but not all, patients at the time of migraine headache (Sicuteri et al., 1962; Curran et al., 1965; Curzon et al., 1969). It thus appears that noradrenergic activity increases before, and in the initial stages of, migraine headache. Published studies agree that the adrenaline level does not alter.

Noradrenaline is contained in neurons of the locus ceruleus, which projects diffusely to the cerebral cortex and also plays a part in the endogenous pain control system. Peripheral actions of noradrenaline include vasoconstriction mediated by alpha receptors and vasodilatation mediated by beta receptors. Noradrenaline also releases free fatty acids, which may in turn release serotonin from platelets. The possible relevance of these functions to the pathophysiology of migraine will be considered later.

Dopamine concentration in platelet-rich plasma increases after migraine headache has been established for an hour or so (Eadie & Tyrer, 1985). Migrainous patients are more susceptible to the emetic effect of apomorphine and the hypotensive effect of bromocriptine, both of which are dopamine agonists (Sicuteri, 1977; Fanciullacci et al., 1980). Dopamine may thus mediate some of the symptoms of migraine, such as nausea and vomiting.

Histamine

Whole-blood histamine is significantly increased after migraine headache (Anthony & Lance, 1971). Receptors responsible for the vasodilator effect of histamine are of the H2 variety in the external carotid circulation of monkey (Lord et al., 1981) and human (Glover et al., 1973) and mainly of the H2 type in the internal carotid circulation of the monkey (Lord et al., 1981). For these reasons, the histamine-2 blocking agent cimetidine has been subjected to controlled trials for the prevention of migraine but has not proven to be effective when administered alone or in combination with a histamine-1 blocking agent (Anthony et al., 1978). This does not exclude the possibility that histamine is released from mast cells in perivascular tissues.

The injection of histamine or the histamine-liberating substance 48/80 into the external carotid artery is said to cause pain (Sicuteri, 1967); thus, liberated histamine may contribute to the vascular component of migraine. However, the infusion of histamine into the internal carotid artery at a rate of 10 to 50 μg/minute does not increase regional cerebral blood flow or cause headache in migrainous subjects (Krabbe & Olesen, 1980). It must be concluded that histamine is of little, if any, importance in the genesis of migraine.

Bradykinin

Bradykinin is a nonapeptide with a vasodilator and hypotensive action that is released by kallikrein from kininogen, an alpha-globulin. Plasma kininogen is diminished at the end of a migraine attack (Sicuteri et al., 1963; Sjaastad, 1970), and the blood level of a bradykinin-releasing enzyme is increased. Kinins are also increased in venous blood (Sjaastad, 1970).

Chapman et al. (1960) found a bradykininlike substance in perivascular tissue during headache, terming it "neurokinin." Sicuteri (1967) has shown that the pain-producing effect of bradykinin injected into a hand vein is potentiated by serotonin. However, the intravenous infusion of bradykinin in humans (Fox et al., 1961) or the intradermal injection of bradykinin into the temporal area (Elkind et al., 1964) does not cause headache.

Prostaglandins

Prostaglandins are long-chain unsaturated fatty acids derived from arachidonic acid with potent constrictor and dilator effects. During migraine headache, plasma levels of PGE_1 do not alter (Anthony, 1976), but the level of PGE_2-like substances has been shown to fall significantly, by 41%, in contrast with its elevation found in cluster headache (Nattero et al., 1984).

The intravenous infusion of PGE_1, into normal subjects has been reported to evoke headache indistinguishable from migraine (Carlson et al., 1968), but the intravenous administration of prostacyclin in migrainous patients caused only a dull headache unlike the subjects' spontaneous attacks (Peatfield et al., 1981a). Nonsteroidal anti-inflammatory agents with prostaglandin antagonist activity are used in the treatment of migraine, but their mechanism of action is uncertain.

Free Fatty Acids

The blood level of free fatty acids increases in fasting patients who subsequently develop headache (Hockaday et al., 1971) and is significantly elevated during migraine headache (Anthony, 1976, 1978). Anthony postulated that free fatty acids might be responsible for the release of serotonin from blood platelets in migraine.

Tyramine and Phenylethylamine

Tyramine is formed from the amino acid tyrosine by decarboxylation, and phenylethylamine is derived from phenylalanine by a similar process. Both substances are present in normal foods—tyramine in old cheeses and gamey meat and phenylethylamine in chocolate. Both have been implicated in "dietary migraine." The controversial literature was reviewed by Kohlenberg (1982), who analyzed the methodology of conflicting studies and concluded cautiously that "the tyramine hypothesis appears to have some validity." Further careful studies are required before these dietary factors can be considered important in the pathophysiology of migraine.

Electrolytes

Sodium and fluid are retained before and during migraine headache (Campbell et al., 1951), but this is probably a secondary phenomenon because the use of diuretics does not prevent attacks (Schottstaedt & Wolff, 1955).

Glucose

Missing a meal may precipitate migraine, possibly because of hypoglycemia (Blau & Cumings, 1966). Migrainous patients have a poor hyperglycemic response to glucagon, suggesting impaired mobilization of liver glycogen (de Silva et al., 1974).

Hormones

Premenstrual migraine recurs each month when plasma estradiol and progesterone levels fall and may be deferred by maintaining an artificially high level of estradiol (Somerville, 1972). Nattero et al. (1979) reported high plasma levels of both hormones in migrainous patients on the 26th day of the menstrual cycle, unlike Somerville, who found that hormonal levels did not differ from those of normal subjects. Mean values of cortisol were not found to be significantly higher in migrainous patients (Ziegler et al., 1979), but the circadian rhythm of its secretion was disturbed.

Immune Complexes

Lord and Duckworth (1977) found breakdown products of the third complement component (C_3) in the plasma of three headache-free patients, each of whom developed a migraine attack within 24 hours, whereas none of the 28 patients without detectable breakdown products had a headache within this period. Immune complexes were present significantly more often at the onset of headache in those patients without prodromal symptoms than in those with classic migraine (Lord & Duckworth, 1978). Jerzmanowski and Klimek (1983) found that the mean value for the C_3 fraction in 54 migrainous patients between attacks was lower than that of 70 control subjects. Other investigations (Moore et al., 1980; Behan et al., 1981) have not found any difference in complement components or immune complexes between the migrainous and the control groups. The possible precipitation of migraine by immune reactions remains an open question.

NEURAL CHANGES IN MIGRAINE

Cortical Events

Lashley (1941) plotted the expansion of his own visual scotoma in migraine and calculated that the visual cortex was being compromised by some process advancing at about 3 mm each minute, a rate corresponding to that of "spreading depression," described in the cortex of experimental animals by Leão (1944). Studies of regional cerebral blood flow in classic migraine indicate that a wave of oligemia sweeps over the cortex slowly at a similar velocity of 2 to 5 mm/minute (Lauritzen et al., 1982). Positron emission tomography has shown that the rate of glucose metabolism in the cerebral cortex diminishes in the early stages of migraine attacks induced by the injection of reserpine (Sachs et al., 1985). This suggests that diminished neuronal activity could possibly be the primary event in causing the neurologic symptoms of migraine, with the diminution in regional cerebral blood flow being secondary to reduced metabolic demand. However, the converse has not been disproved—namely, that vasoconstriction is the primary event since regional cerebral blood flow may be reduced to a critical level in classic migraine (Skyhøj-Olsen et al., 1984).

The contingent negative variation (CNV) is a slow negative potential recorded over the scalp preceding motor activity in a reaction-time task. It is a readiness potential that is thought to be mediated by a central catecholaminergic pathway. The amplitude of the CNV is significantly higher in migraineurs receiving no prophylactic therapy than in patients with tension headache and normal controls, but returns toward normal values when the patients are treated with beta-blockers (Maertens de Noordhout et al., 1985). This increase in CNV, and also in the amplitude of visual evoked potentials recorded in migrainous patients (Gawel et al., 1983), suggests an increased central excitatory state in the cortex itself or in the nonspecific and specific afferent projections to the cortex. Indirect support is given to this view by the findings of Fanciullacci et al. (1974) that migrainous patients are unduly susceptible to hallucinogenic drugs.

Hypothalamus

Premonitory symptoms, such as elation, hunger, thirst, and drowsiness, preceding migraine headache by up to 24 hours suggest a hypothalamic disturbance (Herberg,

1975). The hypothalamopituitary axis appears to be normal in migrainous patients when assessed by conventional tests (Rao & Pearce, 1971). Prolactin secretion is inhibited by tuberoinfundibular neurons using dopamine as a transmitter and is increased by serotonin, probably through a prolactin-releasing factor. A levodopa loading test was found to reduce the prolactin level during attacks of common migraine but to increase it when migraine headache was accompanied by neurologic symptoms and signs (Vardi et al., 1981). This suggests that some factor antagonistic to dopamine, such as serotonin, overcame the inhibitory effect of dopamine in classic migraine. The periodicity of migraine is probably determined by an "internal clock," such as the suprachiasmatic nucleus, that may activate the hypothalamus well in advance of other structures mediating the migraine attack, but proof of this is lacking.

Autonomic Nervous System

Appenzeller et al. (1963) reported that the dilator response of forearm vessels to heat was impaired in migrainous patients, but this was not confirmed by French et al. (1967) or Hockaday et al. (1967). Downey and Frewin (1972) found that resting blood flow in the hand was higher in migrainous patients than in controls and that the reduction in flow to a cold stimulus was reduced.

The pupillary diameter of migrainous patients has been studied by Fanciullacci (1979), who found that oral fenfluramine, which has sympathomimetic properties, induced less mydriasis in migraineurs than in normal controls. Eye drops of guanethidine 5%, a drug that depletes stores of noradrenaline, provoked a greater and more prolonged miosis in migraineurs than in controls, while the instillation of phenylephrine 1%, which causes only a slight dilatation of the normal pupil, produced mydriasis in migrainous patients. Fanciullacci concluded that noradrenaline stores in the iris were depleted and that the receptors were hypersensitive in migraine; curiously however, he observed no difference between sides in unilateral migraine, although Drummond (1986) has recently found consistent pupillary changes on the side of habitual headache. Denervation hypersensitivity of the iris was confirmed by Gotoh et al. (1984), who also demonstrated a decrease in blood pressure overshoot in the Valsalva maneuver and a tendency toward orthostatic hypotension in migrainous patients compared with controls. Sweating of the dorsum of the hand in response to the local intradermal injection of 0.05 ml of pilocarpine 1% was found to be diminished in migrainous patients (Hamada et al., 1985), suggesting a sympathetic deficit without denervation hypersensitivity.

Endogenous Pain Control Pathways

Mayberg et al. (1981) demonstrated that horseradish peroxidase applied to the middle cerebral artery was transported to cells in the Gasserian ganglion that receive afferents from the first division. These trigeminovascular fibers contain substance P, suggesting that they are involved in pain transmission. The spinal tract and nucleus of the trigeminal nerve descend to the second cervical segment of the spinal cord where pain afferents from the second cervical root and from the trigeminal system converge on the same second-order neurons. This "pain center" in the rostral segments of the spinal cord facilitates referral of pain from the front of the head to the neck and vice versa.

Interneurons control pain perception control using enkephalins and possibly gamma amino butyric acid (GABA) as their transmitter substances to gate the inflow from peripheral pain pathways by presynaptic and probably postsynaptic inhibition in the dorsal horn of the spinal cord (Basbaum & Fields, 1978, 1984). These inhibitory interneurons are modulated by monoaminergic pathways descending from the brain stem, which also have a direct effect on dorsal horn cells. The serotonergic pathway passes downwards from the periaqueductal gray matter of the midbrain to nucleus raphe magnus in the midline and also to lateral medullary nuclei (Duggan, 1982) to regulate the discharge of neurons in trigeminal and spinal pain pathways. A complementary noradrenergic tract originates from locus ceruleus in the upper pons and descends in the dorsolateral funiculus of the spinal cord. There is evidence that the electrophoretic administration of serotonin and noradrenaline near the bodies of dorsal horn cells reduces their rate of discharge (Duggan, 1982), but the precise manner in which monoaminergic pathways are effective in pain control is unknown. It appears likely that depletion of monoamines could open the pain control gates and lead to the perception of aching in the head and neck, as postulated by Sicuteri (1976).

How accurately levels of enkephalin and beta-endorphin in blood and cerebrospinal fluid reflect their activity in the central nervous system remains open to question. Fettes et al. (1985) reported that the plasma level of immunoreactive beta-endorphin was significantly low during a headache-free period in patients with classic migraine but not in patients with common migraine and chronic daily headache compared with normal subjects. Baldi et al. (1982) found that plasma beta-endorphin was lowered during attacks of common migraine compared with headache-free periods and with levels in normal controls. This was not confirmed by Bach et al. (1985) who could not demonstrate any differences in plasma beta-endorphin between migraine attacks and headache-free periods. Such negative findings do not, of course, exclude a central dysfunction of the opioid system.

Even in periods of freedom from migraine, migrainous subjects carry with them susceptibility to head pain. Raskin and Knittle (1976) found that cold drinks or ice cream evoked headache in 93% of migrainous patients compared with only 31% of control subjects. In a recent survey (Drummond & Lance, 1984), one third of patients with ice cream headache stated that this pain involved precisely the same part of the head as their habitual migraine headache. Moreover, 42% of migrainous patients are prone to sudden jabs of pain in the head (ice-pick pains), compared with 3% of nonheadache controls (Raskin & Schwartz, 1980). Drummond and Lance (1984) found that ice-pick pains coincided with the site of the customary headache in 40% of patients. The trigeminal pathways may thus become activated spontaneously in paroxysms lasting a fraction of a second (ice-pick pains) or may be activated reflexly for seconds or minutes by sudden cooling of the pharynx (ice-cream headache). This indicates a persisting disinhibition of trigeminal pathways in migrainous patients, suggesting that the trigeminal system could also discharge excessively for hours or days to provide a neural origin for migraine headache.

Brain Stem Control of the Cranial Circulation

The discovery of intrinsic noradrenergic and serotonergic pathways from brain stem to cerebral cortex may prove to be of relevance to the neurologic symptoms and vascular changes of migraine.

Locus Ceruleus

The locus ceruleus (LC) is located near the wall of the fourth ventricle in the upper pons and is the largest collection of noradrenaline-containing neurons in the brain. It receives afferent fibers from insular and visual cortex, amygdala, hypothalamus, brain stem reticular formation, raphe, vestibular nucleus, and tractus solitarius—all areas related to internal and external sensory stimuli or to the affective state. It projects to the cerebral cortex mainly through a dorsal bundle of fibers passing through the septum, turning backwards through the cingulum, and sending lateral projections to all areas of neocortex. In the squirrel monkey, noradrenergic fibers are distributed particularly to layers *III, V,* and *VI* of the visual cortex in contrast with serotonergic fibers from the raphe nuclei, which terminate in layer IV (Morrison et al., 1982) Locus ceruleus also projects to hypothalamus, thalamus, the medial and lateral geniculate nuclei, the facial nerve nucleus, and the spinal nucleus of the trigeminal nerve and spinal cord, predominantly ipsilaterally. The upstream projections seems to be related to the state of awareness, with a subpopulation of LC neurons that switch off just prior to and during the rapid eye movement (REM) phase of sleep (Foote et al., 1983). Maximal activity in LC neurons occurs at times of arousal and vigilance. Their effect on target organs is, in general, to reduce spontaneous activity and enhance the activity evoked by sensory systems. The downstream projection from LC is, at least in part, related to pain control mechanisms.

Hartman et al. (1980) found that electrical or chemical stimulation of LC neurons bilaterally in the monkey decreased cerebral blood flow and increased vascular permeability without associated changes in blood pressure or pulse rate. De la Torre et al. (1977), using the hydrogen washout technique, showed that unilateral stimulation of LC at 1.5/per second reduced rCBF. Goadsby et al. (1982) confirmed that cerebral vascular resistance increased—that is, blood flow fell—by about 20% with low frequency stimulation of monkey LC. On the other hand, external carotid resistance diminished—that is, blood flow increased—as the frequency of LC stimulation increased. The extracranial vasodilator effect was later shown to be mediated by the greater superficial petrosal (GSP) branch of the facial nerve. These changes, which were predominantly ipsilateral, bear a striking resemblance to the vascular changes accompanying classic migraine.

Raphe Nuclei

Serotonin-containing neurons from the midbrain raphe project rostrally in the medial forebrain bundle and are distributed to hypothalamus, dorsal thalamus, and diffusely to the cerebral cortex (Moore et al., 1978). In the visual cortex of the monkey, serotonergic nerve terminals are distributed chiefly to spiny stellate cells of layer IV, the layer that receives incoming geniculocalcarine fibers (Morrison et al., 1982). Nucleus raphe dorsalis and medianus send an ascending serotonergic pathway that innervates blood vessels of the cerebral microcirculation in the rat cortex (Reinhard et al., 1979) and to pial arteries and arterioles (Edvinsson et al., 1983). A serotonergic innervation has also been demonstrated on intrinsic brain stem vessels of monkeys and rats (di Carlo, 1977), on rabbit vertebral arteries (Griffith et al., 1982), and on the vertebrobasilar system of cats (di Carlo, 1981), the latter originating from nucleus raphe pallidus and obscurus in the brain stem.

Stimulation of nucleus raphe dorsalis increases cerebral blood flow in the monkey, and in the cat and the monkey it dilates both internal and external carotid circulations, the latter through connections with the facial (GSP) nerve (Goadsby et al., 1985 b,c). The extracranial vasodilatation is comparable with the reflex effects of LC stimulation. The ascending projections of the midbrain raphe nuclei have been implicated in the control of sleep behavior and neuroendocrine regulation, as have noradrenergic pathways. It appears that catecholaminergic and serotonergic projections from the brain stem exert an influence on both neuronal discharge and vascular supply to the cerebral cortex, although whether these pathways are complementary or at times antagonistic (analogous to sympathetic and parasympathetic autonomic nervous systems) remain to be determined.

The Trigeminovascular Reflex

Thermocoagulation of the gasserian ganglion for tic douloureux, a procedure that would be very painful if the patient were not anesthetized, produces a facial flush in the distribution of the division or divisions coagulated (Drummond et al., 1983). Lambert et al. (1984a) showed that electrical stimulation of the gasserian ganglion diminished carotid resistance and increased blood flow and facial temperature in cats by a reflex pathway traversing the trigeminal root as its afferent limb and the greater superficial petrosal (GSP) branch of the facial nerve as its efferent limb. A minor component of the response, particularly that elicited from the third division, persisted after section of the trigeminal root and may be caused by the antidromic liberation of a vasoactive agent such as substance P (Moskowitz, 1984). The main reflex vasodilator response to stimulation of locus ceruleus, raphe nuclei, or the trigeminal nerve is mediated by the sphenopalatine and otic ganglia and employs vasoactive intestinal polypeptide (VIP) as its neurovascular transmitter (Goadsby & Macdonald, 1985).

A pathway has thus been established that can account for extracranial vascular dilatation accompanying a primary pain-producing excitation of trigeminal pathways, a mechanism that may prove relevant to the vascular changes of migraine. A suitable name for this phenomenon might be the trigeminovascular reflex (Figure 5-1).

THE HUMORAL–VASCULAR THEORY OF MIGRAINE

The humoral–vascular theory postulates that circulating vasoactive amines constrict the cortical microcirculation, thus causing the neurologic symptoms and signs of

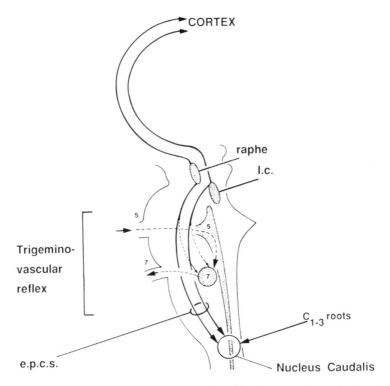

Figure 5-1. Physiologic actions of brain-stem nuclei of possible relevance to the mechanism of migraine.

The raphe nuclei and locus ceruleus (LC) project rostrally to the cerebral cortex to alter the cerebral blood flow and caudally as part of the endogenous pain control system (EPCS).

Fibers carrying pain impulses from the head descend in the spinal tract of the trigeminal nerve to the second and third cervical segments of the spinal cord where afferents from the upper three cervical roots converge on some of the same cells in the nucleus caudalis. Transmission at this synapse is modulated by the endogenous pain control system.

Stimulation of the trigeminal nerve (5) causes an increase in extracranial blood flow through the greater superficial petrosal component of the facial nerve (7). Stimulation of the dorsal raphe nucleus and LC also augments extracranial blood flow through the same pathway, which has been termed the trigeminovascular reflex.

classic migraine and that a subsequent phase of dilatation (predominantly extracranial) is responsible for headache. It has even been suggested that migraine is part of a generalized vasospastic disorder allied to Raynaud's phenomenon and variant angina, but a recent study has shown no link between these syndromes (Corbin & Martyn, 1985).

Dilatation of extracranial, middle meningeal, or cerebral arteries is thought to cause pain in migraine because the vessel wall has been sensitized by the adsorption of serotonin released from platelets and the periarterial accumulation of histamine and bradykinin. Platelet aggregation and the platelet release reaction are caused by a plasma substance of low molecular weight, at present unidentified, which could be one or more of the free fatty acids liberated by catecholamines secreted as part of a response to stress. This would be consistent with the precipitation of migraine by reserpine, which releases monoamines from body stores. Migraine may also be trig-

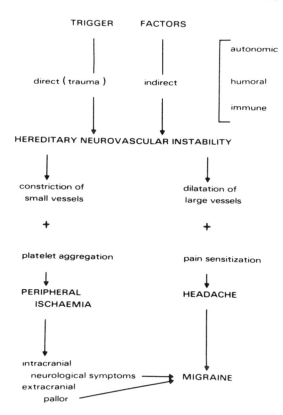

Figure 5-2. An outline of the humoral–vascular theory of migraine. (Reproduced with permission from Lance J.W. (1978). *The Mechanism and Management of Headache,* 3rd ed., p. 173. London, Butterworths.)

gered by vasodilators such as alcohol, monosodium glutamate, and glyceryltrinitrate and by the direct invasion of carotid or vertebral vessels during angiography. There is a latent period of hours, however, before these vascular precipitants result in headache, which leaves ample time for some neural intermediary.

Vomiting is most likely to be cause by the action of dopamine or other catecholamines on the area postrema of the medulla. Vomiting and diarrhea are known to release serotonin from the gastrointestinal tract. This increases blood serotonin to normal levels, thus assisting in a self-cure phenomenon. Noradrenaline and serotonin levels are increased before migraine headache, after which the serotonin level falls. Free serotonin could constrict the microcirculation initially; subsequently, as it is adsorbed to vessels or metabolized, the lowered level could reduce a tonic vasoconstrictor influence and permit the painful dilatation of larger arteries (Figure 5-2). Is the observed drop in serotonin levels sufficient to account for these vascular changes? If one considers the amount of serotonin that has to be infused into the carotid circulation of the anesthetized monkey to produce changes in blood flow comparable with those of migraine, it becomes apparent that the drop in serotonin levels in humans is too small and inconsistent to produce these vascular reactions (Spira et al., 1976). There appears to be no difference between the serotonin receptors of human temporal arteries in migrainous patients and in normal subjects to account for undue susceptibility to changes in serotonin levels (Skarby et al., 1982).

The consistent localization of neurologic phenomena and the alternating pattern of hemicrania are difficult to explain by platelet aggregation and serotonin release. One would have to postulate that this process took place preferentially in specific branches of the carotid or vertebrobasilar tree or that such areas were selectively embolized to produce focal cortical ischemia. If this were the case, why would the ensuing headache appear as often as not on the side inappropriate to that giving rise to the prodromal symptoms (Peatfield et al., 1981b)?

Although some features of the humoral theory (e.g., sensitization of the vessel wall to pain) remain attractive, it is necessary to postulate neural involvement to account for the asymmetry of migrainous symptoms and headache as well as the prompt precipitation of attacks in some patients by an afferent stimulus such as a bright flashing light.

THE NEUROGENIC THEORY OF MIGRAINE

Monoamines have been considered to be the neurotransmitters most likely to be involved in the mechanism of migraine because blood levels of noradrenaline and serotonin fluctuate with the course of headache. Difficulties in sustaining a purely humoral theory of migraine based on sensitization of vessel walls and changes in vasoactivity caused by direct action of monoamines on cranial vessels have already been outlined. The newly acquired knowledge of brain stem monoaminergic nuclei and their influence on cortical activity and cerebral blood flow as well as their participation in the endogenous pain control system makes it feasible to erect a neurogenic hypothesis (Lance et al., 1983) without completely excluding some aspects of the humoral theory.

Because migraine is a familial disorder, there may well be an hereditary anomaly

Figure 5-3. Schema of a neurovascular hypothesis for the mechanism of migraine. The hypothalamus may determine spontaneous cycles of migraine that can be overridden or reset by emotion, stress, excessive afferent input, or a direct blow to the head. The periaqueductal gray matter (PAG) projects downstream to the nucleus raphe magnus (NRM), which inhibits transmission of pain impulses by a serotonergic (S) pathway. Adjacent to PAG is the nucleus raphe dorsalis (NRD), which distributes serotonergic fibers to the cortical microcirculation.

The locus ceruleus (LC) projects down to the upper cervical spinal cord to inhibit pain transmission by a noradrenergic (NA) pathway and also sends noradrenergic fibers to the cortical microcirculation. Stimulation of the trigeminal nerve (CR N 5) or of LC increases extracranial blood flow by connections with the facial nerve (CR N 7) and the greater superficial petrosal nerve, employing VIP as a transmitter agent (x). Pain from the head is mediated by the spinal tract of the fifth nerve, fibers of which synapse on the same second-order neurons as pain afferents from the first to third cervical roots (C1-3). Transmission in this pathway is mediated by an enkephalinergic interneuron (filled circle), which is regulated from the brain stem as described above.

The release of catecholamines from the adrenal gland is caused by stimulation of LC, probably by means of the adjacent nuclei such as nucleus subceruleus. Platelet aggregation and serotonin release is induced by serotonin-releasing factors (SRF), possibly free fatty acids mobilized by NA. Released serotonin may sensitize the vascular walls of branches of the internal carotid (IC) or external carotid (EC) arteries to pain. The postulated sequence of events is outlined in the text. (Reproduced with permission from Lance, J.W. (1982). *The Mechanism and Management of Headache*, 4th ed., p. 170. London, Butterworths.)

of monoaminergic transmission that copes well enough under normal circumstances but is vulnerable to sudden changes in the internal or external environment, to emotional stress, or to overload of afferent systems by excessive glare, noise, smells, or other stimuli. All of these factors are known to impinge on the brain stem monoamine nuclei that project diffusely to the cerebral cortex (Figure 5-3). In addition, internal "clocks," such as the suprachiasmatic nucleus that determines circadian rhythms, probably exert their effect through the monoamine nuclei. For example, the

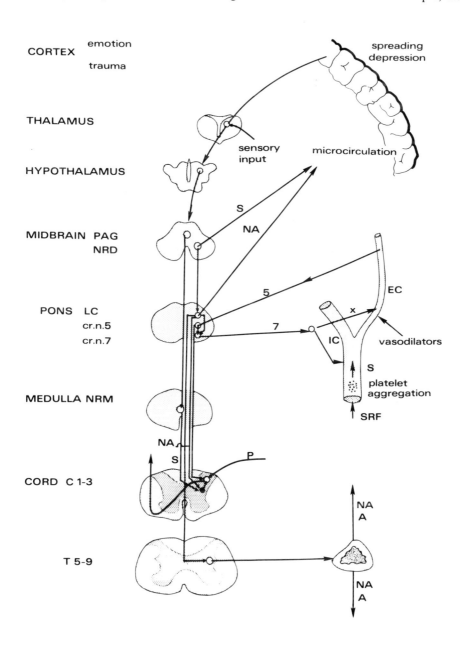

REM phase of sleep is anticipated by a change in discharge rate of a group of neurons in the locus ceruleus (Foote et al., 1983). The premonitory symptoms of elation, hunger, or drowsiness experienced by some migrainous patients presumably reflect changes in hypothalamic function initiated by some internal clock.

If monoaminergic systems were genetically unstable in subjects prone to migraine, trigger factors could induce a phase of excessive neuronal discharge followed by a state of monoamine depletion. Studies in the monkey (Goadsby et al., 1982) have shown that low-frequency stimulation of locus ceruleus diminishes cerebral blood flow by about 20%, an effect blocked by yohimbine (Goadsby et al., 1985a). This fall in flow is similar to that recorded in patients during the prodromal phase of classic migraine. As the frequency of stimulation increases, extracranial vessels dilate—a process mediated by the GSP nerve, which arises from the superior salivary nucleus and runs with the facial nerve to be distributed to peripheral end organs after synapsing in the sphenopalatine and otic ganglia (Goadsby et al., 1984). This induced extracranial vascular dilatation resembles that seen in some patients during classic and common migraine headache. Finally, in a state of monoamine depletion, the pain gate would be opened, giving rise to spontaneous pain in the head and neck. The fact that ice cream headache and ice-pick pains are often referred in migrainous patients to the habitual site of their headache suggests that a segment of the pain control pathway may be defective even in headache-free periods. Some patients complain of a dull ache in certain parts of the head long before a typical migraine headache develops; thus, in some patients spontaneous discharge of trigeminal pain pathways may be the primary event, followed on occasions by increased extracranial blood flow mediated by the trigeminovascular reflex (Lambert et al., 1984a). Because not all phases are present in all patients or in all episodes, one must postulate that "upstream" and "downstream" effects may be independent. A suitable analogy is with the reticular formation in generalized epilepsy in that absences, myoclonic jerks, and akinetic attacks may occur together or independently, depending on whether rostral or caudal projections are excited or inhibited by the epileptic process.

Vascular changes evoked from LC are mainly ipsilateral. One LC has an inhibitory effect on the other (Buda et al., 1975), a reciprocal arrangement that could account for descending impulses from cortex or hypothalamus being transformed into unilateral or alternating symptomatology at the brain-stem level. Stimulation of LC leads to the adrenal gland's secretion of noradrenaline (Goadsby, 1985), which could release free fatty acids and promote platelet aggregation, serotonin release, and sensitization of vessel walls as originally proposed in the humoral theory.

Sensory hyperacuity and the gastrointestinal symptoms of migraine remain to be explained. Locus ceruleus projects to medial and lateral geniculate nuclei and to the insular cortex. If the pain gates are opened by removal of descending inhibition, then sensitivity to light, noise, and smells may be caused by removal of ascending inhibition. Nausea and vomiting can be induced in cats and dogs by the administration of adrenaline or noradrenaline (an effect blocked by yohimbine), probably by action on the area postrema of the medulla (Cahen, 1974). The conclusion that central monoamine systems play a central role in the pathophysiology of migraine is difficult to escape, but the detailed mechanisms and sequence of events remain to be clarified before the treatment of migraine can emerge from its present empirical state.

CONCLUSION

Physiologic and biochemical observations of patients during migraine attacks and experimental findings in animals have led to the accumulation of a lot of data awaiting synthesis. The common ground of the various hypotheses for the mechanism of migraine is the involvement of monoamines, centrally as neurotransmitters, peripherally as humoral agents, or both. This is supported by pharmacologic evidence from the results of treatment. Most effective interval therapy for migraine alters the availability or action of serotonin (e.g., methysergide, pizotifen), noradrenaline (beta-blocking agents), or both monoamines (e.g., amitriptyline, monoamine oxidase inhibitors). Other agents that act directly on vascular smooth muscle, such as the calcium-entry blocking agents, may diminish vasoconstriction, whether produced by humoral agents or by intrinsic monoamine pathways from brain stem to cortex. Non-steroid anti-inflammatory agents presumably suppress the sterile inflammatory responses in vessel walls.

The emphasis placed in this chapter on mechanistic explanations for the phenomena of migraine should not obscure the fact that the vulnerable neurovascular systems described are part of the individuals concerned, responsive to their mental state and their reaction to stress or to sudden change in the internal or external environment. Migraine could thus be considered as an unduly sensitive mechanism for protecting the integrity of the brain. The neurovascular reaction induced by stress may reduce cerebral activity and blood supply with results incidentally detrimental to the patient. The headache itself may be the by-product of such a reaction or a primary event warning of physical or mental stress. In some cases, it may represent a faulty alarm system triggered periodically by some biological clock.

Progress in the understanding of migraine depends not only on improved knowledge of the personality and life-style of the sufferers from this distressing complaint but on meticulous dissection of the neural and vascular mediators of the migraine attack in the hope that the final common pathways can be identified and thus lead to more effective treatment.

REFERENCES

Anthony, M. (1976). Plasma free fatty acids and prostaglandin E in migraine and stress. *Headache 16:*58–63.

Anthony, M. (1978). Role of individual free fatty acids in migraine. *Res. Clin. Stud. Headache 6:*110–116.

Anthony, M. (1981). Biochemical indices of sympathetic activity in migraine. *Cephalalgia 1:*83–89.

Anthony, M., H. Hinterberger, and J.W. Lance (1967). Plasma serotonin in migraine and stress. *Arch. Neurol. 16:*544–552.

Anthony, M., H. Hinterberger, and J.W. Lance (1969). The possible relationship of serotonin to the migraine syndrome. *Res. Clin. Stud. Headache 2:*29–59.

Anthony, M. and J.W. Lance (1971). Histamine and serotonin in cluster headache. *Arch. Neurol. 25:*225–231.

Anthony, M. and J.W. Lance (1975). The role of serotonin in migraine. In *Modern Topics in Migraine* (J. Pearce, ed.), pp. 107–123. Heinemann, London.

Anthony, M. And J.W. Lance (1985). Chronic tension headache and platelet serotonin. *J. Neurology 232* (Suppl.):198 (abstract).

Anthony, M., G.D.A. Lord, and J.W. Lance (1978). Controlled trials of cimetidine in migraine and cluster headache. *Headache 18:*261–264.

Appenzeller, O., K. Davison, and J. Marshall (1963). Reflex abnormalities in the hands of migrainous subjects. *J. Neurol. Neurosurg. Psychiatry. 26:*447–450.

Bach, F.W., K. Jensen, N. Blegvad et al. (1985). Beta-endorphin and ACTH in plasma during attack in common and classic migraine. *Cephalalgia 5:*177–182.

Bakke, M., P. Tfelt-Hansen, J. Olesen, and E. Møller (1982). Action of some pericranial muscles during provoked attacks of common migraine. *Pain 14:*121–135.

Baldi, E., S. Salmon, B. Anselmi et al. (1982). Intermittent hypoendorphaemia in migraine attack. *Cephalalgia 2:*77–81.

Basbaum, A.I. and H.L. Fields (1978). Endogenous pain control mechanisms: Review and hypothesis. *Ann. Neurol. 4:*451–462.

Basbaum, A.I. and H.L. Fields (1984). Endogenous pain control systems: Brainstem spinal pathways and endorphin circuitry. *Annu. Rev. Neurosci. 7:*309–338.

Behan, W.M.H., P.O. Behan, and W.F. Durward (1981). Complement studies in migraine. *Headache 21:*55–57.

Blau, J.N. (1980). Migraine prodromes separated from the aura: Complete migraine. *Br. Med. J. 21:*658–660.

Blau, J.N. and J.N. Cumings (1966). Method of precipitating and preventing some migraine attacks. *Br. Med. J. 2:*1242–1243.

Blau, J.N. and S.L. Dexter (1981). The site of pain origin during migraine attacks. *Cephalalgia 1:*143–147.

Blegvad, N., K. Jensen, J. Fahrenkrug et al. (1985). Plasma VIP and plasma substance P during migraine attack. *Cephalalgia 5 (Suppl.3):*252–253.

Buda, M., B. Roussel, B. Renaud, and J-F. Pujol (1975). Increase in tyrosine hydroxylase activity in the locus coeruleus of the rat brain after contralateral lesioning. *Brain Res. 93:*564–569.

Cahen, R.L. (1974). Emetic effect of biogenic amines. *Res. Clin. Stud. Headache 3:*227–244.

Campbell, D.A., K.M. Hay, and E.M. Tonks (1951). An investigation of salt and water balance in migraine. *Br. Med. J. 2:*1424–1429.

Carlson, L.A., L.-G. Ekelund, and L. Orö (1968). Clinical and metabolic effects of different doses of prostaglandin E in man. *Acta Med. Scand. 183:*423–430.

Carroll, P.R., P.W. Ebeling, and W.E. Glover (1974). The responses of the human temporal and rabbit ear artery to 5-hydroxytryptamine and some of its antagonists. *Aust. J. Exp. Biol. Med. Sci. 52:*813–823.

Chapman, L.F., A.O. Ramos, H. Goodell et al. (1960). A humoral agent implicated in vascular headache of the migrainous type. *Arch. Neurol. 3:*223–229.

Corbin, D. and C. Martyn (1985). Migraine is not a manifestation of a generalized vasospastic disorder. *Cephalalgia 5 (Suppl.3):*458–459.

Couch, J.R. and R.S. Hassanein (1977). Platelet aggregability in migraine. *Neurology 27:*843–848.

Curran, D.A., H. Hinterberger, and J.W. Lance (1965). Total plasma serotonin 5-hydroxyindoleacetic acid and p-hydroxy-m-methoxymandelic acid excretion in normal and migrainous subjects. *Brain 88:*997–1010.

Curzon, G., M. Barrie, and M.I.P. Wilkinson (1969). Relationships between headache and amine changes after administration of reserpine to migrainous patients. *J. Neurol. Neurosurg. Psychiatry. 32:*555–561.

De la Torre, J.C., J.W. Surgeon, and R.H. Walker (1977). Effects of locus coeruleus stimulation on cerebral blood flow in selected brain regions. *Acta Neurol. Scand. (Suppl.) 64:*104–105.

Deshmukh, S.V. and J.S. Meyer (1977). Cyclic changes in platelet dynamics and the pathogenesis and prophylaxis of migraine. *Headache 17:*101–108.

De Silva, K.L., M.A. Ron, and J. Pearce (1974). Blood sugar response to glucagon in migraine. *J. Neurol. Neurosurg. Psychiatry. 37:*105–107.

Di Carlo, V. (1977). Histochemical evidence for a serotonergic innervation of the microcirculation in the brainstem. In *Neurogenic Control of the Brain Circulation* (C. Owman and L. Edvinsson, eds.), pp. 55–58. Pergamon Press, Oxford.

Di Carlo, V. (1981). Serotoninergic innervation of extrinsic brainstem blood vessels. *Neurology (NY) 31(2):*104.

Downey, J.A. and D.B. Frewin (1972). Vascular responses in the hands of patients suffering from migraine. *J. Neurol. Neurosurg. Psychiatry. 35:*258–263.

Drummond, P.D. (1982). Extracranial and cardiovascular reactivity in migrainous subjects. *J. Psychosom. Res., 26:*317–331.

Drummond, P.D. (1987). Pupil diameter in migraine and tension headache. *J. Neurol. Neurosurg. Psychiatry. 50:*228–231.

Drummond, P.D., A. Gonski, and J.W. Lance (1983). Facial flushing after thermocoagulation of the gasserian ganglion. *J. Neurol. Neurosurg. Psychiatry 46:*611–616.

Drummond, P.D. and J.W. Lance (1981). Extracranial vascular reactivity in migraine and tension headache. *Cephalalgia 1:*149–155.

Drummond, P.D. and J.W. Lance (1983). Extracranial vascular changes and the source of pain in migraine headache. *Ann. Neurol. 13:*32–37.

Drummond, P.D. and J.W. Lance (1984). Neurovascular disturbances in headache patients. *Clin. Exp. Neurol. 20:*93–99.

Duggan, A.W. (1982). Brainstem control of the responses of spinal neurones to painful skin stimuli. *TINS 5:*127–130.

Dvilansky, A., S. Rishpon, I. Nathan, Z. Zolotow, and A.D. Korczyn (1976). Release of platelet 5-hydroxytryptamine by plasma taken from patients during and between migraine attacks. *Pain 2:*315–318.

Eadie, M.J. and J.H. Tyrer (1985). *The Biochemistry of Migraine,* p. 65. MTP Press, Lancaster.

Edvinsson, L., A. Deguerce, D. Duverger et al. (1983). Central serotonergic nerves project to the pial vessels of the brain. *Nature 306:*55–57.

Edvinsson, L., R. Uddman, P. Tfelt-Hansen, and J. Olesen (1984). Localization and effect of vasoactive intestinal polypeptide (VIP) and substance P in human temporal arteries. In *Progress in Migraine Research, Vol. 2* (F. Clifford Rose, ed.), pp. 150–154. Pitman, London.

Elkind, A.H., A.P. Friedman, and J. Grossman (1964). Cutaneous blood flow in vascular headache of the migrainous type. *Neurology (Minneap.) 14:*24–30.

Fanciullacci, M. (1979). Iris adrenergic impairment in idiopathic headache. *Headache 19:*8–13.

Fanciullacci, M., G. Franchi, and F. Sicuteri (1974). Hypersensitivity to lysergic acid diethylamide (LSD-25) and psilocybin in essential headache. *Experentia 30:*1441–1442.

Fanciullacci, M., S. Michelacci, C. Curradi, and F. Sicuteri (1980). Hyper-responsiveness of migraine patients to the hypotensive action of bromocriptine. *Headache 20:*99–102.

Fettes, I., M. Gawel, S. Kuzniak, and J. Edmeads (1985). Endorphin levels in headache syndromes. *Headache, 25*:37–39.

Fog-Møller, F., I.K. Genefke, and B. Bryndum (1978). Changes in concentration of the catecholamines in blood during spontaneous migraine attacks and reserpine-induced attacks. In *Current Concepts in Migraine Research* (R. Greene, ed.), pp 115–119. Raven Press, New York.

Foote, S.L., F.E. Bloom, and G. Aston-Jones (1983). Nucleus locus ceruleus: New evidence of anatomical and physiological specificity. *Physiol. Rev. 63*:884–914.

Fox, R.H., R. Goldsmith, D.J. Kidd, and G.P. Lewis (1961). Bradykinin as a vasodilator in man. *J. Physiol. (Lond.) 157*:589–602.

Fozard, J.R. (1982). Serotonin, migraine and platelets. In *Progress in Pharmacology* (P.A. Van Zwietan and E. Schonbaum, eds.). Gustav Fischer Verlag, Stuttgart.

French, E.B., B.W. Lassers, and M.G. Desai (1967). Reflex vasomotor responses in the hands of migrainous subjects. *J. Neurol. Neurosurg. Psychiatry. 30*:276–278.

Gaddum, J.H. and Z.P. Picarelli (1957). Two kinds of tryptamine receptor. *Br. J. Pharmacol. Chemother. 12*:323–328.

Gawel, M., M. Burkitt, and F. Clifford Rose (1979). The platelet release reaction during migraine attacks. *Headache 19*:323–327.

Gawel, M., J.F. Connolly, and F. Clifford Rose (1983). Migraine patients exhibit abnormalities in the visual evoked potential. *Headache 23*:49–52.

Glover, V., R. Peatfield, R. Zammit-Pace et al. (1981). Platelet monoamine oxidase activity and headache. *J. Neurol. Neurosurg. Psychiatry. 44*:786–790.

Glover, W.E., P.R. Carroll, and N. Latt (1973). Histamine receptors in human temporal and rabbit ear arteries. In *International Symposium and Histamine H2 Receptor Antagonists*, pp. 169–174. Smith Kline and French, Welwyn Garden City, England.

Goadsby, P.J. (1985). Brainstem activation of the adrenal medulla in the cat. *Brain Res. 327*:241–249.

Goadsby, P.J., G.A. Lambert, and J.W. Lance (1982). Differential effects on the internal and external carotid circulation of the monkey evoked by locus coeruleus stimulation. *Brain Res. 249*:247–254.

Goadsby, P.J., G.A. Lambert, and J.W. Lance (1984). The peripheral pathway for extracranial vasodilatation in the cat. *J. Autonom. Nerv. Syst. 10*:145–155.

Goadsby, P.J., G.A. Lambert, and J.W. Lance (1985a). The mechanism of cerebrovascular vasoconstriction in response to locus coeruleus stimulation. *Brain Res. 326*:213–218.

Goadsby, P.J., and G.J. Macdonald (1985). Extracranial vasodilatation mediated by vasoactive intestinal polypeptide (VIP). *Brain Res. 329*:285–288.

Goadsby, P.J., R.D. Piper, G.A. Lambert, and J.W. Lance (1985b). The effect of activation of the nucleus raphe dorsalis (DRN) on carotid blood flow. I. The Monkey. *Am J. Physiol. 248*:R257–R262.

Goadsby, P.J., R.D. Piper, G.A. Lambert, and J.W. Lance (1985c). The effect of activation of the nucleus raphe dorsalis (DRN) on carotid blood flow. II. The Cat. *Am. J. Physiol. 248*:R263–R269.

Gotoh, F., T. Kanda, F. Sakai et al. (1976). Serum dopamine B-hydroxylase in migraine. *Arch. Neurol. 33*:656–657.

Gotoh, F., S. Komatsumoto, N. Araki, and S. Gomi (1984). Noradrenergic nervous activity in migraine. *Arch. Neurol. 41*:951–955.

Gouswaard, P., J. Passchier, and A. van Boxtel (1985). Physiological reactions of migraine patients on real-life stress. *Cephalalgia, 5 (Suppl.3)*:30–31.

Gowers, W. (1893). *Diseases of the Nervous System*, Vol. 2, pp. 836–866. P. Blakiston, Philadelphia.

Graham, J.R. and H.G. Wolff (1938). Mechanism of migraine headache and action of ergotamine tartrate. *Arch. Neurol. Psychiatry. 39:*737–763.

Griffith, S.G., J. Lincoln, and G. Burnstock (1982). Serotonin as a neurotransmitter in cerebral arteries. *Brain Res. 247:*388–392.

Hachinski, V.C., J.W. Norris, P.W. Cooper, and J.G. Edmeads (1978). Migraine and the cerebral circulation. In *Current Concepts in Migraine Research* (R. Greene, ed.), pp. 11–15. Raven Press, New York.

Hamada, J., F. Gotoh, Y. Ishikawa et al. (1985). Autonomic nervous function in migraine—quantitative determination of perspiration and retinal vasomotor activity. *Cephalalgia 5 (Suppl. 3):*460–461.

Hanin, B., M.-G. Bousser, J. Olesen et al. (1985). Platelet aggregation study in migraine patients between and during attacks. *Cephalalgia 5 (Suppl.3):*398–399.

Hartman, B.K., L.W. Swanson, M.E. Raichle et al. (1980). Central adrenergic regulation of cerebral microvascular permeability and blood flow, anatomic and physiologic evidence. In *The Cerebral Microvasculature. Advances in Experimental Medicine and Biology 131:*113–126.

Henry, P.Y., J. Vernhiet, J.M. Orgogozo, and J.M. Caille (1978). Cerebral blood flow in migraine and cluster headache. *Res. Clin. Stud. Headache 6:*81–88.

Herberg, L.J. (1975). The hypothalamus and aminergic pathways in migraine. In *Modern Topics in Migraine* (J. Pearce, ed.), pp 85–95. Heinemann, London.

Hockaday, J.M., A.L. Macmillan, and C.W.M. Whitty (1967). Vasomotor-reflex response in idiopathic and hormone-dependent migraine. *Lancet 1:*1023–1028.

Hockaday, J.M., D.H. Williamson, and C.W.M. Whitty (1971). Blood glucose levels and fatty acid metabolism in migraine related to fasting. *Lancet 1:*1153–1156.

Hsu, L.K.G., A.H. Crisp, R.S. Kalucy et al. (1978). Nocturnal plasma levels of catecholamines, tryptophan, glucose and free fatty acids and the sleeping electroencephalographs of subjects experiencing early morning migraine. In *Current Concepts in Migraine Research* (R. Greene, ed.), pp. 121–130. Raven Press, New York.

Humphrey, P.P.A. (1984). Peripheral 5-hydroxytryptamine receptors and their classification. *Neuropharmacology 23:*1503–1510.

Jensen, K., U. Pedersen-Bjergaard, C.Tuxen et al. (1985). Nociception and pressure-pain threshold in the temporal muscle following local injection of bradykinin and serotonin. *Cephalalgia 5 (Suppl.3):*24–25.

Jerzmanowski, A. and A. Klimek (1983). Immunoglobulins and complement in migraine. *Cephalalgia 3:*119–123.

Kalendovsky, Z. and J.H. Austin (1975). Complicated migraine: Its association with increased platelet aggregability and abnormal plasma coagulation factors. *Headache 15:*18–35.

Kerr, F.W.L. (1961a). A mechanism to account for frontal headache in case of posterior fossa tumours. *J. Neurosurg. 18:*605–609.

Kerr, F.W.L. (1961b). Trigeminal and cervical volleys. *Arch. Neurol. 5:*171–178.

Kimball, R.W., A.P. Friedman, and E. Vallejo (1960). Effect of serotonin in migraine patients. *Neurology (Minneapolis) 10:*107–111.

Knapp, R.D. Jr. (1963). Reports from the past 2. *Headache 3:*112–122.

Kohlenberg, R.J. (1982). Tyramine sensitivity in dietary migraine: A critical review. *Headache 22:*30–34.

Krabbe, A.A. and J. Olesen (1980). Headache provocation by continuous intravenous infusion of histamine. Clinical results and receptor mechanisms. *Pain 8:*253–259.

Kruglak, L., I. Nathan, A.D. Korczyn et al. (1984). Platelet aggregability, disaggregability and serotonin uptake in migraine. *Cephalalgia 4:*221–225.

Lambert, G.A., N. Bogduk, P.J. Goadsby et al. (1984a). Decreased carotid arterial resistance in cats in response to trigeminal stimulation. *J. Neurosurg. 61:*307–315.

Lambert, G.A., J.W. Duckworth, N. Bogduk, and J.W. Lance (1984b). Low pharmacological responsiveness of the vertebro-basilar circulation in Macaca nemestrina monkeys. *Eur. J. Pharmacol. 102:*451–458.

Lance, J.W. (1982). *The Mechanism and Management of Headache,* 4th ed. Butterworths, London.

Lance, J.W. and M. Anthony (1966). Some clinical aspects of migraine: A prospective survey of 500 patients. *Arch Neurol. 15:*356–361.

Lance, J.W., M. Anthony, and A. Gonski (1967). Serotonin, the carotid body and cranial vessels in migraine. *Arch. Neurol. 16:*553–558.

Lance, J.W., G.A. Lambert, P.J. Goadsby, and J.W. Duckworth (1983). Brain stem influences on the cephalic circulation: Experimental data from cat and monkey of relevance to the mechanism of migraine. *Headache 23:*258–265.

Lashley, K.S. (1941). Patterns of cerebral integration indicated by the scotomas of migraine. *Arch. Neurol. Psychiatry. 46:*331–339.

Lauritzen, M., M.B. Jørgensen, N.H. Diemer et al. (1982). Persistent oligemia of rat cerebral cortex in the wake of spreading depression. *Ann. Neurol. 12:*469–474.

Lauritzen, M. and J. Olesen (1984). Regional cerebral blood blow during migraine by xenon-133 inhalation and emission tomography. *Brain 107:*447–461.

Lauritzen, M., T. Skyhøj Olsen, N.A. Lassen, and O.B. Paulson (1983a). Changes in regional cerebral blood flow during the course of classical migraine attacks. *Ann. Neurol. 13:*633–641.

Lauritzen, M., T. Skyhøj Olsen, N.A. Lassen, and O.B. Paulson (1983b). Regulation of regional cerebral blood flow during and between migraine attacks. *Ann. Neurol. 14:*569–572.

Leão, A.A.P. (1944). Spreading depression of activity in the cerebral cortex. *J. Neurophysiol. 7:*359–390.

Liveing, E. (1873). *On Megrim, Sick-Headache, and Some Allied Disorders: A Contribution to the Pathology of Nerve-Storms.* J. and A. Churchill, London.

Lord, G.D.A. and J.W. Duckworth (1977). Immunoglobulin and complement studies in migraine. *Headache, 17:*163–168.

Lord, G.D.A. and J.W. Duckworth (1978). Complement and immune complex studies in migraine. *Headache 18:*255–260.

Lord, G.D.A., E.J. Mylecharane, J.W. Duckworth, and J.W. Lance (1981). Effects of histamine H1- and H2-receptor antagonists in the cranial circulation of the monkey. *Clin. Exp. Pharmacol. Physiol. 8:*89–100.

Lous, I. and J. Olesen (1982). Evaluation of pericranial tenderness and oral function in patients with common migraine, muscle contraction headache and "combination headache." *Pain 12:*385–393.

Maertens de Noordhout, A., M. Timsit-Berthier, and J. Schoenen (1985). Contingent negative variation (CNV) in migraineurs before and during prophylactic treatment with beta-blockers. *Cephalalgia 5 (Suppl.3):*34–35.

Mayberg, M., R.S. Langer, N.T. Zervas, and M.A. Moskowitz (1981). Perivascular meningeal projections from cat trigeminal ganglia: possible pathway for vascular headaches in man. *Science 213:*228–230.

Moore, R.Y., A.E. Halaris, and B.A. Jones (1978). Serotonin neurons of the midbrain raphe: Ascending projections. *J. Comp. Neurol. 180:*417–437.

Moore, T.L., R.E. Ryan Jr., D.A. Pohl et al. (1980). Immunoglobulin, complement and immune complex levels during a migraine attack. *Headache 20:*9–12.

Morrison, J.H., S.L. Foote, M.E. Molliver et al. (1982). Noradrenergic and serotonergic fibers innervate complementary layers in monkey primary visual cortex: An immunohistochemical study. *Proc. Natl. Acad. Sci USA 79:*2401–2405.

Moskowitz, M.A. (1984). The neurobiology of vascular head pain. *Ann. Neurol. 16:*157–168.

Mück-Šeler, D., Ž. Deanović, and M. Dupelj (1979). Platelet serotonin (5-HT) and 5-HT releasing factor in plasma of migrainous patients. *Headache 19:*14–17.

Nattero, G., D. Bisbocci, and F. Ceresa (1979). Sex hormones, prolactin levels, osmolarity and electrolyte patterns in menstrual migraine—relationship with fluid retention. *Headache 19:*25–30.

Nattero, G., J.S. Franzone, L. Savi, and R. Cirillo (1984). Serum prostaglandin-like substances in cluster headache and common migraine. In *Progress in Migraine Research Vol. 2* (F. Clifford Rose, ed.), pp. 199–204. Pitman, London.

Norris, J.W., V.C. Hachinski, and P.W. Cooper (1975). Changes in cerebral blood flow during a migraine attack. *Br. Med. J. 3:*676–677.

O'Brien, M.D. (1971). Cerebral blood changes in migraine. *Headache 10:*139–143.

Oleson, J., B. Larsen, and M. Lauritzen (1981a). Focal hyperemia followed by spreading oligemia and impaired activation of rCBF in classical migraine. *Ann. Neurol. 9:*344–352.

Olesen, J., P. Tfelt-Hansen, L. Henricksen, and B. Larsen (1981b). The common migraine attack may not be initiated by cerebral ischaemia. *Lancet 2:*438–440.

Peatfield, R.C., M.J. Gawel, and F. Clifford Rose (1981a). The effect of infused prostacyclin in migraine and cluster headache. *Headache 21:*190–195.

Peatfield, R.C., M.J. Gawel, and F. Clifford Rose (1981b). Asymmetry of the aura and pain in migraine. *J. Neurol. Neurosurg. Psychiatry 44:*846–848.

Pratt, J.M. (1985). Stress-induced superficial temporal artery flow differences between migraine and muscle-contraction headache groups. *Cephalalgia 5 (Suppl.3):*488.

Rao, N.S. and J. Pearce (1971). Hypothalamic–pituitary–adrenal axis studies in migraine with special reference to insulin sensitivity. *Brain 94:*289–298.

Raskin, N.H. and S.C. Knittle (1976). Ice cream headache and orthostatic symptoms in patients with migraine headache. *Headache 16:*222–225.

Raskin, N.H. and R.K. Schwartz (1980). Icepick-like pain. *Neurology 30:*203–205.

Ray, B.S. and H.G. Wolff (1940). Experimental studies on headache. Pain sensitive structures of the head and their significance in headache. *Arch. Surg. 41:*813–856.

Reinhard, J.F. Jr., J.E. Liebmann, A.J. Schlosberg, and M.A. Moskowitz (1979). Serotonin neurons project to small blood vessels in the brain. *Science 206:*85–87.

Rolf, L.H., G. Wiele, and G.G. Brune (1981). 5-hydroxytryptamine in platelets of patients with muscle contraction headache. *Headache 21:*10–11.

Sachs, H., J. Russell, D. Christman, and A. Wolf (1985). Positron emission tomographic studies on induced migraine. *Cephalalgia 5 (Suppl.3):*456–457.

Sakai, F. and J.S. Meyer (1978). Regional cerebral hemodynamics during migraine and cluster headache measured by the ^{133}Xe inhalation method. *Headache 18:*122–132.

Sakai, F. and J.S. Meyer (1979). Abnormal cerebrovascular reactivity in patients with migraine and cluster headache. *Headache 19:*257–260.

Schoenen, J., A. Maertens de Noordhout, and P.J. Delwaide (1985). Plasma catecholamines in headache patients: Clinical correlations. *Cephalalgia 5 (Suppl.3):*28–29.

Schottstaedt, W.W. and H.G. Wolff (1955). Variations in fluid and electrolyte excretion in association with vascular headache of the migraine type. *Arch. Neurol. Psychiatry. 73:*158–164.

Sicuteri, F. (1967) Vasoneuroactive substances and their implication in vascular pain. *Res. Clin. Stud. Headache 1:*6–45.

Sicuteri, F. (1976). Migraine, a central biochemical dysnociception. *Headache 16:*145–159.

Sicuteri, F. (1977). Dopamine, the second putative protagonist in headache. *Headache 17:*129–131.

Sicuteri, F., M. Fanciullacci, and B. Anselmi (1963). Bradykinin release and inactivation in man. *Int. Arch. Allergy 22:*77–84.

Sicuteri, F., G. Franchi, S. Michelacci, and S. Salmon (1962). Aumento della escrezione urinaria dell'acido vanilmandelico, catabolita delle catecolamine durante l'accesso emicranico. *Settim. Med. 50:*13–16.

Sicuteri, F., A. Testi, and B. Anselmi (1961). Biochemical investigations in headache: Increase in hydroxyindoleacetic acid excretion during migraine attacks. *Int. Arch. Allergy 19:*55–58.

Simard, D. and O.B. Paulson (1973). Cerebral vasomotor paralysis during migraine attack. *Arch. Neurol. 29:*207–209.

Sjaastad, O. (1970). Kinin- and histamine-investigations in vascular headache. In *Kliniske Aspekter i Migraeneforskningen,* pp. 61–69. Nordlundes Bogtrykkeri, Copenhagen.

Skarby, T., P. Tfelt-Hansen, F. Gjerris et al. (1982). Characterization of 5-hydroxytryptamine receptors in human temporal arteries: Comparison between migraine sufferers and non-sufferers. *Ann. Neurol. 12:*272–277.

Skinhøj, E. (1973). Hemodynamic studies within the brain during migraine. *Arch. Neurol. 29:*95–98.

Skyhøj-Olsen, T., M. Lauritzen, and N.A. Lassen (1984). Focal ischemia during migraine attacks in patients with classical and complicated migraine. *Acta Neurol. Scand. 69 (Suppl. 98):*258–259.

Somerville, B.W. (1972). The role of oestradiol withdrawal in the etiology of menstrual migraine. *Neurology (Minneap.) 22:*355–365.

Spira, P.J., E.J. Mylecharane, and J.W. Lance (1976). The effect of humoral agents and antimigraine drugs on the cranial circulation of the monkey. *Res. Clin. Stud. headache 4:*37–75.

Sramka, M., G. Brozek, J. Bures, and P. Nadvornik (1977–78). Functional ablation by spreading depression: Possible use in human stereotactic neurosurgery. *Appl. Neurophysiol. 40:*48–61.

Tfelt-Hansen, P., I. Lous, and J. Olesen (1981). Prevalence and significance of muscle tenderness during migraine attacks. *Headache 21:*49–54.

Tunis, M.M. and H.G. Wolff (1953). Long term observations of the reactivity of the cranial arteries in subjects with vascular headache of the migraine type. *Arch. Neurol. Psychiatry. 70:* 551–557.

Vardi, J., S. Flechter, D. Ayalon et al. (1981). L-dopa effect on prolactin plasma levels in complicated and common migrainous patients. *Headache 21:*14–20.

Wolff, H.G. (1963). *Headache and Other Head Pain.* Oxford University Press, New York.

Yamamoto, M. and J.S. Meyer (1980). Hemicranial disorder of vasomotor adrenoceptors in migraine and cluster headache. *Headache 20:*321–335.

Ziegler, D.K., R.S. Hassanein, A. Kodanez, and J.C. Meek (1979). Circadian rhythms of plasma cortisol in migraine. *J. Neurol. Neurosurg. Psychiatry. 42:*741–748.

6

The Treatment of Migraine

DEWEY K. ZIEGLER

There are two difficult problems in comparing migraine treatments. The first problem is defining homogeneous patient groups. It is fairly easy to identify a classic migraine attack by its characteristic preceding neurologic phenomena—usually visual. But attacks called "common migraine" vary to extreme degrees in location of pain, duration, and occurrence of nausea or vomiting. Whether such individual attacks should be called "muscle contraction" or migraine headache is often a matter of arbitrary opinion (Ziegler, 1979). Furthermore, individual patients may have certain characteristics during one attack and strikingly different ones in another.

A related problem is that of measurement. Migraine attacks can be studied in terms of intensity, character, location, duration of pain, frequency of attacks, use of analgesic medication, and occurrence of nausea and vomiting. Unless exactly the same measures have been used in two studies, a comparison is exceedingly complex.

Acute headache attacks that are generally labeled "common" migraine, however, are characterized by various combinations of the following features: (1) pain of moderate to extreme severity, (2) pain on the anterior part of one side of the head, (3) presence of nausea and/or vomiting, (4)photophobia, and (5) pallor and coldness of hands and feet.

The discussion of migraine therapy is best divided into two parts: (1) the treatment of the acute headache attack, and (2) prophylaxis for future attacks.

TREATMENT OF THE ACUTE ATTACK

Differential Diagnosis from Structural Disease

Of first importance in managing the patient with these symptoms is the realization that occasionally they are symptoms not of migraine but of more dangerous conditions—particularly meningeal irritation due to subarachnoid hemmorhage (Kassel et al., 1985). This possibility must be considered in every migraine attack and a decision made (often difficult) as to whether or not to proceed with further diagnostic measures. The subject of differential diagnosis is dealt with elsewhere in this volume, but this particular problem of the acute headache is so prevalent and important that it bears repeating.

Induction of Relaxation

Minimizing stimuli of all kinds, particularly visual ones, is probably the most important initial measure in alleviating the migraine attack. Preferably, patients should retire to a dark, quiet room and try to sleep (see pp. 100–105). Most patients know from long experience that light and noise disturb them. Many, however, are unable or unwilling to cancel their daily activities at the time of an attack. Often these patients, determined to "keeping going," progressively increase their intake of ergotamine and analgesics to override the migraine symptoms. Such behavior, of course, frequently leads to habituation to these drugs—a most dangerous condition. This potential problem must be discussed at length with patients. The physician, while sympathetic, should refuse to be forced to overprescribe.

Conversely, patients should be told that some individuals, particularly those who note the occurrence of their migraine attacks in conjunction with periods of nervous tension, find that they can, at the first warning of an attack, deliberately induce a state of relaxation that can abort the episode (discussed below).

Similarly, some patients find that the use of 40 mg of propranolol at the onset of a migraine attack will abort the attack (Featherstone et al., 1983). This observation is of interest because this drug has been found to be prophylactic and therapeutic for panic and anxiety attacks (Kellner et al., 1974; Easton et al., 1976). Small doses of chlorpromazine have also been reported to accomplish the same purpose. Some patients find that they can prevent an attack from developing without the use of drugs. A variety of techniques of induction of a calm, relaxed mental state are used. Recorded tapes of instruction in muscle relaxation are used by some. Mental imagery of calm scenes can be used. Patients whose migraine headaches come on slowly, usually those whose pain begins in the neck or back of the head and proceeds gradually to a full-blown attack, should be carefully instructed to try these measures. Those who respond are often individuals who recognize that their attacks occur at times of emotional stress.

Ergotamine

Ergotamine is a more or less specific treatment for the acute migraine attack. It is one of several closely related alkaloids that have a remarkably wide spectrum of action, many of which are not fully understood. These actions include constriction of the smooth muscle of blood vessels and the uterus, and neurohumeral effects influencing the action of epinephrine, serotonin, and dopamine. Some alkaloids have definite central nervous system action, particularly on centers for control of the sympathetic nervous system (Berde, 1980). Ergotamine was originally derived from a fungus *(Claviceps purpurea)* on rye. Poisoning with accidental ingestion of excessive amounts of this fungus on grain may have caused unexplained "epidemics" of delirium and convulsions in Europe during the Middle Ages. Some central nervous system toxicity does occur with use of large amounts (Loew et al., 1978).

Ergotamine was found several decades ago to ameliorate the pain of the severe migraine attack. Vasoconstriction, one of the many actions of the drug, has been considered the most important in this context. Ergotamine produces extreme pressor activity in the spinal preparation and produces increased vascular resistance in many arteries but seems to have selective actions in the carotid and basilar system (Mylecharane et al., 1978). An interesting aspect of the vascular phenomenon is that it is amphoteric; that is, vasoconstriction occurs in vessels of low vascular resistance and vasodilation in vessels of high resistance (Berde, 1980). One theory of its effectiveness has been that the pain of migraine is due to vasodilation, and the action of ergotamine one of vasoconstriction of the dilated external carotid arteries. Studies in recent years have cast some doubt on this formulation for at least three reasons: (1) there is doubt as to whether the increased pulsation of the temporal arteries is frequent or severe enough to account for the migraine syndrome (Blau, 1978; Heyck, 1981); (2) changes in cerebral blood flow have indeed been documented in the migraine attack, but they *apparently* occur only in cases of classic migraine (Olesen et al., 1982) whereas the pain is similar in both types; (3) the striking blood flow change during most of the painful period is one of oligemia not hyperenia (Olesen et al., 1981).

Whatever its mechanism, ergotamine is, nevertheless, strikingly successful with many patients.

Whether the administration of ergotamine at a very early phase of the headache is more effective than that given later, during the height of the headache, is not known. Theoretically, if vasospasm plays a part early in the migraine episode, administration of a vasoconstrictor at an early stage should be ineffective. Usually, however, patients state that ergotamine is ineffective if the pain has achieved a certain level.

Currently in America, ergotamine can be administered in one of four ways—orally, rectally, sublingually, and by inhalation. The preferred route for administration ergotamine is determined by several variables: (1) the need for rapid action; (2) the presence or absence of nausea or vomiting; (3) the availability of the preparation; and (4) the patient's preference.

Ergotamine, both in the experimental animal and in man, produces nausea, an unfortunate quality for a drug used to treat pain episodes that are characteristically accompanied by this same symptom.

The usual initial oral dose of ergotamine for adults is 2 mg, usually combined with caffeine, which seems to facilitate absorption. An additional milligram can be taken at half-hour intervals, in the average adult, to a maximum of 5 mg per attack. Patients should be warned to terminate medication with the symptoms of peripheral or coronary vasoconstriction.

Although oral administration of the drug is the most convenient route, clearly patients who are vomiting will not benefit from medication given orally. Nausea itself, in the absence of vomiting, is often accompanied by gastric stasis and will limit absorption.

Sublingual administration is also convenient, but some studies have shown disappointing blood levels with its use, probably because of erratic absorption (Sutherland et al., 1974).

For those patients who can use them, rectal suppositories provide an excellent route for rapid absorption. Insertion of one-half suppository can be tried in patients whose response to ergotamine is unknown. One difficulty is the frequent desirability of prescribing more than one drug rectally, for example, ergotamine and an anti-emetic—an awkward but possible practice.

Inhalation of ergotamine apparently does quickly provide rapid absorption, but many patients are not familiar with this type of drug use. Patients may also easily overdose because inhalation is easy and absorption is excellent (Crooks et al., 1964; Ekbom et al., 1983).

It now seems to be definite that ergotamine is most effective when taken early in the attack and, conversely, as noted, less effective when taken at the height of pain, probably partly because of nausea and impaired absorption.

It has been thought that therapeutic effect parallels blood levels, which are usually low (0.2 to 0.5 mg/ml), although one recent study reported biologically active ergotamine (administered rectally) despite unmeasurable plasma levels (Bulow et al., 1985). One study showed that nausea parallels not ergotamine blood levels but rather delay in treatment. This finding suggests that the initial use in the acute migraine attack, of 3 to 4 mg should be tried (Ala-Hurula, 1982). Another suggestion has been that the initial dose be adjusted according to the response of the patients to amounts needed in previous attacks; that is, if no response had occurred to an initial 1-mg dose, in the next attack the initial dose should be raised to 2 mg, and then subsequently to 3 mg, if necessary (Bradfield, 1976). As a general rule, in any single attack the dosage of ergotamine should be no more than 6 mg, as noted previously, and no more than 12 mg should be used weekly.

Aside from nausea, the most common unwanted and occasionally dangerous side effect of ergotamine is vasoconstriction, which may be difficult to detect in a patient whose migraine attack itself may produce cold, clammy extremities. In addition to the peripheral arteries, dangerous spasm of carotid, coronary, and mesenteric arteries can occur from ergotamine and can lead to gangrene (Fedotin & Hartman, 1970; Benedict & Robertson, 1979; Greene et al., 1977; Connolly, 1978). Individual susceptibility to ergot varies markedly, however, and much smaller amounts, well within the low therapeutic range, have induced ergotism (Enge & Silvertssen, 1965; Benedict & Robertson, 1979; Diamant-Berger et al., 1972).

Those patients most susceptible are those with sepsis, thyrotoxicosis, anemia, and any type of vascular disease. Ergotamine must be used with caution in the elderly and with extreme caution, if at all, during pregnancy because of its oxytoxic action. Ergotism must be treated promptly; possible treatments include sodium nitroprusside, vasodilators, and sympathetic block (Husum et al., 1980; Whitsett et al., 1978; Tfelt-Hansen et al., 1982).

Also to be avoided is the curious "addiction" to ergotamine in which the patient takes large amounts of the drug daily and usually is still afflicted with headaches, often of even greater severity. This pattern of drug taking is difficult to break; severe withdrawal headaches occur, and recidivism is usual (Wainscott et al., 1974; Karoll & Dalessio, 1972).

Ergotamine, as noted earlier, is offered in some preparations with caffeine, which has been shown to enhance gastric absorption (Cafergot). Another preparation contains phenobarbital and belladonna, alkaloids in addition to caffeine (Cafergot P-B).

In patients taking large amounts of these preparations, the pharmacologic effects of these additional compounds are occasionally important (e.g., unpleasant stimulation from caffeine).

Dihydroergotamine (DHE)

Dihydroergotamine is another ergot alkaloid of use in the acute migraine attack. Its probable major current use in medicine is to counteract orthostatic and postoperative hypotension and to prevent embolism (Lubke, 1976; Mantyla et al., 1978; Pedersen & Christianson, 1983; Benowitz et al., 1981). It is a much weaker vasoconstrictor than ergotamine; therefore, dangerous arterial constriction with complications are rare, although they have been reported (Kakkar, 1982; Franco et al., 1978). This substance was demonstrated decades ago to be therapeutic in migraine (Herschberg, 1950; Tillgren, 1947), but its use has been limited probably because parenteral administration is required. Its usefulness despite this limitation has been emphasized recently (Raskin & Raskin, 1984). Its beneficial action is probably due to the selective vasconstrictive action on the capacitance vessels. The drug can be given orally or parenterally. Intravenous use of .5 mg followed by a few subsequent doses at hourly intervals has been recommended (Raskin and Raskin, 1984).

Isometheptene Naveate

This sympathomimetic amine is marketed in a compound with paracetamol and dichloralphenazone. The compound is said to lack the emetic quality of ergotamine and, in one study, was found to be equally effective (Yuill et al., 1972). There has been, however, no reported study of the drug for several years.

Antiemetics

Because both the migraine episode itself and the ergotamine used in treatment may induce nausea, antiemetic agents are usually therapeutic when used early.

Metaclopramide is useful in the migraine attack because it functions as an antinauseant and an antiemetic and also counteracts gastric stasis. The promotion of normal gastric motility is important in the migraine attack because it improves absorption of the active therapeutic agents, for example, analgesics. Blood levels of ingested aspirin have been shown to be higher after use of metaclopramide than without the drug. Ten to 20 mg can be administered intramuscularly or rectally early in the attack and repeated once in a half hour if no benefit results (Tfelt-Hansen et al., 1980). Uncommonly, anxiety, restlessness, and dystonic movements can occur as a side effect. Metaclopramide can be used in a somewhat different way in the many patients who habitually develop nausea or vomiting with attacks and whose headache responds to ergotamine. In these individuals, at the first warning of a migraine attack, 10 mg of Metaclopramide can be taken one-half hour before the use of ergotamine.

Patients should, of course, be warned that judgment must be used so that they do not use the drug indiscriminately for minor headache.

Other antiemetic agents can be used, for example, trimethobenzamide in amounts of 250-mg tablet or suppository. Many of the phenothiazine compounds such as prochlorperazine also have antiemetic properties; they also have the advantage of providing useful sedation, and for migraine patients in severe pain this is important. Occasionally rather high doses under careful monitoring are needed—for example 25 mg of prochloperazine; acute dystonia and hypotension are always risks with these compounds and are not consistently dose related.

Analgesics

Migraine attacks are usually extremely painful and patients devour analgesics with varying degrees of urgency. Most patients, before consulting a physician, try the over-the-counter drugs—aspirin, acetaminophen, and ibuprophen. Aspirin has been shown to be slightly more effective for general pain than acetaminophen; in many studies pain of inflammatory action has been shown to be clearly more responsive to aspirin (Koch-Weser, 1976). In migraine, equivalent doses of the three analgesics seem about equal in effect (Tfelt-Hansen & Olesen, 1980). Occasionally, patients develop the habit of taking huge amounts of these drugs, frequently out of apprehension of attacks. Acetaminophen in very large doses causes severe hepatotoxicity. Hepatic failure can progress to encephalopathy, coma, and death, and maximum onset of liver failure may be delayed for 4 to 6 days after ingestion (Gazzard et al., 1976).

Aspirin itself carries the danger of irritation of gastric mucosa, occasionally causing hemorrhage and anemia with large or abrasive doses.

Of the more potent analgesics, codeine is one of the safest for occasional use. Although it is a narcotic, true addiction with severe withdrawal symptoms is rare, but habituation is common. Dangerous allergy to codeine is not uncommon. Of somewhat equal potency are oxycodone (Percodan) and propoxyphene (Darvon), although for potency equal to that of 60 mg of codeine, probably 90 to 120 mg of propoxyphene is required (Beaver, 1974). One study reported the latter drug somewhat inferior to acetaminophen (Smith et al., 1975). Propoxyphene has been abused for its euphorogenic effect, and addiction can occur. In large doses, furthermore, it can be used as an agent of suicide by causing respiratory depression. Intermittent use of these compounds is permissible for acute migraine attacks, but the danger of habituation is real.

The pain migraine patients suffer often induces physicians to use even more potent analgesics—Dilaudid, meperidine, or morphine. Use of these drugs is more dangerous, however, because migraine is a recurrent condition and once the patient discovers the prompt pain relief and euphoria the drugs produce, he or she may demand such treatment with increasing frequency. The patient also may be unwilling subsequently to try other treatments for an attack, demanding injection of morphine or meperidine for less severe episodes. It is wise to explain this danger to patients who have frequent and severe attacks and persuade them to rely on combinations of adequate amounts of sedatives and less potent analgesics for treatment.

Sedatives

There is no doubt that the use of sedatives concomitant with analgesics increases the effectiveness of the latter. Commercial preparations combining analgesics, caffeine, and a small amount of barbiturate are frequently beneficial in mild attacks. Again, the danger of habituation is real if patients use these drugs in excess. Specifically, patients should not take these drugs on a daily basis.

During attacks of extreme pain, patient need heavier sedation from their medication. Some of the phenothiazine compounds, as noted previously—for example, prochlorperazine—are helpful for this purpose, because in addition to their sedative property they possess strong antiemetic action and do not endanger respiration except when given in massive doses. Several of these agents can be given by suppository. It is well to recall the potential acute side effects of hypotension or acutely occurring dystonic movements, which can occur even after a small dose. The latter reactions can, however, be treated effectively with a parenteral antihistamine or sedative.

The benzodiazepines, such as Diazepam, are also helpful when used with analgesics. They have the advantage of rapid action, short duration of effect, and little hypotensive effect. Because pain raises the resistance of patients to the action of these drugs, they often must be given, in severe attacks, in doses exceeding those generally used for nighttime sedation.

PROPHYLAXIS OF ATTACKS

Avoidance of Precipitating Factors

Many sufferers from migraine are certain that nothing consistently precedes their headache that can be considered a precipitating event. Other patients, however, name factors that are consistently followed by attacks, such as the following:

1. A change in the amount of sleep may bring on an attack. Most commonly the migraine patient, after a week of intense work, will sleep soundly and for a particularly long period on weekend nights and awaken with a severe migraine episode. In a systematic study Sunday was found to be a day of high migraine frequency (Osterman et al., 1981). It is not known, however, whether it is the sleep itself or some other temporal phenomenon that induces the headache. An occasional patient routinely awakens from sound sleep with severe migraine attacks—such awakenings have been demonstrated to occur during periods of REM sleep (Dexter, 1979). Manipulation of sleep hours may be tried in such sleep-locked patients.

2. Hypoglycemic states are often characterized by headache, and even slight drops in blood sugar levels add to other factors in the etiology of the migraine attack; patients should be told not to miss meals. High-protein meals tend to protect against wide swings in blood sugar.

3. In some individuals the use of female sex hormones (birth control pills) seems to precipitate headache, and these compounds must be avoided when possible. Recent literature is summarized in Table 6-1. (Dennerstein et al., 1978).

Table 6-1 Oral contraceptive (OC) pill and headaches[a]

Study	Year	Country	Type	Sample source	No. studied	Effect of contraceptive
Whitty et al.	1966	UK	R	Neurologic clinic	30	↑ severity of migraine. ↑ migraine in days off OC
Nisson et al.	1967	Sweden	R	Contraceptive clinic	281	↑ frequency of headache in 22% ↓ frequency of headache in 14%
Grant	1968	UK	P,12 M	Contraceptive clinic	521	↑ frequency of headache by 13%
Herzberg and Coppen	1970	UK	P,11 M IUD controls	Contraceptive clinic	163	↑ frequency of headache in OC users compared with IUD users
Larson-Cohn and Lundberg	1970	Sweden	P,12 M	Contraceptive clinic	1,676	↑ frequency of migraine by 10% in nonsufferers of migraine ↑ frequency by 18% in migraine sufferers ↓ frequency by 36% in migraine sufferers
Herzberg et al.	1971	UK	P,12 M IUD controls	Contraceptive clinic		↑ frequency of headaches by 20% in those who continued on OC ↓ frequency of headaches by 10% in IUD users

[a]Key to symbols and abbreviations: ↑ = increase; ↓ = decrease; R = retrospective; P = prospective; OC = oral contraceptive pill; M = months.
(From Dennerstein, L., B. Laby, G.D. Burrows, and G.J. Hyman (1978). Headache and sex hormone therapy. *Headache 18*:146–153.)
Whitty, C.W.M., J.M. Hockaday, and M.M. Whitty (1966). The effect of oral contraceptives on migraine. *Lancet 1*:856:858.
Nilsson, A., L. Jacobsen, and C.A. Ingemanson (1967). Side effects of an oral contraceptive with particular attention to mental symptoms and sexual adaptation. *Acta Obstet Gynecol Scand 46*:537–556.
Grant, E.C.G. (1968). Relation between headaches from oral contraceptives and development of endometrial arterioles. *Br Med J 3*:402–405.
Herzberg, B., and A. Coppen (1970). Changes in psychological symptoms in women taking oral contraceptives. *Br J Psychiatry 116*:161–164.
Larsson-Cohn, U., and P.O. Lundberg (1970). Headache and treatment with oral contraceptives. *Acta Neurol Scand 46*:267–278.

4. Whether or not some cases of migraine are due to food allergy is still a debated subject, but controlled studies seem to indicate that for 10 to 20% of migraine patients dietary substances are a provocative factor (Monro et al., 1984). Tyramine has been considered the offending compound, but its administration in controlled studies did not cause headache (Ziegler & Stewart, 1977). The list of food substances that have been implicated is very large, and eliminating all of them would restrict diet considerably. Furthermore, the attention such a complex diet would require might well have the psychological effect of increasing headache. In some cases, patients are convinced that certain foods precipitate attacks—most commonly chocolate, cheese, and red wine.

Study	Year	Country	Type	Sample source	No. studied	Effect of contraceptive
Goldzieher et al.	1971	U.S.	P,6 M Double-blind placebo crossover	Contraceptive clinic	398	↓ in headache frequency for both placebo and OC Significantly more headaches on "Ovulen" than placebo
Carroll	1971	UK	R	Migraine/neurology clinic	290	↑ frequency and/or intensity of migraine in 49%
Cullberg	1972	Sweden	P,2 M Double-blind placebo	Menstruation study	320	No difference in headache frequency between OC and placebo users
Royal College General Practitioners	1974	UK	P,48 M	General practice	46,000	Headache and migraine the most frequent reported symptoms in OC users
Kudrow	1975	U.S.	R	Headache clinic	300	↑ frequency of migraine in hormone takers Discontinuing OC significantly reduced migraine in 70%
Dalton	1976	UK	R	Migraine volunteers	886	↑ frequency of migraine in 34% of OC users and 60% of ex-OC users. OC induced migraine in 5%. Ceasing OC improved migraine in 39% of ex-OC users

Herzberg, B.N., K.C. Draper, A.L. Johnson, and G.C. Nicol (1971). Oral contraceptives, depresssion and libido. *Br Med J* 3:495–500.

Goldzieher, J.W., L.E. Moses, E. Averkin et al. (1971). A placebo-controlled double-blind crossover investigation of the side effects attributed to oral contraceptives. *Fertil Steril* 22:609–623.

Carroll, J.D. (1971). Migraine and oral contraception. In: *Proceedings of the International Headache Symposium*, Sandoz, Basle, 45–46.

Cullberg, J. (1972). Mood changes and menstrual symptoms with different gestagen/estrogen combinations. *Acta Psychiatr Scand (Suppl.)*:236.

Royal College of General Practitioners (1974). *Oral Contraceptives and Health*. Pitman Publishing Corp., London.

Kudrow, L. (1975). The relationship of headache frequency to hormone use in migraine. *Headache* 15:37–40.

Dalton, K. (1976). Migraine and oral contraceptives. *Headache* 15:247–251.

Pharmacologic Prophylaxis of Attacks

At some point it is decided that the patient's headaches are sufficiently severe and frequent to warrant daily prophylactic treatment—frequently with drugs. The patient and physician must always balance the necessity of such treatment against its undesirable features—the possible side effects of any drug used and its expense. At present several classes of drugs exist for which there is some evidence of effectiveness in this role. Only carefully controlled studies can provide good evidence for the usefulness of any drug because the placebo effect in migraine is as significant as in other conditions (Beecher, 1955).

It is wise to remember that textbooks of 80 years ago recommended prophylactic measures that today sound amusing, for example cold water clysters (to remedy constipation), and long sojourn in the mountains or by the sea, galvanic current to the head, and arsenic (Oppenheim, 1900). Before being too amused, one might consider how some of our current measures may sound 100 years hence.

The medications that now appear most useful are the following:

Beta-adrenergic blocking agents—propranolol, timolol, metoprolol, and atenolol.
Tricyclic antidepressants—amitriptyline.
Nonsteroidal anti-inflammatory—naproxen, aspirin.
Anticonvulsant drugs—phenytoin, phenobarbital, and carbamazepine.
Antiserotonin antihistaminic agents—methysergide, cyproheptadine and clonidine.
Calcium-blocking agents—verapamil, nifedipine, and flunarizine.

Drugs in each of these categories often have several pharmacologic effects and which is the effective one is uncertain.

Beta-Adrenergic Blocking Agents

The group of drugs that block the beta-adrenoreceptors has previously had multiple uses in medicine in the treatment of angina pectoris, hypertension, cardiac arrhythmias, thyrotoxicosis, cardiomyopathy, anxiety disorders, glaucoma, and migraine. Some block all beta-adrenoreceptors nonselectively (e.g., propranolol) and others block more selectively, (e.g., metaprolol, which blocks the beta-one receptors).

Propranolol is now considered one of the most useful drugs for those patients who need daily medication to prevent migraine attacks. It has been shown to reduce the number, severity, and duration of attacks (Wideroe & Vigander, 1974; Behan & Reid, 1980). Its usefulness was discovered serendipidously during its use in patients with hypertension. The drug induces a modest degree of bradycardia (usually not a problem) and lowers the blood pressure. The exact mechanism of action in migraine is unknown; speculation is that it modifies or prevents an intermittent vasospasm of intracerebral or extracerebral cranial arteries that may result from episodic disturbed function of the autonomic nervous system. There are several lines of evidence that vasospasm may play a key role in migraine: (1) the occasional occurrence of permanent brain infarction after a migraine attack (Boisen, 1975; Dorfman et al., 1979); (2) the pallor and coldness of the extremities during the attack; (3) the demonstration of diminished cerebral blood flow in classic migraine patients during neurologic aura (Olesen et al., 1982). Propranolol does, however, have central nervous system depressant effects, as noted previously, which may bear on its effectiveness.

The daily dosage of propranolol varies from 80 to 240 mg, in divided doses (twice daily dosage can now be used since a long-acting preparation is available). Dosage can be raised fairly rapidly (over a period of a few weeks), although it is desirable to pause for some weeks after the 120-mg daily dosage to see if this dosage is effective. Because the drug does block adrenergic responses, it is best to avoid it in patients with history of asthma. It also can impair carbohydrate metabolism and mask hypoglycemic responses (Kotler et al., 1966) in diabetic patients, as well as cause a clinically important hypertensive response to hypoglycemia. Huge overdoses have resulted in severe hypoglycemia. Severe adverse reactions are rare; on occasion, however, it can cause dangerous pulmonary edema and hypotension, but almost all patients suffering from these dangerous complications have had acute ischemic heart disease or thyrotoxicosis (Greenblatt & Koch-Weser, 1973).

Indigestion and nausea occur occasionally, apparently relieved by taking medication before meals. Fairly commonly it causes feelings of lethargy and indolence—a different sensation from true sedation. This effect quite possibly lends support to the view that the drug works by means of its effect on the central nervous system. As noted previously, it has been reported to alleviate acute anxiety attacks.

In general, propranolol is a safe agent when used properly; it has been used without harm in migrainous children. Patients given the drug should be warned about hypotension and that, if they discontinue its use, they must do so gradually or cardiac arrhythmias may occur. This rare complication tends to occur chiefly in the elderly if the drug is discontinued abruptly. Occasionally, also, "rebound" headache occurs if the drug is withdrawn quickly.

There has been one report of ergotism in a patient receiving a beta-blocker and taking no more than a therapeutic dose of ergotamine, which suggests a possible interaction (Venter et al., 1984); however, as noted earlier such a complication has occurred without propranolol.

Of the other beta-adrenergic blocking drugs, several have been reported successful in migraine prophylaxis. Timolol, a nonselective beta-blocker, has been reported to be as effective as propranolol in doses of 20 to 30 mg/day. (Tfelt-Hansen et al., 1984; Standnes, 1982). Other selective beta-blockers (e.g., metoprolol) have also been reported effective (Langohr et al., 1985).

These drugs have many pharmacologic properties, and it is not certain which are responsible for the antimigraine effect. Some beta-adrenergic blockers have membrane-stabilizing properties. Some penetrate easily into the central nervous system, and in some patients central nervous system effects occur, for example, insomnia. It has been speculated that antimigrainous efficacy may be a result of central beta-receptor blockage producing a fall in sympathetic outflow. Some of the agents have sympathomimetic action; none of these, however has antimigraine effects. Most of the drugs are also 5-hydroxytryptamine antagonists with activities similar to those of methysergide and cyproheptadine.

A drug without beta-adrenergic properties and used in the treatment of hypertension, clonidine, has been found in a double-blind study to be no more effective in migraine control than a placebo (Langohr et al., 1985). This finding is of interest because it suggests that the beta-adrenergic blocking drugs' antihypertensive effect is produced by a mechanism different from their antimigrainous effect.

Tricyclic Antidepressants

Amitriptyline has been shown to reduce the severity and duration of migraine attacks. There is evidence that, although depression and headache tend to occur in the same population, the therapeutic effect of amitriptyline is not due simply to its antidepressant effect. Many migraine patients without depression respond well to the drug. Its effect on migraine may be produced by the same mechanism that produces its demonstrated analgesic effect in certain pain states of central origin, such as postherpetic neuralgia (Merskey & Hester, 1972; Taub, 1973). The optimal dose varies markedly from one patient to another—usually from 50 to 100 mg daily. It is advisable to start slowly with a 25-mg dose nightly, since some patients develop unpleasent sedation when the drug is first prescribed. Before raising the dosage, it is best to wait 3 to 4 weeks because the drug may not take effect until after such a period. The daily dose can be gradually raised on a twice daily schedule.

Side effects often limit the use of the drug. In some patients it produces sedation. Anticholinergic effects (especially dryness of the mouth) bother some; weight gain, probably due to increased appetite, disturbs others. It should be kept in mind that overdosage of the drug is frequently used for suicide. There is little systematic information about the effectiveness of other tricyclic antidepressant drugs in migraine.

Nonsteroidal Anti-Inflammatory, Prostaglandin-Blocking Drugs

Naproxen sodium is a substance that inhibits platelet function and also inhibits prostaglandin synthesis. Because abnormal platelet aggregation has been shown to accompany migraine, and prostaglandin has been hypothesized to play a part in the attack, it has been introduced as a migraine prophylactic agent. Three controlled studies reported its effectiveness in doses of 550 mg bid (Welch et al., 1985; Ziegler & Ellis, 1985; Lindegaard, 1980). It has been reported chiefly to reduce the severity and duration of attacks, the need for additional medication, and the occurrence of vomiting. The only common side effect has been that of burning sensation of epigastrium. One study noted that the drug did not diminish the frequency of headaches lacking migraine characteristics, which suggests a specificity of action.

There are scattered reports of other drugs with similar pharmacologic actions used as prophylactics against migraine, such as indomethacin (Mathew, 1981). Tolfenaminic acid, as well as fluferaminic acid, have been reported effective in acute attacks.

Anticonvulsant Drugs

It has long been known that seizure disorders are slightly more common in the migrainous population than in the general population. In seizure patients, headache is a frequent symptom, at times occurring shortly before or after the seizure itself. Obvious electroencephalographic (EEG) abnormalities are rare, however, in the adult migraine population, and there are few convincing reports of anticonvulsant drugs being of service prophylactically in adults.

The situation is different with children. Electroencephalographic abnormalities are much more common (Swaiman & Frank, 1978) and migraine seems to occur in children with other paroxysmally occurring disorders—motion sickness, vertigo, abdominal pains, and somnambulism. This cluster of symptoms has been called the periodic syndrome.

Many of these children respond to the use of phenobarbital and/or phenytoin. In one recent uncontrolled study of 62 children and adolescents, EEGs were said to be abnormal in 56%, and almost all patients reported excellent (over 75%) reduction in severity and duration of headache with anticonvulsant treatment. Little is known of the optimum duration of treatment or the long-term prognosis for children so treated (Buda & Joyce, 1979).

Antiserotonin—Antihistaminic Agents

Methysergide Methysergide has been used successfully in prophylaxis of migraine for several decades. It has a variety of pharmacologic actions, among which are serotonin inhibition and mild vasoconstriction. The serotonin inhibition probably accounts for the drug's usefulness in migraine.

The therapeutic dose is usually 6 mg daily by mouth in three divided doses, although some individuals seem to respond to smaller amounts. Occasional individuals cannot tolerate the drug because of development of disturbing subjective sensations; occasionally, hallucinations occur.

Cases have been reported of dangerous vasoconstriction, and the risk is somewhat increased when the drug is used in conjunction with ergotamine (Katz & Vogel, 1967; Kelly, 1965; Joyce & Gubbay, 1982)

The most feared complication of methysergide is fibrosis of the abdominal or pleural cavities, or pericardium. All of these conditions have occurred in patients taking methysergide continuously for extended periods (Elkind et al., 1968; Graham, 1967). If patients are given a ' vacation" from the use of the drug for 2 months after the being on the medication 5 months, this complication can be avoided.

Cyproheptadine This substance has both antiserotonin and antihistaminic properties. Few controlled trials of this drug for headache have been conducted, but some report a definite benefit. The optimum dosage for this purpose is not known but probably varies from 4 to 30 mg a day. The major limiting side effect is sedation (Miller, 1963).

Platelet Aggregation Inhibitor—Aspirin Platelets of migraine patients apparently aggregate abnormally (Couch & Hassanein, 1977). Platelet aggregation is presumably followed by the liberation and destruction of serotonin, a substance whose complex connection to migraine has been studied for decades. Platelet aggregation–inhibiting substances also inhibit the secretion of prostaglandins, which are potent vasodilation substances—and it was demonstrated several years ago that infusion of prostaglandin (PGE), produced migrainelike headache (Carlson, 1968). For these reasons, substances with the property of platelet aggregation inhibition have been tried for prophylaxis of migraine. In one double-blind study aspirin was compared with propranolol; the drugs were reported to give equally useful results (Baldrati et al., 1983). In another study, aspirin was given in a dosage of 325 mg bid combined with dipyramidole. Significant improvement occurred in the treated group overall, but to a greater degree in those with platelet hyperaggregability (Masel et al., 1980).

Calcium Entry-Blocking Agents (CEB)

In recent years these agents have been used in increasing amounts for migraine prophylaxis. Five such compounds have been reported—flunarizine, diltiazem, nifedipine, nimodipine, and verapamil. There are some data on the use of each of these in migraine. Only two, however (verapamil and nifedipine), are currently available in the United States, and neither has been officially approved by the Food and Drug Administration for therapy in migraine.

These drugs interfere with the entry of the calcium ion into the cells of smooth muscle walls; such action prevents the sustained contraction of the muscle. There is

Table 6-2 Comparison of side effects of calcium-blocking drugs

Drug	CNS behavioral/ sedation	Percentage of patients with side effects		
		Muscular	Vascular	Gastric/ constipation
Flunarizine	18	15	0	11
Nimodipine	23	34	6	16
Verapamil	0	0	23	17
Nifedipine	13	0	39	13
Diltiazem	NA	NA	NA	NA

(From Solomon, G.D. (1985). Comparative efficacy of calcium antagonist drugs in the prophylaxis of migraine. *Headache* 25:368–371.)

evidence that they produce arterial dilatation with preferential effect on the intracerebral arteries. The effects on cerebral function after vascular lesions, however, are complex, and there is some evidence that they may affect nonvascular terminals in the brain (Weir, 1984). The drugs are therapeutic in various types of angina pectoris, in cardiac arrhythmias, in hypertension, and in prevention of intracerebral artery spasm secondary to subarachnoid hemorrhage. The question of whether they are effective or to be avoided in acute coronary disease is still disputed.

The effectiveness of these drugs in migraine is thought to be tied in some way to relaxation of arterial walls. There is almost no information on the value of these drugs in migraine prophylaxis compared with that of the other classes of agents so used. Their reported potency seems to rival that of even the most successful—propranolol and methysergide—whereas side effects, particularly those of verapamil, are usually minimal.

All five drugs have been reported, in greater or lesser detail, to reduce significantly the frequency of migraine and in some cases the other parameters by which headache is measured, (e.g., intensity). For four of the drugs this evidence comes from controlled double-blind studies—diltiazem (Louis & Spierings, 1982), verapamil (Solomon et al., 1983), nifedipine (Kahan et al., 1983), and nimodipine (Gelmers, 1983). One report contained information that with nimodipine, more patients benefited from higher doses. The side effects varied markedly but seem to predominantly affect the CNS with nimodipine and flunarizine, whereas nifedipine, verapamil, and probably diltiazem produced vascular and gastrointestinal effects. Side effects occur infrequently with verapamil and usually are not severe (Baky & Singh, 1982). (Table 6-2). For all of these drugs the optimal effect may be delayed several weeks after use of the proper dosage.

Other drugs used with one or more of these agents produce a variety of potentially dangerous interactions. These include cimetidine, digitalis, diuretics, guinidine, phenytoin, and barbiturates (Ahmad, 1984).

These agents seem to hold great promise in this field. At least two studies have attempted to compare their reported efficacy and side effects (Peroutka, 1984; Solomon, 1985). One group concluded that nimodipine and nifedipine were the most selective and potent. It is apparent that more knowledge about the comparative efficacy of these drugs is needed.

Comment

Some general comments and speculations on the pharmacologic prophylaxis of migraine are in order. This subject is particularly difficult to study for two reasons. The natural history of the syndrome is variable in the extreme—attacks decrease in frequency or cease for no obvious reason. Furthermore, migraine is a syndrome particularly subject to the "nonspecific" therapeutic effect of evidence of personal interest by the physician in the efficacy of a drug. In therapeutic trials, then, there is usually a striking reduction in headache during the introductory placebo period. Double-blind controlled studies with placebo should eliminate this problem, but one interesting study using the drug clonidine illustrates the difficulty. Although a controlled study had reported the drug effective, two later double-blind studies could not confirm this result. One of these latter studies (with clonidine) pointed out that the *last* course of treatment, whether placebo or clonidine, tended to be the most effective; this strongly suggests that the physician's demonstrated ongoing interest in the patient was the therapeutic factor rather than the specific drug.

Nevertheless, enough consistency has been found in several agents to warrant their consideration as useful. The striking variety of their pharmacologic effects is of note. Why do drugs with such varying action as beta-adrenergic blocking, inhibition of serotonin action, and cell-reentry calcium blocking all seem to prevent migraine? To date, the answer is not known, although the mechanism of interrelationship has been proposed (Raskin, 1981).

There is little guidance as to which of the several prophylactic agents discussed in the previous pages should be given preferential trial in the individual patient. Rarely has one agent been compared with another in controlled trial. Both propranolol and amitriptyline for example have some tranquilizing action and therefore might be tried early in patients in whom anxiety is associated with migraine. Since amitriptyline has a sedative side effect in some, it might be tried first if the patient has coincident insomnia. Those agents with the more dangerous, albeit rare, toxicity tend to be left for later trial.

How long one should try an agent before pronouncing it ineffective is another problem. Certainly trials of less than a month are inadvisable unless severe side effects attributable to the drug occur. It is important to prevent patients from becoming discouraged and terminating use of a drug before an effective dosage is reached. If nonspecific side effects that are not a result of the drug occur, the patient should be informed that they are not caused by the drug and urged to continue. For most of the drugs used in prophylaxis of migraine, we have no information correlating blood level with clinical effectiveness. In the case of propranolol, at least, there apparently is no such correlation (Cortelli et al., 1985).

To date also almost no information exists as to whether combinations of these agents may be more effective for prophylaxis than a single medication, and, if so, in what kind of patients. Obviously no such information will be available until and unless we know the characteristics of patients who respond to any single medication.

The problem of adverse side effects, for example, in the use of a combined therapy such as the calcium-blocking drug verapamil and the beta-adrenergic blocking drug propranolol, has been addressed occasionally, for example, in the treatment of angina pectoris. No such side effects have been found.

Nonpharmacologic Prophylaxis of Attacks

In many migrainous patients, nonpharmacologic treatment can offer much. Even when drugs are prescribed, much of the therapeutic effect must be ascribed to nonspecific causes. This fact has been demonstrated time and again when, as noted previously, drugs thought to be useful were found in blind and controlled studies to be no more effective than placebo. The placebo is the oldest nonpharmacologic treatment in the armamentarium. It is not unethical for the physician to depend on the placebo effect by encouraging the use of any treatment with words indicating his or her belief in its usefulness.

Nonpharmacologic treatment begins with the doctor–patient relationship established on the first visit of the headache patient to the office. A careful, complete neurologic examination should be followed by an explanation to the patient that there is no evidence of structural disease of the brain. In most patients this can be accompanied by a statement to the effect that the possibility of brain tumor, for example, though not out of the question, is very remote. (A surprising number of patients with headache come to the physician with this unspoken fear.) It is well to follow with a brief explanatory lecture to the effect that migraine is the result of many elements, that "the cause" is not known, but that many frequently important factors are.

It can then be explained that there is often a hereditary tendency for migraine and that the attacks tend to be precipitated in predisposed patients by a variety of stimuli. These stimuli include alcohol, missing meals, bright lights, phases of the menstrual cycle in women, dietary substances, violent exercise, and periods of emotional stress or intense work. At this point it is wise to explain the inextricable connection of mind and body in pain problems to avoid the occasional retort, "My pain is not imaginary." Such a brief introduction to the problem should also include, particularly for young people, an explanation about the unpredictability of the life course of migraine and the usual absence of permanent total remission. This brief lecture should terminate with a request for the patient to ask about anything he or she might not understand or wishes to know. Such requests often elicit concerns, apprehensions, and ideas unsuspected by the physician.

Therapy without drugs is relevant in all phases of the headache problem. In acute migraine attack, as noted previously many patients discover for themselves a warning phase before the full-blown attacks during which he or she can make a conscious effort to "relax" and abort a full attack. This effect is very rare in attacks with definite neurologic aura—visual scotomata, paresthesias, and so on. Some patients however, have a warning consisting of pain in the occipital region, or in neck muscles; the pain then progresses to one side of the head accompanied by nausea, prostration, and other migraine symptoms. As noted above, some patients find that a small amount of medication will abort an attack; others achieve the effect with willed relaxation. Patients can be taught some relaxation techniques, using "autogenic" repetitive phrases, and instructed to retire to a quiet, dark place to use these at the time the warning signs occur. Clearly, this technique is helpful only to certain patients. A major clue as to the identity of such a group of patients is the existence of episodic or persistent, overt anxiety. These individuals will frequently identify the attack as occurring in a stressful situation. They will also occasionally say they feel "tension" in the neck or the back of the head as a prelude to a typical migraine attack, suggesting evolution from a "muscle contraction" headache to migraine.

There are many forms of systematic nondrug prophylactic treatments for recurrent migraine. Studies comparing the effectiveness of formal methods have only recently been made. Much rarer are studies comparing the success of a nonpharmacologic treatment with that of a drug treatment.

There is considerable evidence from psychological testing of headache patients as a group that they have more than normal anxiety and depression (Couch et al., 1975), and psychotherapy is sometimes indicated for those psychiatric symptoms apart from headache. It is, however, particularly difficult in nonpharmacologic treatments to determine if all are equally effective because they share the element of suggestion and induction of relaxation. Several treatments will be discussed.

Formal Psychotherapy

There are a few reports of a variety of psychotherapeutic techniques, from brief therapy to psychoanalysis, proving effective in reducing migraine problems (Brenner et al., 1949). Almost no controlled studies have been done, so judgment as to the usefulness of psychotherapy is, in general, intuitive. Migraine patients who suffer from overt psychiatric symptoms, particularly anxiety or depression, may improve in both areas with such therapy.

Behavior Modification

On the theory that migrainous individuals have a stereotyped disadvantageous reaction to stressful situations, which sets off a chain reaction, patients are taught a course of alterated behavior using a variety of techniques. These include training by audio instruction session in relaxation (discussed below) and a wide variety of self-management techniques to encourage patients to self-confidence and "positive thinking" (Mitchell & White, 1976).

Biofeedback

Voluntary relaxation of muscles obviously can be achieved. A variety of techniques have stemmed from the remarkable demonstrations that experimental animals could "learn" to control certain autonomic functions with conditioning (Miller, 1969). It was postulated that humans could also learn such control given "feedback" concerning their success or failure. It was subsequently discovered that human subjects could learn to raise their hand temperature (Sargent et al., 1973) or cool it (Turin & Johnson, 1976; Kewman & Roberts, 1980) and to affect the pulsation of extracranial arteries (Friar & Beatty, 1976; Knapp, 1982). It has been learned that biofeedback can affect the electroencephalogram in specific ways by (1) altering the alpha rhythm (Mulholland et al., 1983) and (2) reducing epileptiform abnormalities (Findley et al., 1975).

Biofeedback refers to the use of techniques to demonstrate to patients that they have, or have not, succeeded in altering a function. In migraine the two functions most discussed are those of skin temperature of the fingers and contraction of scalp and neck muscle. For raising the finger skin temperature, changes are recorded by a thermal electrode. Similarly, electrodes placed over the scalp or neck musculature record degrees of underlying muscle contraction. In both cases, changes are "fed back" to the patient with either visual or auditory signals.

The theory underlying the emphasis on elevation of finger temperature is that the migraine attack may be initiated or accompanied by constriction of peripheral arteries in the extremities, with accompanying painful dilation of the extracranial arteries—the latter a major tenet of the Wolff theory of etiology of migraine and pain. Raising the skin temperature in the hand might, then, reverse the process.

There is no doubt that many individuals have a remarkable ability to raise their skin temperature and that some of these individuals, concomitantly with such courses of activity, experience improvement in migraine (Diamond et al., 1981). The major problem in evaluating this approach, as in so many treatments, continues to be disagreement over two issues: (1) whether or not the procedure is specific—equal benefit, for example, has been reported from patients who learned to cool their hand temperature (Kewman & Roberts, 1980)—and (2) what element of the treatment is specific—that is, are the "machines" (the demonstration on some type of auditory or visual monitor that success or failure has occurred) necessary (Silver & Blanchard, 1978)? In other words, it might well be that something in the process of teaching patients to raise their finger temperature is therapeutic, but that it makes no difference whether the patient monitors skin temperature or not.

Considerable attention has been paid to this problem. In their 1982 review Blanchard et al. discussed studies of progressive muscle relaxation, transcendental meditation, and other behavioral techniques that had been reported equally effective in migraine, and their own controlled study indicating that relaxation training was at least as effective as skin temperature biofeedback. In a later exhaustive review of more recent controlled studies Holmes and Burish (1983) pointed out the absence of evidence that raising hand skin temperature produces therapeutic results superior to those of relaxation training. The rationale of finger-warming in migraine has also been challenged by the demonstration that this procedure results in no consistent change in cerebral blood flow (Largen et al., 1981) and that temporal artery flow (a decrease in which is postulated to be etiologic in migraine) is actually *increased* with an increase in finger temperature (Price & Tursky, 1976). In their critical review of biofeedback, after a careful analysis of data and methodology, Holmes and Burish (1983) concluded that

> there is no consistent statistically reliable evidence that biofeedback treatment is effective for treating patients suffering from migraine headaches. In many cases the patients undergoing the biofeedback treatment did report declines in headache activity, but those declines were not greater than the declines reported by patients in no-treatment control conditions or in control conditions involving treatments that would not be expected to help, thus suggesting that the effects that have been found with the biofeedback treatment were due to general relaxation and/or placebo effects.

Controversy still persists on this point. One recent study comparing the effectiveness in migraine of techniques of relaxation training, thermal biofeedback, and muscle biofeedback found superior results for the thermal biofeedback of a fairly rapid nature (LaCroix et al, 1983).

Scalp and neck muscle contraction has been found to be greater in migraine patients than in controls, although this finding has been questioned (Passchier et al.,

1984). It might well be that "teaching" patients consistently to relax these muscles would be therapeutic in migraine, and use of this procedure in aborting the acute attack has been mentioned. Many patients (but not all) accept the connection between initiation of migraine and sustained muscle contraction and provide a few regular periods throughout the day in which they concentrate on relaxation.

The question of whether or not biofeedback is therapeutic in muscle contraction headache must also be discussed briefly because the whole concept of muscle contraction causing a specific headache syndrome has recently been called into question. At the very least it is often difficult to determine whether individual attacks are "common migraine" or "muscle contraction." Several studies (Diamond & Montrose, 1984; Philips & Hunter, 1981; Hudzinski, 1983) report that electromyogram (EMG) feedback treatment for these syndromes is indeed effective in prophylaxis against such attacks by reducing their frequency, duration, and severity, or a combination of these parameters. The review quoted above, however, indicates that there is no evidence for specificity of EMG biofeedback in muscle contraction headache.

Hypnosis

Trials of hypnosis in prevention of migraine have been few; successes have been reported most recently in conjunction with the "hand-warming technique" discussed previously (Graham, 1975; Sacerdote, 1978). The usual criticisms of hypnosis apply: (1) it is of limited temporal duration, therefore not optimal for a usually life-long, recurrent condition; (2) it is a "control" exerted on the patient from outside, although it might be argued that use of drugs is subject to the same criticism.

Acupuncture

For centuries the Chinese have needled the skin and subcutaneous tissues of the heads, ears, and other areas of the body for treatment and prevention of a variety of diseases. There are several modifications of this technique—use of low-intensity pulsed electrical stimulation, for example. Benefit has been reported in headache, but few controlled studies have been done (Anderson et al., 1974; Hansen & Hansen, 1985; Loh et al., 1984).

Transcutaneous Nerve Stimulation

The use of low-intensity pulsed electrical stimuli applied to the skin has recently been found therapeutic in some kinds of intractable pain. It has proven successful in postherpetic neuralgia. Such stimulation with scalp electrodes has also recently been reported successful in alleviating the pain of migraine attack (Solomon & Guglielmo, 1985).

SUMMARY

The fields of pharmacologic and nonpharmacologic prophylaxis of migraine present a confusing choice of treatments. In fact, patients receiving drugs also receive nonpharmacologic "treatment" of greater or lesser degree in the form of the physician's attention and support. Many patients who are prescribed drugs also receive much more—discussions of life-style and methods of relaxation, for example. Undoubtedly the interaction of the drug and nondrug treatments is of utmost importance. This important and extremely difficult subject has rarely been evaluated systematically. It may well be that one or more pharmacologic agents are particularly effective in combination with a specific nondrug method.

ACKNOWLEDGMENTS

The author would like to thank Mrs. Patricia Melching and Ms. Althea Ballenger for their help in the typing and preparation of the manuscript.

REFERENCES

Ahmad, S. (1984). Calcium channel blockers and drug interactions. *J. Am. Coll. Cardiol.* 3:1352.

Ala-Hurula, V. (1982). Correlation between pharmacokinetics and clinical effects of ergotamine in patients suffering from migraine. *Eur. J. Clin. Pharmacol.* 21:397–402.

Anderson, D.G., J.L. Jamieson, and S.C. Man (1974). Analgesic effects of acupuncture on the pain of ice water: A double blind study. *Can. J. Psychol. Rev. Can. Psychol.* 28:239–244.

Baky, S.H. and B.N. Singh (1982). Verapamil hydrochloride: Pharmacological properties and rose in cardiovascular therapeutics. *Pharmacotherapy* 2:328–353.

Baldrati, A., P. Cortelli, G. Procaccianti et al. (1983). Propranolol and acetylsalicylic acidecin migraine prophylaxis. *Acta Neurol. Scand.* 67:181–186.

Beaver, W.T. (1974). Are synthetic narcotics adequate substitutes for opium-derived alkaloids? *Adv. Neurol.* 4:519–525.

Beecher, H.K. (1955). The powerful placebo. *JAMA* 159:1602–1606.

Behan, P.O. and M. Reid (1980). Propranolol in the treatment of migraine. *The Practitioner* 224:201–204.

Benedict, C.R. and D. Robertson (1979). Angina pectoris and sudden death in the absence of atherosclerosis following ergotamine therapy for migraine. *Am. J. Med.* 67:177–178.

Benowitz, N., R. Byrd, and J. Rosenberg (1981). Dihydroergotamine therapy for severe orthostatic hypotension. *Clin. Pharmacol. and Ther.* 29:233.

Benson, H.B.P. Malvea, and S.R. Graham (1973a). Physiologic correlates of meditation and their clinical effect in headache: An ongoing investigation. *Headache* 13:23–24.

Berde, B. (1980). *Ergot Compounds and Brain Function: Neuroendocrine and Neuropsychiatric Aspects*, pp. 3–23. Raven Press, New York.

Blanchard, E.B., F. Andrasik, D.F. Neff et al. (1982). Biofeedback and Relaxation Training with Three Kinds of Headache: Treatment Effects and Their Prediction. *J. Consult. Clin. Psychol.* 50:562–575.

Blau, J.N. (1978). Migraine: A vasomotor instability of the meningeal circulation. *Lancet* 2:1136–1139.

Boisen, E. (1975). Strokes in migraine: Report on seven strokes associated with severe migraine attacks. *Dan. Med. Bull.* 22:100–106.

Bradfield, J.M. (1976). A new look at the use of ergotamine. *Drugs 12:*449–453.

Brenner, C., A.P. Friedman, and S. Carter (1949). Psychologic factors in the etiology and treatment of chronic headache. *Psychosom. Med. 11:*53.

Brewis, M.D.C. Poskanzer, C. Rolland, and H. Miller (1966). Neurological disease in an English city. *Acta Neurol. Scand. 42 (Suppl. 24):*64–67.

Buda, F.B. and R.P. Joyce (1979). Successful treatment of atypical migraine of childhood with anticonvulsants. *Milit. Med. 144:*521–523.

Bulow, P., J.J. Ibraheem, L. Paalzow, P. Tfelt-Hansen (1985). Ergotamine tartrate, 1 mg. rectally, is biologically active despite unmeasurable plasma levels. *Cephalalgia 5 (Suppl. 3):*52–53.

Carlson, L.A., L.G. Ekelund, L. Oro (1968). Clinical and metabolic effects of different doses of prostaglandin E_1 in man. *Acta Med. Scand. 183:*423–430.

Connolly, E.S. (1978). Transient ischemic attacks secondary to internal carotid artery spasm in ergotism. *Neurosurgery 2:*171.

Cortelli, P. T. Sacquegna, F. Albani, et al. (1985). Propranolol plasma levels and relief of migraine. Relationship between plasma propranolol and 4-Hydroxypropranolol concentrations and clinical effects. *Arch. Neurol. 42(1):*46–48.

Couch, J.R., D.K. Ziegler, R.S. Hassanein (1975). Evaluation of the relationship between migraine headaches and depression. *Headache 15:*41–50.

Couch, J.R. and R.S. Hassanein (1977). Platelet aggregability in migraine. *Neurology 27:*843–848.

Couch, J.R. and R.S. Hassanein (1979). Amitriptyline in migraine prophylaxis. *Arch. Neurol. 36:*695–699.

Crooks, J., S.A. Stephen, and W. Brass (1964). Clinical trial of inhaled ergotamine tartrate in migraine. *Br. Med. J. 1:*221–224.

Dennerstein, L., B. Laby, G.D. Burrows, and G.J. Hyman (1978). Headache and sex hormone therapy. *Headache 18:*146–153.

Dexter, J.D. (1979). The relationship between Stage III + IV + REM sleep and arousals with migraine. *Headache 19:*364–369.

Diamant-Berger, F., A. Pasticier, C. Haas et al. (1972). Arteriospasme pegeneralise severe apres dose therapeutique minime d'ergotamine. *Sem. Hop. Paris 48:*3395–3399.

Diamond, S., J. Diamond-Falk, J.W. Largen (1981). *Treatment of Migraine,* pp. 37–65. Spectrum, Jamaica, New York.

Diamond, S. and D. Montrose (1984). The value of biofeedback in the treatment of chronic headache: A four-year retrospective study. *Headache 24:*5–18.

Dorfman, L.J., W.H. Marshall, and D.R. Enzmann (1979). Cerebral infarction and migraine: Clinical and radiologic correlations. *Neurology 29:*317–322.

Easton, J.D. and D.G. Sherman (1976). Somatic anxiety attacks and propranolol. *Arch. Neurol. 33:*689–691.

Ekbom, K., A. Krabbe, G. Paalzow et al. (1983). Optimal routes of administration of ergotamine tartrate in cluster headache patients. A pharmacokinetic study. *Cephalalgia 3:*15–20.

Elkind, A.H., A.P. Friedman, A. Bachman et al. (1968). Silent retroperitoneal fibrosis associated with methysergide therapy. JAMA 206:1041–1044.

Enge, I. and E. Silvertssen (1965). Ergotism due to therapeutic doses of ergotamine tartrate, *Am. Heart J 70:*665–670.

Featherstone, H.J. (1983). Low dose propranolol therapy for aborting migraine. *West. J. Med. 138:*416–417.

Fedotin M.S. and C. Hartman (1970). Ergotamine poisoning producing renal arterial spasm. *N. Engl. J. Med. 283:*518–520.

Findley, W.W., H.A. Smith, M.D. Etherton (1975). Reduction of seizures and normalization of the EEG in a severe epileptic following sensorimotor biofeedback training: Preliminary study. *Biol. Psychol. 2:*189–203.

Franco, A., P. Boulard, and C. Massot (1978). Acute ergotism by dihydroergotamine-triacetyloleandomycin *Nouvelle Presse Medicale 7:*205.

Friar, L.R. and J. Beatty (1976). Migraine: Management by trained control of vasoconstriction. *J. Consult. Clin. Psychol. 44:*46–53.

Gannon, L. and R.A. Sternback (1971). Alpha enhancement as treatment for pain: A case study. *J. Behav. Ther. Exp. Psychiatry 2:*209–213.

Gazzard, B.G., M. Davis, J. Spooner et al. (1976). Why do people use parocetamol for suicide? *Br. Med. J. 1(6003):*212–213.

Gelmers, H.J. (1983). Nimodipine, a new calcium antagonist in the prophylactic treatment of migraine. *Headache 23:*106–109.

Graham, G. (1975). Hypnotic treatment for migraine headaches, *Int. J. Clin. Exp. Hypn. 23:*165–171.

Graham, J.R. (1967). Cardiac and pulmonary fibrosis during methysergide therapy for headache. *Am. J. Med Sci 254:*23–24.

Green, J.E. (1976). A survey of migraine in England, 1975–1976. In *Migraine News,* The Migraine Trust, London.

Greenblatt, D.J. and J. Koch-Weser (1973). Adverse reactions to Propranolol in hospitalized medical patients: A report from the Boston Collaborative Drug Surveillance Program. *Am. Heart J. 86:*478–484.

Greene, F.L. S. Ariyan, and H.C. Stansel Jr. (1977). Mesenteric and peripheral vascular ischemia secondary to ergotism. *Surgery 81(2):*176–179.

Hansen, P.E. and J.H. Hansen (1985). Acupuncture treatment of chronic tension headache— a controlled cross-over trial. *Cephalalgia (Oslo) 5:*137–142.

Herschberg, A.D. (1950). Treatment of migraine attacks by dihydroergotamine. *Presse Med. 58:*651.

Heyck, H. (1981). *Headache and Facial Pain.* Year Book Medical Publishers, Georg Thieme Verlag, Stuttgart.

Holmes, D.S. and T.G. Burish (1983). Effectiveness of biofeedback for treating migraine and tension headaches: A review of the evidence. *J. Psychosom. Res. 27:*515–532.

Hudzinski, L.G. (1983). Neck musculature and EMG biofeedback in treatment of muscle contraction headache. *Headache 28:*86–90.

Husum, B.P. Berthelsen, P. Metz, and J.P. Rasmussen (1980). Different approaches to the treatment of ergotism: A review of three cases. *Angiology 31(9):*650–653.

Joyce, D.A. and S.S. Gubbay (1982). Arterial complications of migraine treatment with methysergide and parenteral ergotamine. *Br. Med. J. 285:*260–261.

Kahan, A., A. Weber, B. Amor et al. (1983). Nifedipine in the treatment of migraine in patients with Raynaud's phenomenon. *N. Engl. J. Med. 308:*1102–1103.

Kakkar, V.V. (1982). Ergotism and heparin-dihydroergotamine. *Lancet 2:*96–97.

Karoll, R.P. and D.J. Dalessio (1972). Chronic headache and depression (leading to ergot habituation and analgesic abuse). *JAMA 221:*923.

Kassell, N.P., G.L. Kongable, J.C. Torner et al. (1985). Delay in referral of patients with ruptured aneurysms to neurosurgical attention. *Stroke 16:*587–590.

J. Katz, and R.M. Vogel (1967). Abdominal angina as a complication of methysergide maleate therapy. *JAMA 199:*124–125.

Kellner, R., A.C. Collins, R.S. Shulman, D. Pathak (1974). The short-term antianxiety effects of propranolol HCL. *J. Clin. Pharmacol. 5:*301–340.

Kelly, R.E. (1965). Methysergide and coronary thrombosis. *Practitioner 195:*565–566.

Kewman, D. and A.H. Roberts (1980). Skin temperature biofeedback and migraine headaches. A double-blind study. *Biofeedback Self Regul. 5:*327–345.

Knapp, T.W. (1982). Treating migraine by training in temporal artery vasoconstriction and/or cognitive behavioral coping: A one-year follow-up. *J. Psychosom. Res. 26:*551–557.

Koch-Weser, J. (1976). Drug therapy. *N. Engl. J. Med. 295:*1297–1300.

Kotler, M.N., L. Berman, and A.H. Rubenstein (1966). Hypoglycaemia precipitated by propranolol. *Lancet 2:*1289–1290.

LaCroix, M., M.A. Clarke, J.C. Bock et al. (1983). Biofeedback and relaxation in the treatment of migraine headaches: Comparative effectiveness and physiological correlates. *J. Neurol., Neurosurg. Psychiatry 46:*525–532.

Langohr, H.D., W.D. Gerber, E. Koletzki et al. (1985). Clomipramine and metoprolol in migraine prophylaxis. A Double blind crossover study. *Headache 25:*107–113.

Largen, J.W., R.J. Mathew, K. Dobbins, and J.L. Claghorn (1981). Specific and non-specific effects of skin temperature control in migraine management. *Headache 21:*36–44.

Lindegaard, K.F., L. Ovrelid, and O. Sjaastad (1980). Naproxen in the prevention of migraine attacks: A double-blind placebo-controlled crossover study. *Headache 20:*96–98.

Loew, D.M., E.R. van Duesen, and W.R. Meier (1978). *Ergot Alkaloids and Related Compounds*, pp. 421–439. Springer-Verlag, New York.

Loh, L., P.W. Nathan, G.D. Schott, and K.J. Zilkha (1984). Acupuncture versus medical treatment for migraine and muscle tension headaches. *J. Neurol. Neurosurg. Psychiatry 47:*333–337.

Louis, P. and E.L. Spierings (1982). Comparison of flunarizine and pizotifen in migraine treatment: A double-blind study. *Cephalalgia 2:*197–203.

Lubke, K.O. (1976). A controlled study with dihydergotamine on patients with orthostatic dysregulation. *Cardiology 61 (Suppl 1):*333–341.

Mantyla, R., T. Kleimola, and J. Kanto (1978). The pharmacokinetica of dihydroergotamine in the beagle. *Int. J. Clin. Pharmacol. Biopharm. 16:*124–128.

Masel, B.E., A.L. Chesson, B.H. Peters et al. (1980). Platelet antagonists in migraine prophylaxis. A clinical trial using aspirin and dipyridamole. *Headache 20:*13–18.

Mathew, N.T. (1981). Indomethacin responsive headache syndromes. *Headache 21:*147–150.

Mendelson, G., T.S. Selwood, H. Kranz et al. (1983). Acupuncture treatment of chronic back pain. A double blind placebo-controlled trial. *Am. J. Med. 74:*49–55.

Merskey, H., R.A. Hester (1972). The treatment of chronic pain with psychotropic drugs. *Postgrad. Med. J. 48:*594–598.

Miller, J. (1963). A serotonin antagonist cyproheptadine. II. The treatment of vascular-type and pruritus. *Ann. Allergy 21:*588–592.

Miller, N.E. (1969). Learning of visceral and glandular responses. *Science 163:*434–445.

Mitchell, K.R. and R.G. White (1976). Control of migraine headache by behavioral self-management: A controlled case study. *Headache 16:*178–184.

Monro, J., C. Carini, and J. Brostoff (1984). Migraine is a food-allergic disease. *Lancet 2:*719–721.

Mulholland, T., D. Goodman, and R. Boudrot (1983). Attention and regulation of EEG alpha-attenuation responses. *Biofeedback Self Regul. 8:*585–600.

Mylecharane, E.J., P.J. Spira, J. Misbach et al. (1978). Effects of methysergide, pizotifen and ergotamine in the monkey cranial circulation. *Eur. J. Pharmacol. 48:*1–9.

Olesen, J., B. Larsen, and M. Lauritzen (1981). Focal hyperemia followed by spreading oligemia and impaired activation of rCBF in classic migraine. *Ann. Neurol. 9:*334–352.

Olesen, J., M. Lauritzen, P. Tfelt-Hansen et al. (1982). Spreading cerebral oligemia in classical and normal cerebral blood flow in common migraine. *Headache 22:*242–248.

Oppenheim, H. (1900). *Disease of the Nervous System*, pp. 748–759. J.B. Lippincott, Philadelphia.

Osterman, P.O., K.G. Lovstrand, P.O. Lundberg (1981). Weekly headache periodicity and the effect of weather changes on headache. *Int. J. Biometeord. 25:*39–45.

Passchier, M.S., H. van der Helm-Hylkema, J.F. Oriebeke (1984). Psychophysiological characteristics of migraine and tension headache patients. Differential effects of sex and
pain state. *Headache 24:*131–139.

Pedersen, B. and J. Christiansen (1983). Thromboembolic prophylaxis with dihydroergota-
mine-herparin in abdominal surgery. A controlled randomized study. *Am. J. Surg
145:*788–790.

Peroutka, S.J., S.B. Banghart, and G.S. Allen (1984). Relative potency and selectivity of
calcium antagonists used in the treatment of migraine. *Headache, 24:*558–558.

Philips, C. and M. Hunter (1981). The treatment of tension headache—I. Muscular abnormality and Biofeedback. *Behav. Res. Ther. 19:*485–498.

Price, K.P., B. Tursky (1976). Vascular reactivity of migraneurs and nonmigraneurs: A comparison of responses of self-control procedures. *Headache 16:*210–217.

Raskin, N.H. (1981). Pharmacology of migraine. *Ann. Rev. Pharmacol. Toxicol. 21:*463–
477.

Raskin, N.H. and K.E. Raskin (1984). Repetitive intravenous dihydroergotamine for the treatment of intractable migraine. *Neurol (Suppl. 1)34:*245.

Sacerdote, P. (1978). Teaching self-hypnosis to patients with chronic pain. *J. Human Stress
4:*18–21.

Sargent, J.D., E.E. Green, and E.D. Walters (1973). Preliminary report on the use of autogenic feedback training in the treatment of migraine and tension headaches. Psychosom. Med. 35:129–135.

Silver, B.V. and E.B. Blanchard (1978). Biofeedback and relaxation training in the treatment
of psychophysiological disorders: Or are the machines really necessary? *J. Behav. Med.
1:*217–239.

Smith, M.T. H.M. Levin, W.W. Bare et al. (1975). Acetoaminophen extra strength capsules
versus propoxyphene compound-65 versus placebo: A double-blind study of effectiveness and safety. *Curr. Ther. Res. 17:*452–459.

Solomon, G.D. (1985). Comparative efficacy of calcium antagonist drugs in the prophylaxis
of migraine. *Headache 25:*368–371.

Solomon, G.D., J.G. Steel, and L.J. Spaccavento (1983). Verapamil prophylaxis of migraine:
A double-blind, placebo-controlled study. *JAMA 250:*2500–2502.

Solomon, S. and K.M. Guglielmo (1985). Treatment of headache by transcutaneous electrical
stimulation. *Headache 25:*12–15.

Standnes, B. (1982). The prophylactic effect of timolol versus propranolol and placebo in
common migraine: Beta blockers in migraine. *Cephalalgia 2:*165–170.

Sutherland, J.M., W.D. Hooper, M.J. Eadie, and J.H. Tyrer (1974). Buccal absorption of
ergotamine. *J. Neurol. Neurosurg. Psychiatry 37:*1116–1120.

Swaiman, K.F. and Y. Frank (1978). Seizure headaches in children. *Dev. Med. Child Neurol.
20:*580–585.

Taub, A. (1973). Relief of postherpetic neuralgia with psychotropic drugs. *J. Neurosurg.
39:*235–239.

Tfelt-Hansen, P. and J. Olesen (1980). Paracetamol (acetaminophen) versus acetylsalicylic
acid in migraine. *Eur. Neurol. 19:*163–165.

Tfelt-Hansen, P., J. Olesen, A. Aebelholt-Krabbe et al. (1980). A double blind study of
metoclopramide in the treatment of migraine attacks. *J. Neurol. Neurosurg. Psychiatry
43:*369–371.

Tfelt-Hansen, P. J.R. Ostergaard, I. Gothgen et al. (1982). Nitroglycerin for ergotism experimental studies in vitro and in migraine patients and treatment of an overt case. *Eur.
J. Clin. Pharmacol. 22:*105–109.

Tfelt-Hansen, P., B. Standnes, P. Kangasneimi et al. (1984). Timolol vs propranolol vs placebo in common migraine prophylaxis: A double-blind multicenter trial. *Acta Neurol. Scand. 69*:1–8.

Tillgren, N. (1947). Treatment of headache with dihydroergotamine tartrate. *Acta Med. Scand. (Suppl. 196–198)*:222–228.

Turin, A. and W.G. Johnson (1976). Biofeedback therapy for migraine headaches. *Arch. Gen. Psychiatry 33*:517–519.

U.S. Vital and Health Statistics (1981). *Headache as the Reason for Office Visits, National Ambulatory Medical Care Survey: United States, 1977–78.* Washington, D.C., U.S. Department of Health & Human Services, Public Health Service, pp. 1–6.

U.S. Vital and Health Statistics (1978). Acute conditions, incidence and associated disability, United States, July 1976–June 1977. Series 10(125):1–66.

Venter, C.P., P.H. Joubert, and A.C. Buys (1984). Severe peripheral ischaemia during concomitant use of beta blockers and ergot alkaloids. *Br. Med. J. 289*:288–289.

Wainscott, G., G. Volans, and M. Wilkinson (1974). Ergotamine-induced headaches. *Br. Med. J. 2*:724.

Weir, B. (1984). Calcium antagonists, cerebral ischemia and vasospasm. *Can. J. Neurol. Sci. 11*:239–246.

Welch, K.M.S., D.J. Ellis, and P.A. Keenan (1985). Successful migraine prophylaxis with naproxen sodium. *Neurol. 35*:1304–1310.

Whitsett, T.L., W.S. Myers, and J.M. Hartsuck (1978). Nitropresside reversal of ergotamine-induced ischemia. *Am. Heart J. 96*:700.

Wideroe, T.-E. and T. Vigander (1974). Propranolol in the treatment of migraine. *Br. Med. J. 2*:699–701.

Yuill, G.M., W.R. Swinburn, and L.A. Liversedge (1972). A double-blind crossover trial of isometheptene mucate compound and ergotamine in migraine. *Br. J. Clin. Pract. 26*:76–79.

Ziegler, D.K. and R. Stewart (1977). Failure of tyramine to induce migraine. *Neurology 27*:725–726.

Ziegler, D.K. (1979). Headache syndromes: Problems of definition. *Psychosomatics 20*:443–447.

Ziegler, K.D. and D.J. Ellis (1985). Naproxen in prophylaxis of migraine. *Arch. Neurol. 42*:582–584.

7

Cluster Headache:
Diagnosis, Management, and Treatment

LEE KUDROW

Cluster headache is known by many names. It was first described by Eulenburg (1874) and Romberg (1840), independently, and later by Harris (1926). Cluster headache is often referred to as "migrainous neuralgia," after Harris (1936). Horton et al. (1939), however, popularized the condition when he described it as a new syndrome. Ekbom (1947) was the first to report the periodic nature of cluster headache. This "clustering" pattern, noted by Kunkle et al. (1954), gave the term *cluster headache* to the disorder (Table 7-1).

CLASSIFICATION

There are two major types of cluster headache. (Subtypes or variations are not discussed here.) The episodic type is the most common, constituting 80% of all cases. Episodic cluster headache is defined by periods of susceptibility to headache, called "cluster periods," alternating with periods of refractoriness, called "remissions."

Chronic cluster headache is the term used when remissions have not occurred for at least 12 months. Other characteristics of chronic cluster, such as increased frequency of attack and decreased responsiveness to prophylactic drug therapy, distinguish it from episodic cluster. Approximately 50% of chronic cluster patients have never experienced remissions. The term *primary cluster* is used for this type. Secondary chronic types have, in the past, experienced remission but have become chronic (Ekbom & Olivarius, 1971). Despite the distinction between primary and secondary chronic cluster, there appears to be little difference—either therapeutically or prognostically—between the two types.

Chronic paroxysmal hemicrania, or Sjaastad's syndrome was first described in 1974 (Sjaastad & Dale, 1974). At this time it is considered by many to be a variant of cluster headache. There appear to be sufficient differences, however, to consider chronic paroxysmal hemicrania quite separately from cluster (Sjaastad et al., 1980).

Table 7-1 Cluster headache—eponyms, misnomers, and other appelations

| Authors | Date | Nomenclature | |
		Eponyms	Other names
Romberg	1840	Description only	
Möllendorff	1867		Red migraine
Eulenburg	1878		Angioparalytic hemicrania
Sluder	1910	Sluder's syndrome	Sphenopalatine neuralgia Lower-half headache
Bing	1913	Bing's headache Bing's syndrome	Erythroprosopalgia
Harris	1926		Migrainous neuralgia
Harris	1936		Ciliary neuralgia
Vail	1932		Vidian neuralgia
Gardner et al.	1947		Greater superficial petrosal neuralgia
Horton et al.	1939 1952	Horton's headache Horton's syndrome	Erythromelalgia Histaminic cephalgia
Kunkle et al.	1952		Cluster headache

(From Kudrow, L. (1979). Cluster headache: Diagnosis and management. *Headache 19*:143.)

In chronic paroxysmal hemicrania, attacks are quite frequent: more than 10 attacks per day. The duration of the attacks is short: 10 to 30 minutes. Response to indomethacin is dramatic, whereas usual anticluster agents are of little value (Sjaastad & Dale, 1974).

THE CLUSTER ATTACK

The cluster attack is stereotyped by specific signs, symptoms, emotions, and behavior. The following is a firsthand account of such an episode (Kudrow, 1980, pp. 25–27):

Following a period of perhaps several hours of feeling quite elated and energetic, I experienced a fullness in my ears, somewhat more on the right side than the left, and having a character similar to that which occurs during rapid descent in an airplane or elevator. I then became aware of a dull discomfort, an extension of ear fullness at the base of my skull—further extending over the entire head, on both sides, though somewhat more on the right. At this point, two or three minutes have elapsed; seemingly short but long enough for me to know that a ''cluster'' has indeed begun and will ultimately get worse. Such anticipation causes me considerable consternation regarding any decision to continue my activities, or cancel plans and find a place to be alone; giving way to a slowly increasing anxiety, fear, panic, and withdrawal. I become aware of myself ''listening'' for changes in my head. Is the cluster prematurely aborting itself, progressing further, or unchanging? A sudden stab, only fleeting, strikes my temple, then again—

somewhere near the apex of my skull and upper molars in my face, always on the right side. It strikes me again, deep into the skull base, and as quickly, changes location to a small area above my eyebrow. My nose is stuffed and yet runs simultaneously. If I could sneeze I feel the attack would end. Yet in spite of all tricks, I find myself unable to induce sneezing. While the sharp stabs continue in this fashion, a slow crescendo of dull pain presents itself in an area of a hand's length and breadth over the eye and temporal region. The pain area narrows into a smaller area, and yet, as if magnified, enlarges in intensity. I find myself bending my neck downward, though slightly, as if my head is being gently pushed from behind. My neck, up to the base of my skull, is tight and feels as if I were wearing a neck collar. I feel compelled to remove my tie and loosen my shirt collar even though I know that it will not offer me even a modicum of relief.

In an effort to alter this persistent discomfort, I drop my head between my legs while seated. My face and eyes seem to fill with fluid, but the pain remains unchanged. Despite my suntan, as I look into the mirror, a gaunt, sickly, pale face peers back. My right lid is only slightly drooping and the white of my eye is charted with many red vessels, giving the eye an over-all color of pink. Right and left pupils appear equal and constricted, as is usual for light-eyed people. Having difficulty standing in one place too long, I leave the mirror to continue alternating my pacing and sitting.

As usual, I am struck with the additional fear that the pain will never end, but dismiss it as impossible since even if that were the case, I would surely kill myself.

The pain, now located somewhere behind my eye and slightly above it, worsens. The pain is best described as a "force" pushing with such incredible power through my eye that my head appears to be moving backward, yielding to its resistance. The "force" wanes and waxes, but the duration of successive exacerbations seem to increase. The cluster attack is at its peak which is celebrated by an outpouring of tears from only my right eye. I have now been in cluster for thirty-five minutes—ten minutes at its peak.

My wife peeks into the room where I hold forth. I look up and see her expression of pity, frustration, and helplessness. She sees my tortured face as I have seen it in the mirror at this stage before; a drooling mouth, agape, gray face wet on one side, an almost closed eyelid, and smelling of pain and anguish. She closes the door and leaves, feeling hurt for me, anger for the stupidity of medical science, and guilt—since deep within her mind is the suspicion that she is the cause for my suffering.

I cry for her, but cry more for myself. The pain is so incredible. Suddenly I am overwhelmed by a fury. I lift a chair high over my head and crash it to the floor. With a doubled fist I strike the wall. The pain persists.

Waning periods soon become longer in duration and I allow myself to suspect that the peak is behind me—but cautiously, since I have been too often disappointed.

Indeed, the pain is ending. The descent from the mountain of pain is rapid. The "force" is gone. Only severe pain remains. My nose and eye continues to run. The road back, as with all travel, covers the same territory, but faster. Stabbing, easily tolerated pain is felt. Then gone. Dull, aching fullness, neck stiffness, all disappear, replaced in turn by a welcome sensation of pins and needles over the right scalp area—similar to the way one's leg feels after it has been "asleep." Thus my head has awakened after a nightmare of torment.

Eye and nose dry, I let out a sigh. I collect my pile of wet tissues that are strewn all over the floor and deposit them in a wastepaper basket. The innocent chair, now up-righted, I rub my slightly bruised fist.

Thus, having ended the battle and cleaned up its field, I open the door and enter my pain-free world—until tomorrow.

Table 7-2 Several reports on the incidence of cluster
headache and migraine

Authors	No. of patients		Ratio
	Migraine	Cluster	Migraine:cluster
Lieder	52	4	13.0:1
Carroll	89	16	5.6:1
Balla & Walton	399	28	14.3:1
Ekbom	400	16	25.0:1
Lance et al.	612	13	47.1:1
Heyck	1890	48	39.4:1
Friedman	2667	237	11.3:1
Kudrow	2835	425	6.7:1

(From Kudrow, L. (1979). Cluster headache: Diagnosis and management. *Head-ache 19*:144.)

PREVALENCE

The prevalence rate of cluster headache in a general population is unknown. Estimates have been offered, however, based on populations in headache clinics (Table 7-2). These have varied from prevalence rates of 0.04% (Heyck, 1975) to 1.5% (Kudrow, 1980, pp. 10–20).

Sex, Age, and Race

Cluster headache is predominantly a male disorder. Male to female ratios of clinic populations range from 4.5:1 to 6.7:1 (Ekbom, 1970a; Friedman & Mikropoulos, 1958; Kudrow, 1980; Lance & Anthony, 1971a; Lovshin, 1961). The mean age of onset, approximately 27 to 30 years, varies little between clinic populations (Ekbom, 1970a; Friedman & Mikropoulos, 1958; Kudrow, 1980). The range varies widely, however, from the age of 1 year (Kudrow, 1980) to the late 60s (Table 7-3).

Lovshin (1961) reported that black patients appeared to be overrepresented within the Cleveland Clinic's population of patients with cluster headache. Our own clinic survey supports this finding (Kudrow, 1980).

CLINICAL PICTURE

Cluster periods, defined as those periods during which attacks occur, generally last between 6 and 12 weeks. Remission periods have an average duration of approximately 12 months. There may be considerable variation. Attacks occur with a frequency of approximately one to three times a day, each lasting about 45 minutes.

Table 7-3 Male:female ratio and mean age at onset of cluster
headache

Authors	Date	No. of patients	Onset Age	Range	Ratio M:F
Friedman & Mikropoulos	1958	50	28	11–44	4.5:1
Ekbom	1970	105	27.5	10–61	5.6:1
Lance & Anthony	1971	60		8–62	6.5:1
Kudrow	Present	425	29.6	1–63	5.1:1

(From Kudrow, L. (1979). Cluster headache: Diagnosis and management. *Headache 19*:144.)

They are unilateral, oculotemporal, or oculofrontal in location, excruciating in severity, and boring and nonthrobbing in character. The associated symptoms are also
unilateral and consist of lacrimation, rhinorrhea, or nasal stuffiness, and partial Horner's syndrome, which includes unilateral ptosis and miosis.

The frequency with which partial Horner's syndrome is observed during cluster
attacks has been reported separately by Ekbom (1970a), Lance (1978), and Kudrow
(1979) (Table 7-4).

Characteristically, vasodilator medications such as nitroglycerin and histamine will
induce cluster attacks. Ekbom (1968) was able to induce an acute cluster attack in
all of his subjects diagnosed as having cluster headache using 1 mg of nitroglycerin
sublingually. Often, but not always, alcohol induces an acute cluster attack while the
patient is in an active cluster period. Attacks are commonly induced on awakening
from a nap in the afternoon or from sleep during the night—most commonly, approximately 90 minutes after falling asleep.

PERIODICITY

The onset of cluster periods has been reported by Ekbom (1970a) and others to occur
with seasonal periodicity. Specifically, spring and autumn are seasons of high inci-

Table 7-4 Frequency of ptosis and/or miosis in cluster
headache clinic populations

Investigators	Year	Frequency (%) of partial Horner's Temporary	Permanent
Ekbom	1970	69	5.7 (ptosis) 6.7 (miosis)
Lance & Anthony	1971	32	Rare
Kudrow	1981	60	0.5

(From Kudrow, L. (1982). Cluster headache. Clinical, mechanistic, and treatment aspects. *Panminerva Med. 24*:47.)

Table 7-5 Physical characteristics often observed among cluster males

Facial
Ruddy complexion
Deep furrows
"Orange peel" skin
Telangectasia
Narrowed palpebral fissures
Asymmetric creases
Broad chin, skull
Leonine appearance
General
Rugged appearance
Tall, trim
Obesity rare
Hazel eye color (1/3)

(From Kudrow, L. (1979). Cluster headache: Diagnosis and management. *Headache 19*:145.)

dence. Lance (1978) did not find this to be the case; among his patients who associated their cluster periods with seasons, the distribution was equally divided among all four seasons.

More curious is the attack periodicity in cluster headache. As noted earlier, an individual often awakens with an attack from a nap, or about 2 hours after falling asleep; it strikes especially during relaxation. The circadian accuracy in which these attacks occur is not at all understood. Attacks that occur 24 hours apart frequently recur at exactly the same time. Attacks that occur twice a day are generally 12 hours apart but, more important, again at the same time of day.

PHYSICAL CHARACTERISTICS

Graham (1969) noted that a great many individuals with cluster headache had specific facial features. He described them as having a "leonine" appearance, deep skin furrows (especially the nasolabial and glabellar folds) and forehead wrinkles. He also described the presence of telangiectasia, often observed across the bridge of the nose. We have also noted, as had Dr. Graham, that there appears to be narrowing of the palpebral fissures. Quite often there are asymmetrical skin wrinkles and "orange-peel" thick skin—in all, the appearance of an alcoholic. However, Graham states that some of his patients who were nondrinkers had the typical cluster facies (personal communication). He found that, although women did not have all these characteristics, they were somewhat masculine looking. We have noted rather similar appearances among some of our women patients with cluster headache, many, however, appearing quite feminine. Moreover, we have found that a number of our male patients had characteristics more descriptive of acromegaly (Table 7-5).

On the average, males with cluster headache are 3 inches taller than matched male controls (Kudrow, 1974; Schele et al., 1978). In our clinic population, hazel eye

Table 7-6 Cluster headache compared with noncluster and general population groups

Group	Disorder incidence (%)				
	Migraine		Ulcer	C.H.D.	H.B.P.
	M	F	M	M	M
Cluster	10.9	52.4	21.0	7.6	3.4
Noncluster			10.7[a]	3.6	8.6
U.S. population	4.0	16.0[a]	10.0[a]	3.0	10.0

[a] $P < 0.5$.
(From Kudrow, L. (1979). Cluster headache: Diagnosis and management. *Headache 19*:145.)
C.H.D. = coronary heart disease
H.B.P. = high blood pressure

color occurred three times more frequently than in controls. Patients with cluster headache smoked more often and smoked more cigarettes per day than controls. Use of alcohol was significantly greater in the cluster group. Hemoglobin levels have been reported to be higher among patients with cluster headache (Graham et al., 1970; Kudrow, 1974), although in a more recent survey no significant differences were found between cluster and control groups (Kudrow, 1980 pp. 39–52).

ASSOCIATED DISORDERS

An increased incidence of peptic ulcer disease has been reported by Ekbom (1970b), Graham (1972), and others. We found a 21% incidence of duodenal ulcer disease in our male cluster population—twice that of controls (Kudrow, 1976a).

The incidence of coronary artery disease among our cluster patients was higher than that of controls, but not significantly. Graham believes that a significant difference would have been reached had our cluster and control groups been older (personal communication).

Hypertension was negatively associated with the cluster headache group. This lower frequency, however, was not significant.

The incidence of migraine among cluster women was over 50%, consistent with the results of Lance and Anthony (1971b). This incidence is two to three times that expected for the general female population. Among cluster males, a higher, but not significantly higher frequency of migraine was found (Kudrow, 1976a) (Table 7-6).

PSYCHOPERSONALITY FACTORS

Contrary to earlier reports, recent Minnesota Multiphasic Personality Inventory (MMPI) studies by Kudrow and Sutkus (1979) and others (Cuypers et al., 1981); (Andrasik et al., 1982) have demonstrated no evidence of neuroses or other psychopathology in cluster headache populations.

DIFFERENTIAL DIAGNOSIS

Only a few conditions can possibly be confused with cluster headache. These include migraine, trigeminal neuralgia, temporal arteritis, pheochromocytoma, and Raeder's paratrigeminal syndrome (Table 7-7).

Migraine

Characteristically, migraine attacks occur with a frequency of one to three times a month, often associated with menstrual periods. Each attack may last from 1 to 3 days, with some variation; pain develops slowly over a period of several hours. In 80% of cases the headache is unilateral, involving the region of the temporal artery and extending over the hemicranial area. Often, the pain is described as throbbing and is associated with nausea, vomiting, photophobia, and sonophobia. Not infrequently, strong odors are poorly tolerated during the headache phase. Paresthesias, hot-and-cold sensations, orthostatic lightheadedness, and anorexia may also be experienced..In classic migraine, a visual prodrome lasting approximately one-half hour precedes the headache phase.

Trigeminal Neuralgia

Trigeminal neuralgia occurs with equal frequency in men and women, generally in older age groups. The pain of trigeminal neuralgia is characterized as severe, razor sharp, electriclike, or cutting. It is precipitated by the touching of trigger zones on the face, ipsilaterally. These zones are most commonly found in an area around the nasolabial folds, but may occur anywhere from the chin to the forehead. Activation of the trigger site may result from the slightest touch, including even a gentle breeze across the face. Most frequently, the act of eating, chewing, or shaving triggers the attack. The attack begins with a slight sensation of gentle jabbing over the involved site followed by a sensation of lightning tics that last from seconds to minutes. The attack may begin abruptly with warning sensations. Among other differentiating features, attacks of trigeminal neuralgia are not likely to occur in the middle of the night, awakening the patient from sleep, as is seen in cluster headache.

Temporal Arteritis

Temporal arteritis generally affects older age groups. The arteries most typically affected are the superficial, temporal, vertebral, and ophthalmic. Other arteries such as the internal carotid and the central retinal are also affected, although less frequently. The disease is self-limiting but may cause blindness if untreated. In approximately 50% of cases, a nonspecific aching or stiffness of the neck, shoulders, or hip girdle precedes the onset of head pain by several months (polymyalgia rheumatica). The head pain is described as persistent, waxing and waning throughout the day, unilat-

Table 7-7 Differential diagnosis of cluster headache

Conditions resembling cluster	Timing	Frequency	Duration	Location	Intensity	Character	Associated signs and symptoms
Migraine	Often menstrual	1–2/month	1–2 days	Unilateral, fronto-temporal, temporo-parietal	Moderate to severe	Throbbing	Nausea, vomiting, photophobia, sonophobia
Trigeminal neuralgia	No pattern	Several/day	Seconds to minutes	Unilateral, 5th nerve distribution	Severe	Electric, lancinating, nonthrobbing	Trigger zones on face
Temporal arteritis	No pattern	Persistent	——	Unilateral, temporal	Severe	Burning, throbbing, nonthrobbing	Chewing claudication, tender and torturous temporal artery, elevated ESR,[a] polymyalgia
Pheochromocytoma	Mornings, often on awakening	Daily to monthly	Less than 1 hour	Bilateral, occipital	Severe in supine position	Throbbing	Sweating, pallor, tachycardia with rise in blood pressure
Raeder's syndrome	Often awakens from sleep	Persistent	Persistent	Unilateral, supraocular	Severe	Burning throbbing, nonthrobbing	Partial Horner's syndrome
Cluster	Occurs with regularity, often awakens from sleep	1–3/day	30–90 minutes	Unilateral, oculofrontal, temporal	Excruciating	Nonthrobbing, boring	Unilateral lacrimation, rhinorrhea, injection, partial Horner's, cannot lie down

[a]ESR = erythrocyte sedimentation rate.
(From Kudrow, L. (1983). Cluster headache: New concepts. *Neurol. Clin. 1*:374.)

eral in location, and related to the distribution of the superficial temporal artery. It is severe, burning, and throbbing in the early course of the disease and nonthrobbing later. The superficial temporal artery is generally tender on palpation and reveals a marked firmness and tortuosity. Claudication upon chewing is frequently experienced and is an important feature. The sedimentation rate is generally elevated quite markedly, and the finding of giant cells on temporal artery biopsy is diagnostic of this condition.

Pheochromocytoma

The paroxysmal hypertensive episode seen in pheochromocytoma is associated with release of catecholamine followed by head pain, pallor, tachycardia, and profuse sweating. The pain may be described as paroxysmal, rapid in onset, and severe. It often awakens the patient during early morning hours or is commonly induced during exertion. Headaches are characterized as throbbing and almost always bilateral and occipital in location. Coughing, sneezing, bending, and straining may aggravate the pain. Attacks may occur with a daily to monthly frequency, generally lasting less than 1 hour.

Raeder's Paratrigeminal Syndrome

The pain of Raeder's syndrome is persistent and may last from weeks to months. During the first 2 weeks the patient is likely to be awakened in the middle of the night with severe, unilateral, supraorbital pain of a burning, throbbing, or nonthrobbing character. Late in the course, the pain is less severe but continuous. Drooping of the ipsilateral eyelid associated with miosis is an accompanying feature. Anhydrosis is not a typical feature of this disorder. Several features causing confusion with cluster headache include partial Horner's syndrome, severe and burning ipsilateral supraorbital pain, and pain awakening the patient in the middle of the night. Unlike with cluster headache, however, the duration of pain is constant.

MECHANISMS

Genetics and Family History

The frequency of familial migraine among patients with cluster headaches differs little from that of control populations. Reports have varied from between 15 and 34% (Ekbom, 1970a; Kudrow, 1980; Kunkle et al., 1954; Lance, 1978). The frequency of familial cluster headache among patients with cluster headache in our series was only 3.4% (Kudrow, 1980). A search for human leukocyte antigen (HLA) specificity in a population of 25 male patients with cluster headache revealed no significant differences for HLA frequency (Kudrow, 1978a). This negative finding was corroborated by Cuypers and Altenkirch (1979). It may be concluded, therefore, that if genetic factors are associated with cluster headache, such an association is outside the HLA histocompatibility antigen system.

Vascular Changes

Following their initial observations of patients with cluster headache, Horton et al. (1939) concluded that dilatation of the external carotid artery caused the symptoms of cluster headache. Further, Horton believed that this dilatation was mediated by intrinsic blood histamine. Horton noted that during the attack patients often exhibited enlarged temporal arteries, compression of which relieved the pain. He also observed an ipsilateral flush during the attacks associated with an increase in skin temperature of 1 to 2°C. It should be noted, however, that Ekbom and Kudrow (1979) have not found flushing to be a characteristic of cluster headache; in fact, ipsilateral pallor was more frequently observed.

Because of the retro-orbital location of pain, investigations in recent years turned to possible changes in the internal carotid artery. Broch et al. (1970) could find no blood-flow changes between contralateral and ipsilateral internal carotid arteries after placing flowmeters on these vessels during cluster attacks. It should be noted that placement of the flowmeter probes were quite proximal (1 cm cranial to the carotid sinus) and could conceivably have been insensitive to more distal carotid artery changes.

Sjaastad et al. (1974) measured cutaneous blood flow by an isotope washout method on symptomatic and contralateral sides of the forehead on six patients during attack and interval phases of cluster periods. Although the lowest cutaneous blood-flow values were found on the ipsilateral side during attacks, the differences were not significant. Conversely, dynamic tonometry revealed increased pulse synchronous amplitudes on the symptomatic side during attacks. The researchers concluded that, although this evidence did not allow for deductions regarding total blood flow through the eye, vasoconstriction occurring in more distal segments of the intraocular vessels could induce proximal vasodilatation as an effort to overcome increased resistance to blood flow.

Contrary to these observations, during a fortuitous angiographic examination of a patient experiencing an acute attack of cluster headache, Ekbom and Greitz (1970) noted a segmental luminal narrowing of the ipsilateral internal carotid artery in the region of the carotid canal. They also found a significant dilatation of the ipsilateral ophthalmic artery.

In view of Ekbom and Greitz's findings, we studied supraorbital and frontal artery blood-flow changes in patients with cluster headache using Doppler-flow velocity examinations and facial thermography (Kudrow, 1979). Our Doppler-flow velocity results, later corroborated by Nattero et al. (1980), revealed decreased supraorbital artery flow velocity ipsilaterally. Facial thermography consistently revealed decreased temperatures over the supraorbital area (Kudrow, 1979), corroborating the thermographic findings of Friedman and Wood (1976), and Lance and Anthony (1971a).

Cerebral blood flow appears to be increased during an attack of cluster headache. Norris et al. (1976) first reported increased values for cerebral blood flow in a patient during a cluster attack. Sakai and Meyer (1978), in a rather extensive study, presented their findings on cerebral blood flow. During the cluster attack there was a significant increase in cerebral blood flow in both hemispheres; however, cerebral blood flow in the contralateral hemisphere was even greater than that for the ipsilateral side. In contrast to these studies, Henry et al. (1978) could not show changes in cerebral blood flow in three patients with cluster headaches. Further, Aebelholt et al. (1983) found no significant increase in cerebral blood flow by tomographic determinations.

Biochemical and Hormonal Changes

Consistent with the suspicions of Horton (1952) that histamine played a major role in cluster headache, Sjaastad (1970) found an increased urinary output of histamine in three of six patients during cluster attacks. Subsequently, Sjaastad and Sjaastad (1977) determined urinary excretion of labeled histamine and its metabolites in cluster headache following oral and subcutaneous administration of radioactive histamine. With the exception of one patient who was diagnosed as having chronic paroxysmal hemicrania, the results in all the patients were normal. Anthony and Lance (1971) obtained blood histamine levels from 20 patients with cluster headache during 22 attacks. Histamine levels were found to be higher during headache periods than during preheadache periods in 19 out of 22 attacks. The mean increase was 20.5%; this difference was highly significant. The importance of these changes in histamine levels is questionable, however, since in a series of patients later studied by Anthony et al. (1978) the frequency of cluster attacks was not decreased after prophylactic administration H_1 and H_2 receptor antagonists. Similar negative results were obtained in a more recent multicenter study by Graham, Kudrow, and Diamond (unreported, 1980) in which a total of 60 patients witt cluster headache treated prophylactically with H_1 and H_2 receptor blockers showed no significant improvement compared with those treated with placebos.

Plasma testosterone and luteinizing hormone (LH) levels were found to be significantly reduced in a population of patients with cluster headache during periods of cluster compared with periods of remission (Kudrow, 1976b). Subsequently, Nelson reported that testosterone values were abnormally low in 22% of patients with cluster headache but that approximately the same frequency of abnormal values was found in a classic migraine group (Nelson, 1978). More recently, Klimek (1982) further corroborated low testosterone levels in patients with cluster headache but found that plasma testosterone levels were similarly depressed in patients with trigeminal neuralgia and reticular pain syndromes. He concluded that the lowering of plasma testosterone levels observed in patients with cluster headaches is more a function of pain than of a process involving hypothalamic–pituitary axis dysfunction. Pollari et al. (1983) could find no abnormal levels of testosterone or LH in cluster headache males before or after LH-releasing hormones stimulation. They concluded that no substantial impairment of pituitary gonadotropic function occurred in their cluster population.

Autonomic Nervous System Pathways

Kunkle (1959) proposed that cluster headache attacks result from parasympathetic storms involving the 7th and 10th cranial nerves. Indeed, he found acetylcholinelike substances in the cerebrospinal fluid in 4 of 14 patients with cluster headaches. Gardner et al. (1947) were also of the opinion that cluster headaches resulted from parasympathetic activation, specifically mediated through the greater superficial petrosal nerve. Section of the greater superficial petrosal nerve in patients resulted in partial success in 50% and an excellent outcome in 25%. Stowell (1970) suggested that cluster headache was produced by efferent impulses from the greater superficial petrosal nerve, arising in the parasympathetic nuclei of the hypothalamus. He further reported that section of the greater superficial petrosal nerves in 32 patients with cluster headache had a successful outcome in 28 patients. Recurrence, however, was noted in 53.6% of the patients in 3 years postoperatively. One patient, in whom Sachs (1968) sectioned the nervus intermedius, remained free of clusters during a 10-year follow-up period.

In view of the finding of bradycardia during cluster headache in some patients—and in one case, an associated systolic and diastolic hypertension, Bruyn et al. (1976) hypothesized that cluster headache attacks are associated with central alpha-adrenergic paroxysms (both excitatory and inhibitory). Kudrow (1983) recently proposed that the carotid body may play a major role in the pathogenesis of cluster headache. It was suggested that throughout the course of the cluster period, chemoreceptor activity may be blunted by central inhibition of the sympathetic and dysinhibition of parasympathetic efferent pathways. The manifestation of these changes would probably occur during sleep, exaggerating the physiologic depression of respiration associated with sleep. Thus, sleep apnea and hypoxemia may result, and may indeed be an associated feature of the cluster period. In the presence of impaired peripheral receptor responsivity, events such as REM-associated inhibition of respiratory muscle function, NREM-bradycardia, and hypoventilation, vasodilators, and altitude hypoxia may cause hypoxemia and hypercarbia. It was suggested that these events precede and herald the onset of the cluster attack. When oxygen desaturation exceeds threshold limits of chemoreceptor activity, chemoreceptors would be unusually excited, as seen in denervation supersensitivity responses. This may be the consequence of the buildup of stored chemoreceptor activating neurotransmitters. This proposal also presumes that inhibitory mechanisms of chemoreceptor activity may be blocked.

Upon activation of the chemoreceptors, afferent impulses reach the nucleus solitarius in the medulla and through interconnections are further transmitted to the respiratory center, dorsal motor nucleus, and salivary nucleus. This may result in efferent stimulation of the motor nerves of respiration via reticulospinal pathways in the spinal cord and of the vagus and seventh cranial nerves, respectively. As has been postulated by others, stimulation of the seventh cranial nerve may be responsible for the autonomic nervous system symptoms that are associated with the cluster attack. Indeed, in a subsequent study in which 10 cluster patients were subjected to nocturnal polysomnography, six were found to have sleep apnea, as defined by standard criteria (Kudrow et al., 1983).

TREATMENT OF CLUSTER HEADACHE

The selection of particular drugs for the treatment of cluster headache depends on compatibility with other medications, history of untoward reactions or poor respon-

Table 7-8 Prophylactic agents in episodic cluster headache

Conditions	Drug of choice	Common contraindications and side effects[a]
Age		
Under 30	Methysergide (2 mg 3 to 4 times a day)	Cardiac and peripheral vascular disorders, extremity or chest pain, GI effects, paresthesias
30–45	Prednisone (tapering off from 40 mg/day for 3 weeks)	Ulcers, diverticulosis, HBP, diabetes, infection
Over 45	Lithium carbonate (300 mg 2 to 4 times a day)	Diuretic or low-salt therapy, tremor, GI effects
Other		
Attacks in sleep	Ergotamine tartrate (2 mg on retiring)	See methysergide effects

[a]GI = gastrointestinal; HBP = high blood pressure.
(From Kudrow, L. (1983). Cluster headache: New concepts. *Neurol. Clin. 1*:379.)

siveness, and the health of the patient. Drug selection will also depend on the type of cluster headache, its frequency, the timing of attacks, and the patient's age.

In all cases, patients are instructed to avoid afternoon naps and alcoholic beverages, including wine or beer. Alcohol will, in most instances, induce acute attacks during an active period but not during remissions. Dietary influences, with the exception of alcohol, appear to have little importance in cluster headache. Since light glare seems to be poorly tolerated during active periods, patients are advised to wear sunglasses and to avoid facing outside windows when seated indoors.

Bursts of anger, prolonged anticipation, excitement, and excessive physical activity are to be avoided, since cluster attacks are apt to occur in the relaxation period that follows. We have also observed that prolonged or sustained periods of anger, hurt, rage, or frustration experienced during remission periods are often associated with a new onset of a cluster period (Kudrow, 1980).

Not infrequently, cluster periods begin after an alteration in the sleep–wake cycle. Vacation trips, work changes, new occupations, postsurgical periods, completion of university studies, and so on are conditions commonly associated with onset of a cluster period. Although many variables are associated with such changes in lifestyle, alterations of sleep–wake patterns that often accompany these changes may be the most important.

Prophylactic Medication

Methysergide, steroids, lithium, and ergotamine are used prophylactically (Table 7-8).

Methysergide

In patients under 30 years of age, prophylactic treatment with methysergide is recommended. It is less likely to be of benefit at older ages or in patients who have used methysergide for several previous series. Methysergide is prescribed in a dosage schedule of 2 mg three to four times a day. The most common side effects are gastrointestinal disturbances, paresthesias of the lower extremities, and leg pain. In the presence of such symptoms discontinuation is recommended. Complications include retroperitoneal, endomyocardial, or pulmonary fibrosis, as reported by Graham (1965), Graham and Parnes (1965), and Kunkel (1971). Methysergide is contraindicated in coronary artery disease or peripheral vascular disease.

Steroids

Between the ages of 30 and 45 years, individuals who have used methysergide for several cluster series are likely to have become refractory. Therefore, prednisone prophylaxis is the treatment of choice. Prednisone is prescribed at 40 mg per day in divided doses for a period of 5 days and is tapered off over a period of 3 weeks. It is contraindicated in patients with hypertension, peptic ulcer disease, diabetes, current infection, and diverticulosis. Prior to Jammes's controlled study (1975) of prednisone prophylaxis in cluster headache, the use of steroids was noted in the medical literature in several instances (Friedman & Mikropoulos, 1958; Graham, 1976; Horton, 1952; MacNeal, 1978). In our own series of 77 patients with episodic cluster headache (Kudrow, 1978b), therapy with prednisone resulted in a marked relief in 76.6%, partial improvement in 11.7%, and no significant improvement in 11.7%. Of 15 patients with chronic cluster headache, 40% had obtained marked improvement.

Lithium

Lithium carbonate, 300 mg twice to four times a day, is our first choice of treatment in patients with chronic cluster or in those with episodic cluster who are over the age of 45. Ekbom (1974) was the first to report the beneficial effects of lithium prophylaxis in cluster headache. Encouraged by his results, our clinic evaluated the efficacy of lithium in 32 patients over a 32-week period (Kudrow, 1977). Of 28 patients completing the study, 42% obtained improvement ranging between 60 to 90%. Fifty-four percent obtained a greater than 90% improvement, and only one patient was considered unimproved. Subsequent studies by Mathew (1978) and Savoldi et al. (1978) reported similar results.

Side effects are not common after the first day of treatment. In higher doses of 900 mg a day or more, tremor is a common side effect. Toxicity may be avoided by preventing blood levels above 1.2 mg/dl.

Ergotamine

Oral ergotamine is an effective prophylactic agent in cluster headache. For patients who experience one attack daily, particularly during sleep-time hours, ergotamine, 2 mg taken orally at least 2 hours before the expected attack, is the recommended treatment.

Symptomatic Treatment

Oxygen inhalation is the most effective and safest method of aborting acute cluster headaches (Table 7-9). It is similar to ergotamine in its effectiveness as an abortive

Table 7-9 Effects of oxygen inhalation on acute attacks in episodic and chronic cluster groups

Sex and type of cluster	N	Benefited	
		N	Percent
Males			
Episodic	26	21	(80.8)
Chronic	19	13	(68.4)
Subtotal	45	34	(75.6)
Females			
Episodic	7	5	(71.4)
Chronic	0	0	(0)
Subtotal	7	5	(71.4)
Total	52	39	(75.0)

(From Kudrow, L. (1981). Response of cluster headache attacks to oxygen inhalation. *Headache 21*:2.)

agent and has the additional advantage of having neither side effects nor conditions that contraindicate its use. We had systematically evaluated a population of 55 patients with cluster headache for symptomatic response to oxygen inhalation (Kudrow, 1981). Of 33 patients thus treated, 80.8% of males and 71.4% of females were significantly benefited. Of the males with chronic cluster headache, 68.4% achieved success. In all, 75% of the patients obtained significant responses. The method of oxygen treatment is as follows: 100% oxygen is administered through a face mask at a rate of 7 liters per minute with the patient assuming a sitting position. The patient is instructed to breathe the oxygen at a normal rate for no longer than 15 minutes, but may stop treatment within this time once the attack has been relieved.

The mechanism by which oxygen inhalation interrupts the cluster attack is unknown; however, encouraged by our clinical results, Sakai and Meyer (1979) studied changes in cerebral blood flow during oxygen inhalation. They demonstrated that 100% oxygen administered during the attack promptly reduced cerebral blood flow and pain. The beneficial effect of oxygen inhalation may, however, be due to its inhibitory action on activity of the carotid body, as described recently. (Kudrow, 1983).

Where ergotamine is preferred, sublingual or inhalant preparations are recommended. They should be used at the very onset of the attack. Sublingual preparations may be repeated only once or twice after 15-minute intervals. Inhalants may be used three times in 5-minute intervals for a given attack. In general, use of ergotamine should be limited to a maximum of 4 mg per 24-hour periods.

REFERENCES

Aebelholt Krabbe, A., L. Henriksen, and J. Olesen (1983). Tomographic determination of cerebral blood flow during attacks of cluster headache. *Proceedings of the 12th Meeting of the Scandinavian Migraine Society*, p. 10. Helsinki, June 17–18.

Andrasik, F., E.B. Blanchard, J.G. Arena et al. (1982). Cross-validation of the Kudrow-Sutkus MMPI classification system for diagnosing headache type. *Headache 22:2–5.*

Anthony, M. and J.W. Lance (1971). Histaminic and serotonin in cluster headache. *Arch. Neurol. 25:225–231.*

Anthony M., G.D.A. Lord, and J.W. Lance (1978). Controlled trials of cimetadine in migraine and cluster headache. *Headache 18:261–264.*

Broch, A., I. Hørven, H. Nornes et al. (1970). Studies of cerebral and ocular circulation in a patient with cluster headache. *Headache 10:1–13.*

Bruyn, G.W., B.K. Bootsma, and H.L. Klawans (1976). Cluster headache and bradycardia. *Headache 16:11–15.*

Cuypers, J. and H. Altenkirch (1979). HLA antigens in cluster headache. *Headache 19:228–229.*

Cuypers, J., H. Altenkirch, and S. Bunge (1981). Personality profiles in cluster headache and migraine. *Headache 21:21–24.*

Ekbom, K. (1968). Nitroglycerin as a provocative agent in cluster headache. *Arch. Neurol. 19:487–493.*

Ekbom, K. (1970a). A clinical comparison of cluster headache and migraine. *Acta Neurol. Scand. (Suppl. 41) 46:1–48.*

Ekbom, K. (1970b). Pattern of cluster headache with a note on the relation to angina pectoris and peptic ulcer. *Acta Neurol. Scand. 46:225–237.*

Ekbom, K. (1974). Litium vid kroniska symptom av cluster headache. *Preliminart Meddelande Pousc. Med. 19:*148–156.

Ekbom, K., and T. Greitz (1970). Carotid angiography in cluster headache. *Acta Radiol. (Diagn.) (Stockholm) 10:*177–186.

Ekbom K., and L. Kudrow (1979). Facial flush in cluster (Editorial). *Headache 19:47.*

Ekbom, K., and B. de F. Olivarius (1971). Chronic migrainous neuralgia-diagnostic and therapeutic aspects. *Headache 11:97–101.*

Ekbom K.A. (1947). Ergotamine tartrate orally in Horton's "histaminic cephalgia" (also called Harris' "ciliary neuralgia"). *Acta Psychiatr. Scand. (Suppl.) 46:*106–113.

Eulenburg, A. (1874). *Lehrbuch der nervenkrankheiten 2. Au Fl. II Teil,* p. 264. Hirschwald, Berlin.

Friedman, A.P., and H.E. Mikropoulos (1958). Cluster headache. *Neurology 8:653–663.*

Friedman, A.P. and E.H. Wood (1976). Thermography in vascular headache. In *Medical Thermography* (S. Uema, ed.), pp. 80–84. Brentwood Publishers, Los Angeles.

Gardner, W.J., A. Stowell, and R. Dutlinger (1947). Resection of the greater petrosal nerve in the treatment of unilateral headache. *J. Neurosurg. 4:*105–114.

Graham, J.R. (1965). Possible renal complications of Sansert (methysergide) therapy for headache. *Headache 5:*12–14.

Graham, J.R. (1969). Cluster headache. Presentation at the International Symposium on Headache, Chicago.

Graham, J.R. (1972). Cluster headache. *Headache 11:175–185.*

Graham, J.R. (1976). Cluster headache. In *Pathogenesis and Treatment of Headache* (O. Appenzeller, ed.), pp. 93–108. Spectrum, New York.

Graham, J.R. and L.R. Parnes (1965). Possible cardiac and renovascular complications of Sansert therapy. *Headache 5:*14–18.

Graham, J.R., A.Z. Rogado, M. Rahman, and I.V. Gramer (1970). Some physical, physiological and psychological characteristics of patients with cluster headache. In *Background to Migraine* (A.L. Cochrane, ed.). p 38–51 Heinemann, London.

Harris, W. (1926). *Neuritis and Neuralgia.* Oxford University Press, London.

Harris, W. (1936). Ciliary (migrainous) neuralgia and its treatment. *Br. Med. J. 1:457–460.*

Henry, P.Y., J. Vernhiet, J.M. Orgogozo et al. (1978). Cerebral blood flow in migraine and cluster headaches. *Res. Clin. Stud. Headache 6:*10–16.

Heyck, H. (1975). In: Der kopschmerz, 4th ed. p. 114. George Thieme Verlag, Stuttgart.

Horton, B.T. (1952). Histaminic cephalgia. *Lancet 72:*92–98.

Horton, B.T., A.R. MacLean, and W.M. Craig (1939). A new syndrome of vascular headache: Results of treatment with histamine: Preliminary report. *May. Clin. Proc. 14:*257–260.

Jammes, J.L. (1975). The treatment of cluster headache with prednisone. *Dis. Nerv. Syst. 36:*375–376.

Klimek, A. (1982). Plasma testosterone levels in patients with cluster headache. *Headache 22:*162–164.

Kudrow, L. (1974). Physical and personality characteristics in cluster headache. *Headache 13:*197–201.

Kudrow, L. (1976a). Prevalence of migraine, peptic ulcer, coronary heart disease and hypertension in cluster headache. *Headache 16:*66–69.

Kudrow, L. (1976b). Plasma testosterone levels in cluster headache: Preliminary results. *Headache 16:*28–31.

Kudrow, L. (1977). Lithium prophylaxis for chronic cluster headache. *Headache 17:*15–18.

Kudrow, L. (1978a). HL-A antigens in cluster headache and classical migraine. *Headache 18:*167–168.

Kudrow, L. (1978b). Comparative results of prednisone, methysergide, and lithium therapy in cluster headache. In *Current Concepts in Migraine Research,* (R. Greene, ed.), pp. 159–163. Raven Press, New York.

Kudrow, L. (1979). Thermographic and Doppler flow asymmetry in cluster headache. *Headache 19:*204–208.

Kudrow, L. (1980). *Cluster Headache: Mechanisms and Management,* pp. 10–150. Oxford University Press, London.

Kudrow, L. (1981). Response to cluster headache attacks to oxygen inhalation. *Headache 21:*1–4.

Kudrow, L. (1983). A possible role of the carotid body in the pathogenesis of cluster headache. *Cephalalgia 3:*241–247.

Kudrow, L., D.J. McGinty, E.R. Phillips, and M. Stevenson (1983). Sleep apnea in cluster headache. *Proceedings of the 12th Scandinavian Migraine Society Meeting,* p. 56, Helsinki, June 17–18.

Kudrow, L. and B.J. Sutkus (1979). MMPI pattern specificity in primary headache disorders. *Headache 19:*18–24.

Kunkel, R.S. (1971). Fibrotic syndromes with chronic use of methysergide. *Headache 11:*1–5.

Kunkel, R.S. and D.F. Dohn (1974). Surgical treatment of chronic migrainous neuralgia. *Cleve. Clin. Q. 41:*189–192.

Kunkle, E.C., J.B. Pfeiffer, Jr., W.M. Wilhoit et al. (1954). Recurrent brief headache in "cluster" pattern. *Trans. Am. Neurol. Assoc. 77:*240.

Kunkle, E.C. (1959). Acetylcholine in the mechanism of headaches of the migraine type. *Arch. Neurol. Psychiatry 84:*135.

Lance, J.W. (1978). *Mechanisms and Management of Headache,* 3rd ed. Butterworths, London.

Lance, J.W. and M. Anthony (1971a). Thermographic studies in vascular headache. *Med. J. Aust. 1:*240.

Lance, J.W. and M. Anthony (1971b). Migrainous neuralgia or cluster headache? *J. Neurol. Sci. 13:*401–414.

Lovshin, L.L. (1961). Clinical caprices of histaminic cephalgia. *Headache 1:*3–6.

MacNeal, P.S. (1978). Useful therapeutic approaches to the patient with "problem headache." *Headache 18:*26–30.

Mathew, N.T. (1978). Clinical subtypes of cluster headache and response to lithium therapy. *Headache 18:*26–30.

Nattero, G., L. Savi, and G. Pisanti (1980). Doppler flow velocity in cluster headache. *International Congress, Headache '80,* Florence, Italy.

Nelson, R.F. (1978). Testosterone levels in cluster and non-cluster migrainous headache patients. *Headache 18:*265–267.

Norris, J.W., V.C. Hachinski, and P.W. Cooper (1976). Cerebral blood flow changes in cluster headache. *Acta Neurol. Scand. 54:*371–374.

Pollari, A., G. Bono, G. Murialdo et al. (1983). Gonadotropic function in cluster headache. *Proceedings of the 12th Meeting of the Scandinavian Migraine Society,* Helsinski, June 17–18, p. 58.

Romberg, M.H. (1840). *A Manual of Nervous Diseases of Man* (Trans.). E.H. Sievering, London Sydenham Society, London.

Sachs, E., Jr. (1968). The role of the nervous intermedius in facial neuralgia: Report of four cases with observations on the pathways for taste, lacrimation, and pain in the face. *J. Neurosurg. 23:*54–60.

Sakai, F. and J.S. Meyer (1978). Regional cerebral hemodynamics during migraine and cluster headaches measured by the 133 Xe inhalation method. *Headache 18:*122–132.

Sakai, F. and J.S. Meyer (1979). Abnormal cerebrovascular reactivity in patients with migraine and cluster headache. *Headache 19:*257–266.

Savoldi, F., G. Bono, G.C. Manzoni, G. Micieli et al. (1983). Lithium salts in cluster headache treatment. *Cephalalgia 3 (Suppl. 1):*79–84.

Schele, R., B. Ahlborg, and K. Ekbom (1978). Physical characteristics and allergy history in young men with migraine and other headaches. *Headache 18:*80–86.

Sjaastad, O. (1970). Kinin-OG histaminiunders ø kelser ved migrene. In *Kliniske Aspecter i Migrene Forshningen.* pp. 61–69. Norlundes Bogtrykkeri, Copenhagen.

Sjaastad, O., R. Apfelbaum, W. Caskey and et al. (1980). Chronic paroxysmal hemicrania (CPH): The clinical manifestations: A review. *Ups. J. Med. Sci. (Suppl.) 31:*27–33.

Sjaastad, O. and I. Dale (1974). Evidence for a new (?) treatable headache entity. *Headache 14:*105–108.

Sjaastad, O., K. Rootwelt, and I. Hørven (1974). Cutaneous blood flow in cluster headache. *Headache 13:*173–175.

Sjaastad, O., and Ø.V. Sjaastad (1977). Histamine metabolism in cluster headache and migraine. *J. Neurol. 216:*105–117.

Stowell, A. (1970). Physiologic mechanisms and treatment of histaminic or petrosal neuralgia. *Headache 9:*187–194.

8

Chronic Paroxysmal Hemicrania (CPH) and Similar Headaches

OTTAR SJAASTAD

CHRONIC PAROXYSMAL HEMICRANIA

Chronic paroxysmal hemicrania (CPH) was first described by Sjaastad and Dale (1974). It is probably a rare headache. Around 80 cases have been published or reported to us, but since such cases are published only exceptionally nowadays, the real number of diagnosed and treated cases may be several times this number.

Clinical Appearance

Clinically, CPH has many features in common with cluster headache, that is, the severity and unilaterality of the headache, and the accompanying phenomena, such as nasal stenosis/rhinorrhea, tearing, and conjunctival injection. Furthermore, both headaches usually lack typical visual phenomena such as scotomas and scintillations.

It presently is felt that CPH represents a distinct entity for several reasons (Sjaastad & Dale, 1976): (1) in contrast with cluster headache, *females* seem predominantly to be affected in CPH ($P < 0.0002$, binominal test); (2) the number of daily headache attacks generally tends to be much higher in CPH than in cluster headache, that is, usually an *individual* maximum of more than 15 attacks per 24 hours. This figure may have to be lowered considerably, however; (3) indomethacin has a prompt, dramatic, and rather selective effect in CPH, while its effect in cluster headache is generally weak or nonexistent.

There are other differences between CPH and cluster headache. The attacks tend to be shorter in CPH (mean 13.7 ± 7.6 minutes (SD)) than in cluster headache (49.0 ± 35.5 minutes) (Russell 1984). Nocturnal attacks certainly occur in CPH and are characteristic of this headache, but the attacks do not seem to show a nocturnal preponderance, as in cluster headache.

Another clinical feature that may seem to afford a distinction between CPH and cluster headache in some cases is the "mechanical precipitation of attacks": some

CPH patients may bring on attacks by certain movements of the neck, mainly flexion and rotation. However, considerably more than 50 % of the CPH patients are unable to precipitate attacks in this way.

The cluster phenomenon itself may not be a major distinction between CPH and cluster headache. First, the episodic form of cluster headache in a number of cases becomes chronic (the *secondary* chronic form). Next, an episodic as well as a chronic form seem to exist in CPH. The chronic stage in CPH was first discovered. Later, it was shown that there is a stage prior to the chronic one with only periodic symptoms, that is, a prechronic stage. Thus, although the terminology is different, because of a difference in the sequence of discoveries, the phenomena themselves may be essentially the same. And even in the chronic stage of CPH there is a clear fluctuation in attack severity—a "modified cluster pattern".

Whether or not *all* cases in the pre-CPH stage will eventually develop the chronic form is not known. It may be that cases in the pre-CPH stage are rather more common than is presently believed. There also seem to be cases without a prechronic stage (Bogucki et al., 1984). The cases that have reached the chronic stage (i.e., $>\frac{1}{2}$ year with continuous headache attacks) may appear to stay that way. The mean age of onset of the chronic stage may seem to conform well with the mean age of onset of cluster headache (i.e., around 30 years); however, the variation may be marked.

The pain in attacks of CPH is excruciatingly severe at its maximum, but there is a continuous fluctuation between the severe and the moderate attacks and during the latter, the pain may not be too severe to prevent the patient from working. Between attacks, there may be a continuous, sore feeling in the usually painful areas, that is, the ocular-periocular areas, the forehead, and temporal area, and also the aural-retroaural areas, neck, and shoulder. The maximum usually occurs in the frontal area. The pain usually has a piercing, boring, and clawlike character, but in the initial stages, especially of the precipitated attacks, it may be pulsating.

This clinical headache can be removed by the continuous medication with indomethacin, provided the dosage is adequate (Sjaastad & Dale, 1974). The dosage is easily titrated and may vary greatly, even intraindividually (i.e. from $\leq$25–250 mg per day). The dosages will have to be changed according to the fluctuating severity of the attacks. A slight sore feeling may persist even on this therapy, but the attacks disappear. No cases of tachyphylaxis to indomethacin have been reported. Indomethacin is remarkably well tolerated over years, and we have not had to stop treating any of our cases permanently because of dyspepsia, although periods with moderate symptoms have occurred.

Differential Diagnoses

CPH may first and foremost, be confounded with two types of headaches—other unilateral headaches and other headaches responding to indomethacin. CPH responds to indomethacin in an absolute way and presently only one other headache is known to do so: hemicrania continua (Sjaastad & Spierings, 1984). In the latter headache there are no attacks but only a steadily continuing headache; the headache is moderate and not accompanied by the autonomic phenomena.

The other indomethacin-responsive headaches respond only partly to indomethacin and differ clearly from CPH in their clinical pattern: *"jabs and jolts" syndrome* (Sjaastad et al., 1980), with short-lived pains (i.e., usually lasting for a second or a few seconds) appearing in various locations or sometimes in a strictly localized area. Jabs and jolts may occur as a solitary phenomenon or in connection with other headaches, such as migraine and cluster headache. The "ice-pick pain" (described by Raskin & Schwartz, 1980) is probably similar or identical, although it is only described in connection with migraine and has no established indomethacin effect. "Exertional headache" also responds to indomethacin, but usually only partially.

Chronic, unilateral headaches without sideshift consist mainly of the following differential diagnostic possibilities: cluster headache, cervicogenic headache (see elsewhere), and in a few instances, migraine. When one takes the duration of pain, accompanying symptoms, sex, and other factors into consideration, the differential diagnosis should not present any great obstacle.

Pathogenesis

Intraocular pressure and pulse-synchronous (corneal indentation pulse) amplitudes increase during attack compared with the preattack phase, and clearly more so on the symptomatic than on the nonsymptomatic side (Hørven & Sjaastad, 1977). The abruptness with which this occurs strongly indicates that the pressure increase is due to intraocular vasodilatation. The corneal temperature also increases, most markedly on the symptomatic side, which may fit with the vasodilatation theory. If thymoxamine (an alfa-receptor blocking agent) is applied topically as eye drops, the increase in intraocular pressure during attack is no longer evident. It may, therefore, seem as though the signal to the eye is influenced by sympathetic nerves.

The question then arises whether these changes are restricted to the ocular area or are more extensive.

A quantitative study of various parameters demonstrates increased nasal secretion and tearing bilaterally during attacks, and most marked on the symptomatic side. Sweating in the forehead was increased on the symptomatic side in some cases, but not in all. Forehead sweating on the symptomatic side clearly increased following heating in CPH—the opposite of what occurs in cluster headache. Conversely, forehead sweating increased more on the symptomatic side with administration of pilocarpine in cluster headache but not in CPH. This indicates that there are *fundamental* differences in pathogenesis between CPH and cluster headache.

To find out whether these changes in autonomic parameters are confined to the external head/face area, cerebral blood flow (electromagnetic flowmetry and intraarterial xenon method) and intraarterial blood pressure were measured during and between attacks. No definite attack-induced changes were found.

Attacks can be precipitated by applying pressure against certain particularly sensitive points in the neck and by neck flexion. Rubbing or obstructing the flow in the common or internal carotid artery on the symptomatic side does not initiate an attack. The impulse from the neck to the eye logically appears to be neurogenic, since it may take only a few seconds from the start of the precipitation procedure until the tears appear and the intraocular pressure is found to be increased on the symptomatic side.

The autonomic phenomena (e.g., the sweating) are not *caused* by the pain; neither is the pain caused by the autonomic phenomena. In some precipitated attacks, the onset of the pain may be delayed by 30 seconds or more whereas the ipsilateral forehead sweating may appear some time before the pain. If atropine is administered systemically prior to attacks, the autonomic phenomena—that is, sweating, nasal secretion, and tearing—are more or less abolished, but the pain of the attack persists.

A dichotomy between pain and autonomic phenomena can thus be obtained. The attack seems to generate from a locus from which both pain and the various other phenomena can be generated.

The neck thus seems to play a significant part in attack generation. There, nevertheless, seems to be a clear influence of central mechanisms. Thus, nocturnal attacks partly appear in close connection with REM-phase sleep. Furthermore, forehead sweating produced by heat stimuli seems to be delayed compared with that in controls, and when it first appears it may be most irregular, appearing in bursts; these phenomena are hard to reconcile with a solitary "peripheral" mechanism and strongly suggest a "central" dysregulation.

CPH can therefore probably be viewed as a disorder in its own right, closely related to cluster headache, but nevertheless distinct from it, because of its different clinical pattern, different treatment, and partially a different pathogenesis.

ATYPICAL CLUSTER HEADACHE AND "INDOMETHACIN-RESPONSIVE HEADACHE"

The term *atypical cluster headache* was first used by us (Hørven & Sjaastad, 1977) to describe patients exhibiting a symptomatology strongly *reminiscent* of cluster headache, but with atypical clinical features. The name contains the term *cluster headache*. Thus, the link to the cluster headache syndrome must be a strong one; otherwise the use of this term would be meaningless. In the reported cases, the supplementary tests—intraocular pressure, CIP (corneal indentation pulse)-amplitude, and corneal temperature measurements—clearly indicate a link to ordinary cluster headache. In addition, these cases exhibited atypical traits: The group, for example, included cases with marked interparoxysmal EEG-changes as well as a case with recurring bouts of recurring homolateral retrobulbar neuritis, Hageman trait deficiency, and a bleeding tendency. No attempt has been made to classify these cases more subtly.

Unfortunately, the use of this term seems to have gone astray in some circles in recent years. In some materials, more than half of the patients do not have unilateral headache, night attacks are not part of the picture, and nausea and vomiting occur more frequently than lacrimation. Obviously, therefore, the link, if any, to cluster headache is fragmentary. The usage of this term in connection with such ill-defined and vague headaches is ill-conceived and should be abandoned before too much harm is done. Used in the *original* way, this term may still be admissible.

Several separate headache forms respond to indomethacin, some in an *absolute* way—CPH and hemicrania continua—and others only partially—jabs and jolts syndrome and exertional headache.

The two headache forms hemicrania continua and CPH differ distinctly clinically. CPH logically belongs to the cluster headache syndrome (Sjaastad, 1986). Hemicrania continua and the other headaches that only partly respond to indomethacin do not appear to belong in this category. Almost the only thing CPH and hemicrania continua have in common is their response to indomethacin, and that is not enough to justify a grouping.

REFERENCES

Bogucki, A., R. Szymanska, and W. Braciak (1984). Chronic paroxysmal hemicrania: Lack of pre-chronic stage. *Cephalalgia 4*, 187–189.

Hørven, I. and O. Sjaastad (1977). Cluster headache syndrome and migraine. Ophthalmological support for a two-entity theory. *Acta Ophthalmol. (Kbh)* 55:35–50.

Raskin, N.H., and R.K. Schwartz (1980). Icepick-like pain. *Neurology 30*:203.

Russell, D. (1984). Chronic paroxysmal hemicrania: severity, duration and time of occurrence of attacks. *Cephalalgia* 4:53–56.

Russell, D. and L. Storstein (1984). Chronic paroxysmal hemicrania: Heart rate changes and EEG rhythm disturbances. A computerized analysis of 24 h ambulatory EEG recordings. *Cephalalgia* 4:135–144.

Sjaastad, O., R. Apfelbaum, W. Caskey, B. Christoffersen, et.al. (1980). Chronic paroxysmal hemicrania (CPH): The clinical manifestations. A review. *Upsala J Med Sci.* 31:27–35.

Sjaastad, O. and I. Dale (1974). Evidence for a new (?) treatable headache entity. *Headache 14*:105–108.

Sjaastad, O. and I. Dale (1976). A new (?) clinical headache entity "chronic paroxysmal hemicrania" 2. *Acta Neurol Scand.* 54:140–159.

Sjaastad O. and E.L.H. Spierings (1984). "Hemicrania continua." Another headache with absolute indomethacin response. *Cephalalgia* 4:65–70.

Sjaastad, O. (1986). Chronic paroxysmal hemicrania. In *Handbook of clinical neurology,* Vol. 4(48) (P.J. Vinken, G.W. Bruyn, and H.L. Klawans, eds.), pp. 257–266. Elsevier, Amsterdam.

9

Toxic Vascular Headache

JOHN STIRLING MEYER
DONALD J. DALESSIO

This category commonly used in classifying headaches, includes a large number of systemic conditions that are usually associated with bilateral and symmetrical, throbbing, vascular headache. There is a great deal of evidence that these headaches are due to painful dilation of the cephalic vasculature of brain and scalp combined. This subject will be reviewed in detail here, including certain classic experiments performed by Harold Wolff and his colleagues, as they remain basic for understanding the pathogenesis of head pain of vascular etiology.

The most common type of vascular headache, familiar to almost everyone, is that which accompanies fever and which usually becomes more intense as the fever rises. This headache is almost certainly due to congestion of the vessels of the brain and scalp. During stepwise hyperthermia in the monkey, both internal (+42%) and external carotid blood flow (+25%) progressively increase as body temperature is raised from 36 to 41° C. (Meyer and Handa, 1966). Cerebral oxidative metabolism likewise increases and is the cause of increased blood flow and delirium that eventually will result if temperature continues to rise. It has also been shown that in human patients treated with fever therapy, cerebral blood flow increases if effective fever is produced (Heyman et al., 1950). This subject will be discussed in more detail later. Other common causes of toxic vascular headaches include hangover headaches after excessive alcohol ingestion, those associated with respiratory and metabolic acidosis, hypoxia, hypoglycemia, and reactions to many medications. In all of these conditions clinical or experimental evidence shows increased cerebral or cephalic blood flow that documents the accompanying cerebral vascular congestion, and this is the essential cause of vascular headache. These common forms of headache will be discussed later.

Histamine, which is released into the circulation in many allergic and toxic states, increases cerebral blood flow and causes a predictable headache in almost all subjects. Conversely, antihistaminics decrease the cerebral blood flow (Amano & Meyer 1982) and tend to alleviate toxic vascular headache, as do many cerebral vasocontictor agents including aspirin, indomethacin, and other nonsteroidal anti-inflammatory agents. Because histamine has been considered an important etiologic metabolite in relation to a majority of toxic vascular headaches, it has been studied extensively as a model of vascular headache, particularly by Harold Wolff; this will be discussed later in this chapter.

Another biological substance that predictably produces characteristic pounding headaches of the vascular type is the prostaglandin PGI_2, or prostacyclin. This ubiquitous vascular prostaglandin is metabolized from arachidonic acid by means of the enzyme cycloxygenase by all vascular endothelium. Prostacyclin is the most potent cerebral vasodilator substance known. It greatly increases cephalic blood flow, and inhibition of its synthesis by nonsteroidal anti-inflammatory agents, such as indomethacin, greatly reduces cerebral blood flow and relieves vascular headache (Amano & Meyer, 1982). Intravenous administration of prostacyclin rapidly produces a typical pulsatile and pounding vascular headache, associated with nausea and vomiting (Szczeklik & Gryglewski, 1979).

CLINICAL USE OF HISTAMINE AS AN EXPERIMENTAL MODEL OF TOXIC VASCULAR HEADACHE

The response of the cephalic vascular system to histamine is to produce a characteristic headache in a predictable manner. When histamine is administered intravenously, in a dose of 0.1 mg, this provides a suitable model in human volunteers for studying toxic vascular headache. This subject will therefore be reviewed in detail. Analysis of toxic vascular headaches were made possible through observations that when this chemical agent was injected in tests of gastric function, headache often resulted, especially if histamine was injected intravenously. It has been noted in human subjects during neurosurgical procedures, as well as in experimental animals, that injections of histamine dilate cerebral arteries. It was postulated, therefore, that there was some relationship between these observations and the vascular nature of the headache produced. Indeed, some physicians, at one time, advocated repeated intravenous infusions of histamine in those suffering from vascular headache in an attempt to "desensitize" individuals from "histamine cephalalgia," which was thought at that time to be the etiologic nature of many vascular headaches including cluster and migraine headache. This approach to treatment has generally been abandoned.

To ascertain experimentally the role of cephalic blood vessels in the genesis of headache, the agent used to produce head pain must regularly produce headache in human volunteers and be otherwise innocuous, its action should be short-lived and components of its action measurable. Histamine fulfills these requirements, since its effects on the intracranial blood vessels are measurable, the induced headache is predictable and effects of histamine on blood pressure and cerebrospinal fluid pressure are measurable.

It was observed that after injections of histamine the amplitude of intracranial pulsations increased (Pickering & Hess, 1933: Weiss et al., 1932). If this increase in intracranial pulsation represents an increased effect of cardiac systole on dilated cerebral arterial walls, then concurrent measurements of cerebral blood flow (CBF) and amplitude of intracranial pulsations should show this relationship. In other words, if histamine dilates cerebral vessels, after its injection a fall in blood pressure and temporary decrease in CBF should occur as a result of impaired autoregulation, with a slight diminuation in the amplitude of pulsation, followed by restoration of blood pressure with greatly increased CBF and large increases in the amplitude of the intracranial pulsations. Experiments with cats by Wolff and colleagues confirmed these relationships.

A needle inserted into the cisterna magna was connected with a Frank capsule. Moving bromide paper in a camera recorded the waves made by a beam of light reflected from the capsule. Through a hole in the parietal portion of the skull, a thermocouple was submerged beneath the surface of the brain. A stopper snugly fitting about the connections of the thermocouple sealed the hole in the skull.

It was observed that shortly after the injection of histamine and coincident with the fall in systemic arterial blood pressure there was a decrease in cerebral blood flow with but little change or a slight fall in the amplitude of the intracranial pulsations. However, with the restoration of the blood pressure there was an increase in cerebral blood flow. Moreover, the amplitude of the intracranial pulsations considerably exceeded their original height.

It may be concluded, therefore, that the increased amplitude of intracranial pulsations after injections of histamine actually represents an increase in stretch of dilated intracranial vessels with each cardiac systole, and that dilatation itself is not sufficient to increase the amplitude and blood flow if there is at the same time a fall in blood pressure. However, vasodilatation plus a normal systemic arterial pressure will cause both increased cerebral blood flow and increased amplitude of intracranial pulsations. These considerations become particularly significant when one recalls that the dural vessels, the dural sinuses, and the larger pial vessels are important pain-sensitive structures.

The Headache Experimentally Induced by Histamine

Because the increase in amplitude of intracranial pulsations is an expression of changes in pressure in the intracranial and intraspinal arteries, it seemed reasonable to use it as a means of studying the relation of cerebral vessels to headache produced by an experimental agent such as histamine. Information about this relationship has been obtained in human experiments in which, by means of a needle in the lumbar sac, the amplitude of the intracranial pulsations was ascertained and its relation to headache produced by histamine analyzed in the following manner (Clark et al., 1936a,b).

Method

The subjects of these observations were patients on whom it was necessary to perform lumbar puncture for diagnostic purposes and several healthy volunteer adults. The results in the former differed in no wise from those in the latter. With the subject lying on his left side, a lumbar puncture was made and the needle connected with a Frank capsule by means of a column of sterile physiologic solution of sodium chloride contained in metal and heavy rubber tubing. For comparison, and to obtain a record of actual changes in arterial pulsations, simultaneous photographs were taken of the changes in the pulsations in the temporal artery. For this purpose another Frank capsule was connected with a tambour on the temporal pulse by an air

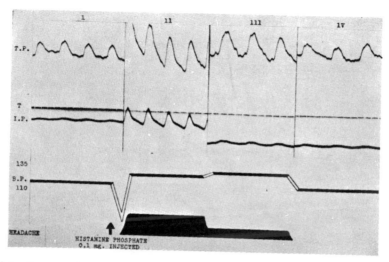

Figure 9-1. Representative sections from a photographic record of the temporal pulse and intracranial pulsations during headache produced by histamine in a subject, with the duration of the headache, the variations in blood pressure, and the injection of histamine indicated diagrammatically. The time was recorded, in this instance, on the same line as the temporal pulse.

system. The two capsules were arranged so as to reflect horizontal beams of light into the camera, which contained a moving strip of bromide paper. In this way changes in pressure within the subarachnoid space were recorded simultaneously with changes in the amplitude of the temporal pulse. Cerebrospinal fluid pressure was taken frequently by a manometer, which could be connected or disconnected from the system by a stopcock. A device recording time at 0.2-second intervals also made a record directly on the moving paper. Readings for blood pressure were made at frequent intervals.

The camera was started and a record taken of the resting stage in each subject. Histamine acid phosphate (0.1 cc of a 1:1000 solution) was then injected into the median basilic vein of the left arm. The exact moment of the injection as well as the moment of each reading of the blood pressure and each sensation experienced by the subject was signaled directly on the photographic record by tapping the time recorder. The camera was run continuously from the initial resting stage through the administration of the injection and the beginning of the headache and until the headache had completely disappeared. The recorded pulsations representing the changes in pressure in the subarachnoid space produced by intracranial and intraspinal pulsations will, for the sake of brevity, be referred to throughout as "intracranial pulsations."

In 19 subjects the effects of the injection of histamine were investigated. Sixteen technically satisfactory experiments were obtained on 11 subjects, and 14 technically satisfactory single injections of histamine in 9 subjects.

Figure 9-1 shows a series of sections taken from the record of a typical experiment. In I the temporal pulsations and the intracranial pulsations as recorded from the pulsatile expansions in the lumbar arachnoid space are minimal in the resting stage; in II the intracranial and temporal pulsations are at their greatest amplitude and the headache is maximal, while the arterial pressure after a fall has returned to slightly above the original resting level; in III the brain and temporal pulses are subsiding and the headache is growing less intense, while the arterial pressure remains at about the same level; in IV the pulsations are once more minimal and the headache has entirely disappeared.

In Figure 9-2 are shown the results of continuous infusion of histamine. At I is shown the

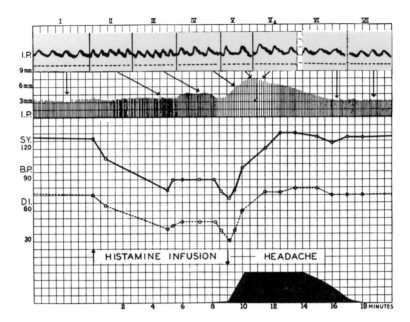

Figure 9-2. Diagrammatic and photographic representation of the course of events in the experiment in which histamine acid phosphate (0.1 mg/minute) was infused continuously during 9 minutes. Systolic blood pressure is indicated by the heavy black line SY, and diastolic pressure by the broken line DI. At I.P. the variations in rate and amplitude of the intracranial pulsation are represented and the top line I.P. is made up of approximately corresponding sections from the photographic record of the intracranial pulsation. Arrows point from the photographed intracranial pulsation to the corresponding pulsation represented diagrammatically. It should be noted that the slow rate of pulsation during the height of the headache and at the maximum amplitude of oscillation is exceptional to this case. The pulse rate is usually more rapid during the height of the headache.

height of the intracranial pulsations before injections of histamine; while at II and III are seen the pulsations after the infusion of histamine has started (0.1 mg of histamine acid phosphate per minute). It is to be noted that the amplitude of the intracranial pulsations is but slightly increased during the period of infusion of histamine; the blood pressure falls and continues at a low level. The small intracranial pulsations and low blood pressure continue as long as the intravenous infusion persists. At IV, the cessation of the infusion and the rise in blood pressure, the intracranial pulsations increase in magnitude and the headache begins. It reaches its maximum at V and persists for the usual length of time after histamine has been injected. At VI the headache is disappearing; at VII it is gone.

Great increase in intracranial pressure played no part in the production of the headache following injection of histamine. In fact, the pressure of the cerebrospinal fluid was in no case elevated to more than 300 mm of water, and the peak pressure usually occurred from 10 to 20 seconds before the onset of the headache. When the headache was of maximum intensity and the intracranial pulsations were maximal, the cerebrospinal fluid pressure was falling toward the resting level or had reached it. Pickering and Hess (1933) made similar observations and inferences.

The effect of increased intracranial pressure on the headache produced by histamine was ascertained in four experiments on 1 of the 19 subjects by the procedure of raising the cerebrospinal fluid pressure to 500 or 600 mm of water by injection of physiologic solution of sodium chloride into the lumbar arachnoid space. Pickering and Hess's observation that the headache was relieved by this procedure was confirmed, but the relation of the improvement to the amplitude of the intracranial pulsations could not be satisfactorily determined with our technique.

In 3 of the 19 subjects the effect of another important cerebral vasodilator which seldom produces headache was ascertained, namely, carbon dioxide. In one subject, the change in the height of the amplitude of the intracranial pulsations after breathing 5% carbon dioxide and 95% oxygen was in one instance from 3.3 to 4.4 mm (+ 33%) and in another from 2.9 to 4.6 mm (+ 57%). There was a sensation of fullness in the head but not true headache or pain. In this same subject, however, histamine produced an increase of amplitude of 100 % and at this point definite (although moderate) headache was experienced. With the administration of 10 % carbon dioxide and 90 % oxygen, the change in the magnitude of the intracranial pulsations was in another subject from 3.9 to 9.3 mm (+ 141%), in another from 3.4 to 9.4 mm (+ 170%), in a third from 3.9 to 10.3 mm (+ 164%). The feeling of fullness in the head was more pronounced, but headache was not experienced. Histamine was not used on this subject.

Clearly the threshold for headache in the first subject (who experienced headache with an increase of 100%) was much lower than that in the second (who had no headache with an increase of 170%). But of paramount importance is the fact that headache did not occur in the first subject with an increase of 57% (carbon dioxide) but did occur when the increase reached 100% (histamine).

Comment

The results reported demonstrate that the intensity of the headache produced by histamine is proportional to the degree of dilatation and stretch of the intracranial vessels and the perivascular tissue. The evidence at hand does not indicate that stretch of the meninges as the result of great increases in intracranial pressure was an important factor in the production of the headache. Pickering and Hess (1933) drew similar inferences from their experiments and supported this view by indicating that raising the arterial pressure or lowering the cerebrospinal fluid pressure during the headache intensified the pain. Conversely, lowering arterial pressure or raising cerebrospinal fluid pressure decreased it; these observations were confirmed by us.

The following explanation of these effects is offered. During the usual state of contraction of the walls of intracranial blood vessels, cardiac systole is reflected as a minor change in the intracranial pressure: the elastic contracted muscle resists pressure changes and absorbs the impact. It has been shown in other vascular beds and can be postulated here that under these circumstances a certain number of afferent impulses arise from the vessel walls with each systole. When the vessels are distended, however, as after injection of histamine, the number of impulses arising from their walls greatly increases, accentuated with each systole (Bronk, 1935). Moreover, the ability of the now hypotonic walls of the vessels to absorb changes in pressure is much reduced and the variations in pressure within the vessels are thus more directly transmitted to sensory end-organs in and about their walls and to the subarachnoid space. The resulting unusual flood of afferent impulses causes pain.

Cranial Arteries Chiefly Involved in Experimentally Induced Histamine Headache

That the headache experimentally induced by histamine is linked with changes in intracranial circulation follows from the previous comment, but the vascular branches chiefly involved must now be defined. Pickering and Hess (1933) suggested, on the basis of their carefully conceived and conducted experiments, that "the disturbance producing the histamine headache arises in the dura matter" and that "the vessels concerned would be the meningeal arteries." Evidence from the experiments to be presented below make it seem unlikely that the dural arteries are primarily responsible for the histamine headache. Pickering (1939) seems subsequently to have accepted the view that the distention of pial arteries was responsible for the headache.

To obtain further information concerning the contribution to pain made by specific cranial arteries in headache and concerning the nerve pathways that conduct these impulses, the following analysis was reported by Schumacher et al. (1940).

SERIES I

Superficial Tissues of the Scalp

The following procedure was performed on 15 patients. All afferent nerves from the scalp on one side were blocked from the midfrontal to the postparietal region with a 1% solution of procaine. This was done by infiltrating the tissues with procaine hydrochloride in a line extending from the middle forehead and temple, extending to the vertex.

Experiment 1. Four subjects received intravenous injections of histamine phosphate, 0.1 mg, immediately after the local analgesia had been produced. The subsequent histamine headache was severe, generalized, and of equal intensity and distribution on the two sides of the head.

Experiment 2. In 11 subjects subsequent injection of air into the subarachnoid space of the lumbar region for encephalographic study was accompanied by headache, which was of the same distribution and intensity on the two sides of the head. The unilateral analgesia had no appreciable influence on the headache of the corresponding side.

These observations indicate that the headache resulting from histamine and from injection of air into the subarachnoid space does not depend on the integrity of superficial sensation.

Temporal, Frontal, and Supraorbital Arteries

Effect of a tight head bandage Pickering and Hess (1933) reported that in their series a tight bandage about the head, interfering with the circulation to the scalp, did not alter the intensity or quality of the histamine headache. Experiments done in the laboratory of the New York Hospital, however, indicate that some modification in the intensity and the distribution of the headache may occur as a result of this procedure.

Experiment. A sphygmomanometer cuff with a firm bandage fitted over it was applied about the head of three subjects. Histamine phosphate was then injected intravenously, and when the headache had made itself manifest, the cuff was inflated to well above the systolic blood pressure (200 mm Hg). The then tight and uncomfortable cuff caused the histamine headache to be imperceptible, considerably diminished, or indistinguishable from the discomfort produced by the tight band. With release of the pressure of air in the cuff the histamine headache again became apparent and seemed to have its former intensity.

In the light of the hypothesis advanced by Hardy, Wolff, and Goodell (1940) that the threshold of sensation to a given pain is raised by the introduction of a second pain, these data may not be interpreted as signifying that the diminution of headache by a tight bandage is due to the obstruction of scalp arteries, which thus prevents painful dilatation. It was demonstrated by these investigators in experiments on three subjects that if a painful stimulus produced by the concentrated thermal radiation from a 1000-watt lamp was allowed to fall on the forehead during the histamine headache it was possible, by increasing the intensity of the secondarily induced pain, to reach a level that made the underlying headache imperceptible. In short, a secondarily induced pain of graduated intensity approximating that of the histamine headache diminished the intensity of the latter. This will be alluded to later in discussing which arteries are chiefly responsible for the intensity of histamine headache.

The effect of a tight bandage may thus have two explanations: (1) painful dilatation of scalp arteries is prevented, and (2) what is more likely, the threshold of pain is raised by application of the tight and slightly painful bandage.

Direct manipulation of arteries of the scalp In order to learn more about the role of the superficial arteries in headache produced by histamine, further experiments were performed as follows.

Experiment 1. In five subjects the effect of manual obliteration of the temporal artery on the histamine headache was investigated. In two subjects the obliteration seemed to reduce the intensity of the headache on that side; in three subjects it had little or no effect. Pressure on the nearby structures had no effect.

Experiment 2. In one subject, the entire frontal, temporal, and parietal areas on the right side of the scalp were thoroughly infiltrated with a 1% solution of procaine hydrochloride, the frontal, temporal, and supraorbital arteries themselves being thus surrounded with the analgesic. This resulted in analgesia over the entire left side of the head in an area bounded by the nose, the ear, and the vertex. Subsequent intravenous injections of 0.1 mg of histamine phosphate produced severe headache in the frontotemporal region, bilaterally, with no perceptible difference on the two sides.

Experiment 3. In four patients ligation of the superficial temporal artery on one side did not alter the quality of the histamine headache on the two sides of the head (see following section on middle meningeal arteries).

Experiment 4. Histamine phosphate was injected directly into the temporal artery in two subjects. In the first subject the agent was injected into the artery through the intact skin; in the other the right temporal artery was surgically exposed and the histamine was injected directly into its lumen. The results by the two methods were identical. The observations on the second subject follow.

The right temporal artery, after surgical exposure, was suitably held by means of a ligature placed about it. Manipulation of the artery was painful. Pulling the artery from below upward, while it was being immobilized in preparation for insertion of the needle, caused pain in the upper teeth. When the artery was pulled down from the temple the pain was felt in the temple, deep behind, and in the eye. Inserting the needle into the artery was very painful. The pain that resulted from spreading the tissues in the neighborhood of the artery was also intense.

When 0.1 mg of histamine phosphate was injected into the temporal artery, the first sensation was unilateral diffuse burning in the temporal bone (21 seconds after injection). The pain became more severe and was soon of a dull aching nature and more widespread than that due to the puncture of the artery. This sensation was followed by the usual taste (after 26 seconds) and then by a slight decline in the intensity of the headache (after 36 seconds). A unilateral flush, heretofore barely perceptible, now (after 44 seconds) became readily visible, persisting for 3 minutes. The headache then returned in greater intensity (after 50 seconds), to remain unilateral and in the general area mentioned, namely, the temporal and parietal regions. It became a deeper, poorly localized headache, but remained unilateral; it was dull and throbbing, but still not severe. It covered the right temporoparietal region, extending upward about two thirds of the way to the vertex, posteriorly to the anterior border of the occipital area, and anteriorly to the lateral margin of the frontal area. After 2 minutes the deeper component increased in intensity and was felt also in the frontal region. Most of the pain remained unilateral, but later (2½ minutes) there was slight headache on the other side. The deep, aching, throbbing pain was still present in the temporoparietal and frontal regions on the side of the injection. The scalp in the region of the injection was "sore" to pressure, and compression of the temporal artery here increased the pain, but reduced it in the remainder of the involved area. The headache was gone 3½ minutes after the injection.

These experiments suggest that the temporal artery, possibly also the frontal, supraorbital, and occipital arteries, may participate in the headache produced by histamine.

It seems probable from the data presented that the contribution of the extracranial arteries does not determine the intensity of the histamine headache. Though local headache was produced by direct injection into the temporal artery, it must be remembered that a comparatively high concentration of histamine was permitted to act directly on the arterial wall, and that extreme stretching probably occurred. Under such circumstances, an artery known to be sensitive to pain might well give rise to local headache. But during generalized headache following injection of histamine into the antecubital vein, in the absence of such extreme local dilatation of extracranial arteries, it is doubtful that the contribution made by these arteries predominates.

Middle Meningeal Arteries

Inferences concerning the contribution to histamine headache by pain impulses from the middle meningeal artery were drawn from experiments on seven subjects who had incomplete rhizotomy of the trigeminal nerve for tic douloureux.

In all seven New York Hospital patients the approach to the gasserian ganglion and its root included ligation and section of the middle meningeal artery and destruction, over 1 to 2 cm, of the periarterial nerve fibers. (The fact that "bleeding back" occurred demonstrated that the ligated arteries were subsequently filled with blood). If, therefore, in these subjects there was no difference in an induced histamine headache on the two sides, the inference could be drawn that the middle meningeal artery did not make a perceptible contribution to the pain of the histamine headache. The interval between ligation and injection of histamine varied in the seven cases, but in no instance was it great enough to afford regeneration of the sensory fibers.

Experiment 1. Histamine was administered intravenously. The headache that resulted was equal on the two sides of the head. Moreover, for four of the seven patients the operative approach involved ligation of the ipsilateral temporal artery. As indicated in experiment 3, above, these four subjects did not differ in their reactions to histamine in any way from the others, who had the temporal artery intact.

Though the pain contributed by the middle meningeal arteries is not as great as was first suggested by Pickering and Hess (1933), one may not infer that they are not involved. It is evident, however, that the absence of a pain-sensitive middle meningeal artery on one side does not appreciably decrease the intensity of the headache. Also, the contribution of pain from the temporal artery can similarly be considered imperceptible.

The evidence just presented suggests that the dural arteries are not the major contributors to the pain of histamine headache. It also adds further weight to the opinion previously expressed regarding the minor role of the extracranial arteries. Observations of Northfield (1938) support these views. After injection of histamine into the internal carotid artery in six cases, that investigator obtained homolateral headache in five cases and no headache in one. After injection of histamine into the external carotid artery in six cases, headache was absent in five and was faint and generalized in one.

Effect of Increasing the Intracranial Pressure

The following experiments are based on the assumption that certain of the cranial arteries, by virtue of their location, can be supported extramurally by increasing the cerebrospinal fluid pressure, thereby diminishing their amplitude of pulsation and thus reducing headache.

The large cerebral arteries at the base of the brain, notably those forming the circle of Willis and its branches, are obviously susceptible to extramural compression by increase in cerebrospinal fluid pressure. Extracranial (scalp) arteries, of course, are outside the direct influence of changes in intracranial pressure. The effect on dural arteries will be considered subsequently.

A method has therefore been devised to increase cerebrospinal fluid pressure rapidly by connecting the subarachnoid space with a high column of fluid (sterile physiologic solution of sodium chloride) in order to observe the effect of such increase in pressure on the intensity of the headache. As has been stated, the experiments rest on the premise that reduction in headache by this means is due to increased support of stretched cranial arteries. In headache due to dilatation of cranial arteries, reduction in pain would indicate that intracranial arteries are responsible, whereas no change in intensity would bespeak an extracranial origin.

On 13 patients in whom spinal puncture was necessary for diagnosis, the effect of increasing intracranial pressure on headache induced by histamine was investigated.

Severe headache was induced within 60 seconds by the intravenous administration of 0.10 to 0.15 mg of histamine phosphate. Such a headache reached its maximum intensity quickly, remaining there for 5 to 8 minutes in most instances, after which it gradually subsided and was gone within 10 to 12 minutes.

Method. In the experiments on subjects with histamine headache, the level of the column of fluid was elevated 800 to 1000 mm above the spinal canal. A clamp was removed from the connecting tube when it was desired to increase the cerebrospinal fluid pressure rapidly and was replaced when further increase in pressure was no longer desired. To reduce pressure rapidly, the clamped tube was disconnected and the fluid allowed to flow freely from the subarachnoid space. Pressure readings by means of the usual glass water manometer were taken at intervals.

Shortly after the onset of headache, and approximately at the time when it reached its maximum intensity, the pressure was suddenly raised as described to 800 to 1000 mm of physiologic solution of sodium chloride. If headache subsequently was abolished, the fluid was then allowed to flow from the subarachnoid space until the pressure was greatly reduced. If headache recurred, the pressure was again raised until the headache was eliminated. This sequence of events was repeated as often as the duration of a given histamine headache permitted.

Results. Of the 13 subjects, there were two from whom adequate information could not be obtained, owing to apprehension or difficulty in understanding. In 11 the headache was elim-

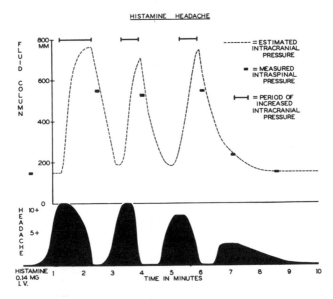

Figure 9-3. Abolishing effect of repeated experimental increases in the intracranial pressure on a headache induced by the intravenous injection of 0.14 mg of histamine phosphate.

inated or grew less when the intracranial pressure was increased. In 7 of the latter there was a constant relationship between increase in cerebrospinal fluid pressure and abolition of the headache. In these subjects there was always a recurrence of severe headache following rapid reduction in pressure. In the other four patients, because of distracting paresthesias or insufficient severity of the headache, the relation of increase in pressure to decrease in intensity of headache was not clearly defined, but in three of the four subjects headache recurred when the pressure was diminished.

In seven headaches induced by histamine the pain was abolished 14 times, each time by increasing the cerebrospinal fluid pressure, and was brought back in every instance by an immediately ensuing reduction in the pressure. In two of the seven subjects headache was abolished once and recurred once on decreasing pressure. In three it was abolished and allowed to recur twice. In two headaches, pain was abolished and reinduced by this procedure three times (Figure 9-3). Furthermore, in none of these seven induced headaches was there an instance in which increase in pressure failed to eliminate the pain.

The average initial pressure, measured before the headache was induced, was 145 mm of solution of sodium chloride. The average manometric pressure at which headache was eliminated was 480 mm of solution of sodium chloride (with a range of 350 to 550 mm). The average pressure on return of headache was 190 mm (with a range of 185 to 240 mm). Cerebrospinal fluid pressure after each increase in pressure was rapidly reduced until the headache returned to its former severity. The average amount of fluid removed to reach this state was 12 cc (with a range of 8 to 15 cc).

The average time from the moment of increasing the cerebrospinal fluid pressure to the first definite awareness of reduction in the headache was 35 seconds (with a range of 15 to 90 seconds). The average time from the moment of increase in pressure to elimination of the headache was 70 seconds (with a range of 25 to 120 seconds). The average length of time required for headache to recur (from the moment that pressure began to fall) was 45 seconds (with a range of 15 to 90 seconds).

Cerebral Arteries

By a process of elimination, it is possible to infer that the cerebral arteries are the chief sources of histamine headache. This view is based, in summary, on the following data that have been presented: (1) demonstration of afferent nerves on the larger cerebral vessels, especially those near the base of the brain (Levine & Wolff, 1932); (2) observed cerebral vasodilatation following injections of histamine (Wolff, 1938); (3) abolition of histamine headache following elevation of intracranial pressure (Pickering & Hess, 1933; Clark et al., 1938ab); (4) ineffectiveness of blocking afferent impulses from the superficial tissues of the scalp in diminishing histamine headache; (5) ineffectiveness of anesthetizing the extracranial arteries themselves; (6) lack of proof that compressing the arteries of the scalp reduces the intensity of histamine headache; (7) lack of appreciable decrease in histamine headache on one side following ligation of the middle meningeal or the temporal artery, or both arteries, on that side; and (8) development of homolateral histamine headache following the injection of the internal carotid artery.

The evidence thus far adduced indicates that many cranial arteries participate in headache but that the cerebral arteries are the chief contributors to the pain of histamine headache and determine its intensity. The question as to which cerebral arteries are implicated may now be considered further.

That the circle of Willis at the base of the brain and the proximal portions of its main branches are pain sensitive has been demonstrated on patients during cerebral exposure under local anesthesia. Furthermore, the pain is intense, definite, and constantly localized. The branches of these vessels become insensitive as they spread over the convexity or become intracerebral arteries and arterioles.

Stimulation of the internal carotid and of the anterior, middle, and posterior cerebral arteries causes pain within, behind, or over the eye as far medial as the midline and as far lateral as the temporal region. Stimulation of pontile and internal auditory branches from the basilar artery causes pain behind the ear. Faradic stimulation of the vertebral and the basilar artery and the posterior inferior cerebellar branches near their origin causes pain in the occipital and the suboccipital regions.

The headache due to histamine is distributed to a variable degree in different persons over the areas just described. It is usually worse in the frontal and the temporal region, but sometimes begins in the occipital and the suboccipital area and moves forward. It is to be expected, therefore, that histamine headache arises from branches of several main arteries to the intracranial cavity: namely, the vertebral arterial branches of the subclavian artery; the basilar artery, which is derived from a confluence of the two vertebral arteries; the posterior cerebral arteries, resulting from a bifurcation of the basilar artery; and, finally, the middle and anterior branches of the internal carotid artery.

In short, it has been demonstrated that the arteries of the scalp are capable of contributing to headache experimentally induced by histamine and that the contribution made by them may vary in different persons, the implication of these arteries possibly adding to the distribution of the headache. Furthermore, evidence has been presented to show that the cerebral arteries are important sources of headache experimentally induced by histamine and that in the absence of pain contributions from the extracranial and dural arteries the intensity of the histamine headache is not diminished. It seems probable that the large arteries at the base of the brain, which include the internal carotid, the vertebral, the basilar artery, and the proximal portions of their branches, are the primary sites of origin of pain in the headache resulting from histamine.

SERIES II

Pain Pathways Involved in Distention of Cerebral and Pial Arteries

In the following experiments designed to demonstrate these pain pathways, headaches were induced by intravenous administration of histamine in subjects who had previously had section of various cranial and cervical nerves. Most of the patients had had partial or complete section of the sensory root of the fifth cranial nerve for trigeminal neuralgia. Others had had section of the 7th, 8th, 9th or 10th cranial nerve. Also studied were patients who had had section of cervical dorsal roots, patients who had disease of the bulb and of the cervical region of the cord, and those who had had section of the sympathetic trunk.

Based on common knowledge concerning the distribution of pain fibers to the skin over the head and neck, the assumption was made that the face and head as high as the vertex are supplied chiefly by the fifth cranial nerve and that the back of the head and neck are supplied chiefly by the second and third cervical nerves. Analgesia in these regions was assumed to be due to destruction of the aforementioned respective pathways or their nuclei. Though other afferent pathways are believed to carry pain fibers from the head, such as the first cervical and the 11th and 12th cranial nerves from the occiput, and the 7th, 9th, and 10th cranial nerves from the region in and just behind the ear, interruption of these pathways did not result in demonstrable analgesia. In these experiments, therefore, anatomic inferences as to which pathways were interrupted were based, whenever possible, on surgical visualization rather than on the area of analgesia (Ray, 1954).

Pickering and Hess (1933) reported that in normal subjects headache induced by histamine affects both sides of the head equally; this we have confirmed. It usually begins in the forehead just above the orbits, occasionally in the temples and while remaining maximal there, sometimes spreads over the vertex and frequently into the occipital region as it increases in severity. It may, however, begin in the occiput and move forward (Figure 9-4).

In this study, subjects with unilateral analgesia were chiefly employed. Thus, the normal side served as a suitable control for the abnormal side in each case. Because in the normal person headache induced by histamine was symmetric and equal on the two sides, the following assumption was made: if headache failed regularly to be induced in an analgesic area on one side of the head but occurred regularly in the corresponding area on the opposite intact side, the absence of headache on the analgesic side was due to the interruption of the afferent pathway conducting impulses interpreted as headache in that region of the head (Schumacher et al., 1940).

Method. Areas of anesthesia over the face, scalp, and neck of the subject were carefully mapped out and recorded. Perception of pin prick and of cotton wool was routinely tested, as

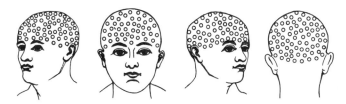

Figure 9-4. Site of headache, indicated by circles, following the injection of histamine in a normal person.

was also sensation of the cornea. The subject then lay on a stretcher in preparation for an intravenous injection of 0.1 mg of histamine phosphate.

In order to be sure that the cranial arteries were stretched adequately during the experiments, photographic records of the pulsations of these arteries were made during each induced headache (Clark et al., 1936ab).

Several control records of pulsations of the normal temporal artery with control readings of the pulse and blood pressure were made. After administration of the histamine, while the arterial puslations were being recorded and frequent readings of the pulse and blood pressure were being made, the subject was interrogated repeatedly as to the site and intensity of the headache. After subsidence of the headache, the experience was again carefully reviewed with the subject. In all cases of induced histamine headache, the photographic record indicated substantial increase in the amplitude of pulsations of the temporal artery.

This series of experiments was performed on 20 subjects, who were separated into several groups according to the afferent pathways interrupted. The location of the histamine headache in each of these groups was as follows:

Partial section of the sensory root of the fifth cranial nerve with no analgesia. In one subject an incomplete rhizotomy of the fifth cranial nerve had been performed, with resultant abolition of tic douloureux. Subsequently, no analgesia could be demonstrated. After injection of histamine the man had severe bifrontal headache.

Partial section of the sensory root of the fifth cranial nerve with unilateral analgesia of the lower part of the face. Six subjects had unilateral loss of cutaneous sensation in the lower portion of the face due to partial section of the sensory root of the fifth cranial nerve on one side, the outermost fibers of the root having been cut. After intravenous injection of histamine, all these persons had bilateral headache. In three it occurred only in the frontal region, but in two it involved the entire head (frontal, temporal, parietal, and occipital areas; Figure 9-5). The sixth patient had headache which was confined to the center of the front of the head, extending somewhat to both sides.

Complete section of the sensory root of the fifth cranial nerve with unilateral analgesia of the whole face and anterior half of the scalp. In eight subjects, as a result of complete section of the sensory root of the fifth cranial nerve, hemianalgesia of the face and of the anterior half of the scalp (including corneal anesthesia) was found. In seven of these subjects, headache was not induced in the frontotemporoparietal region of the head on the side on which the nerve had been cut, but was present elsewhere in the head (Figure 9-5). In three of the seven it was induced only in the frontotemporoparietal region of the opposite side; in the remaining four it occurred both in the frontotemporoparietal region of the opposite side

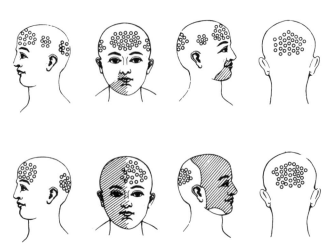

Figure 9-5. Areas of headache following the injection of histamine, and of analgesia to pin prick in a person who first had partial section and then complee section of the sensory root of the fifth cranial nerve.

and in the back of the head on both sides. The eighth subject had headache in the frontoparietal region on both sides, being more severe on the side on which the nerve had been cut.

Pickering and Hess (1933) induced headache with histamine in three patients in whom by surgical intervention cutaneous sensation over the area of distribution of the trigeminal nerve was completely abolished on one side. In all three, headache was confined to the side of the head on which normal innervation was preserved.

Northfield (1938) likewise injected histamine into seven subjects who had had complete section of the sensory root of the trigeminal nerve on one side. In three persons, the resulting headache was restricted to the forehead and temple of the opposite side and the back of the head on both sides. In two subjects headache was distributed over both sides of the front of the head, and in one of these it was worse on the side of the operation. In the remaining two persons no headache occurred, but in one of these injection of 10 cc of air into the lumbar theca produced bilateral headache in the back of the head, later involving only the front and side of the head on the normal side.

A comparison of the results described by Pickering and Hess (1933) and by Northfield (1938) with those obtained by us in cases of complete section of the sensory root of the trigeminal nerve shows incomplete agreement. In seven of eight subjects in the series reported here, headache could not be induced in the analgesic region on the denervated side. Pickering and Hess found this to be true of all their three subjects. Northfield, however, obtained similar results for only three of seven subjects. Of the remaining four subjects, two had headache on the denervated side and two had none at all. The results for the latter may be omitted from consideration on the basis of an insufficient histamine effect; unless a headache is actually induced by an adequate intravenous amount of histamine, it is not possible to draw inferences as to the effect of interruption of a given afferent pathway on the site of headache. Northfield found, nevertheless, that in one of these two subjects headache produced by another means, namely, the injection of air into the spinal subarachnoid space, resulted in pain on only the normally innervated side of the front of the head and on both sides of the back of the head. Thus, in Northfield's series, four of six subjects had no pain in the denervated area but had it elsewhere in the head whereas two also had headache on the denervated side.

In combining the results of our investigations with those of the other workers, it is seen that

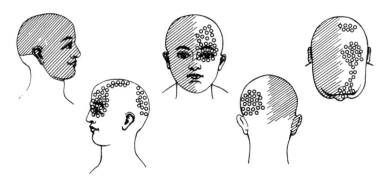

Figure 9-6.   Sites of headache in a person in whom a lesion of the brain stem has produced complete hemianalgesia.

of a total of 17 subjects with complete section of the sensory root of the trigeminal nerve, 14 experienced no headache in the frontoparietal region on the side of the root section after injection of histamine, though all experienced it in other parts of the head.

Lesion of the brain stem and upper part of the cervical region of the cord, with hemianalgesia of the head.

Lesion of the brain stem and upper part of the cervical region of the cord, with hemianalgesia of the head.   One subject had hemianalgesia of the face, forehead, and scalp, including the occipital region, as a result of an injury to the head. The lesion involved, among other structures, the descending sensory nucleus of the trigeminal nerve, including the upper cervical sensory levels of the cord. On injection of histamine this subject had severe headache in the frontal and occipital areas on the normal side but none on the analgesic side (Figure 9-6).

Multiple section of the roots of the cervical and cranial nerve with hemianalgesia of the head.   Two subjects with extensive infiltration of carcinoma (into the orbit and jaw, respectively) had had several nerves sectioned because of intractable pain. Both had had complete unilateral section of the sensory root of the fifth cranial nerve, the ninth cranial nerve, and the sensory roots of the second and third cervical nerves. In addition, one had section also of the 10th cranial nerve and of the sensory root of the 1st cervical nerve. In neither was the pain induced by the carcinoma completely abolished. In each, pain was present on the denervated side of the head before the experiment was begun. The pain seemed to become worse after the administration of histamine, though the induced headache was felt also on the other side of the head. Cooperation was poor, and the reports were difficult to evaluate.

Syringomyelia with unilateral occipital analgesia.   In one patient occipital hemianalgesia had resulted from syringomyelia. After injection of histamine, headache occurred "in the center of the back of the head" and slightly in the front of the head, but was most intense in the back on the normal side. On the analgesic side of the back of the head pain was absent.

Headache following the injection of histamine was absent on one side of the back of the head in two subjects with lesions of the cervical portion of the cord and occipital analgesia (including the subject with complete hemianalgesia of the head mentioned above). This evidence suggests that the cervical nerves are afferent pathways for impulses giving rise to occipital headache.

It is relevant to consider further the afferent pathway for some of the painful impulses from the occiput and the posterior fossa. Stimulation of the dural arteries of the posterior fossa, with faradic current, causes pain to be experienced in the occiput. Similarly, stimulation of the vertibral artery and the proximal segment of the posterior inferior cerebellar artery gives rise to pain in the occiput and subocciput. The proximal segments of the pontile and the internal auditory artery are supplied by fibers, stimulation of which causes pain behind the ear. Section of cranial and cervical nerves followed by stimulation of pain-sensitive structures in the posterior fossa indicated further that these structures are supplied chiefly by branches of the 9th and 10th cranial nerves and the first three cervical nerves.

Section of the seventh cranial nerve. In one patient extirpation of an acoustic neurinoma on the left side involved section of the left seventh and eight cranial nerves close to the brain stem. The operation required a transverse incision across the back of the head at the level of the external occipital protuberance. At the time of this experiment the patient had complete anesthesia of the occipital region from the external occipital protuberance to the vertex, left nerve deafness, and complete palsy of the left side of the face. The headache following intravenous injection of histamine was severe, bilateral, and equal on the two sides and was limited to the frontotemporal region.

This observation demonstrated that the seventh cranial nerve does not play a major part in conduction of the pain impulses resulting from effects of histamine on cranial arteries, since severe frontal and temporal headache was experienced by the subject when the nerve was sectioned close to the brain stem. This face is of interest, because it has been shown that afferent nerves from the pial arteries enter the brain stem through the seventh cranial nerve. Apparently, this nerve is not an important afferent path for pain.

The effect of section of the eighth cranial nerve can be waived in a discussion of histamine headache, since it has been repeatedly demonstrated that no pain results from stimulation of the central end of this nerve.

Section of the glossopharyngeal nerve. In one subject the glossopharyngeal nerve had been sectioned as a therapeutic measure for anomalous tic douloureux. After section, the patient was relieved on the symptoms and had poorly defined analgesia in the back of the throat and over the tonsil. Intravenous injection of histamine phosphate was associated with the usual generalized headache, which did not differ on the two sides of the head.

It may be inferred, therefore, that the glossopharyngeal nerve does not play a major role in conveying impulses essential to the headache experimentally induced by histamine.

It is, however, impossible to exclude both the seventh and the ninth cranial nerves, as taking no part in conduction of pain, for, according to the hypothesis stated previously, the absence of minor contributions to the headache could not be appreciated if the most intense contribution, conveyed along other pathways, was still present.

Section of the sympathetic trunk. One subject, who had had bilateral section of the cervical portion of the sympathetic trunk at the stellate ganglion for Raynaud's disease, experienced severe and generalized headache after injection of histamine. A second patient, who had had bilateral section of the second and third thoracic white rami communications, in addition to transection of the thoracic portion of the sympathetic trunk beneath the third ganglion, also had generalized headache after injection of histamine.

Although Dandy (1931) produced termination of severe hemicrania in two patients by resecting the inferior cervical and the first thoracic ganglion on the side of the pain, both Northfield (1938) and Pickering and Hess (1933), on injecting histamine into patients after this operation, found that resection of the ganglia did not modify the usual distribution of the headache experimentally induced by histamine.

The fact that the patients with unilateral analgesia in the occipital and suboccipital regions have less or no pain in these regions after administration of histamine suggests that the sensory roots of the upper cervical nerves (1st, 2nd, and 3rd) and the 9th and 10th cranial nerves are afferent pathways for these sensations. However, section of the 5th, 7th, 9th, and 10th cranial nerves and the sensory roots of the 1st, 2nd, and 3rd cervical nerves did not eliminate the headache due to histamine or that due to invasion of the skull and dura by carcinoma. Also, section of the seventh or the ninth cranial nerve alone failed to diminish perceptibly the headache experimentally induced by histamine. It is therefore evident that the afferent pathways are numerous, and that to ascribe the entire function of the sensation of headache to one or another nerve is an unjustified simplification.

Other Headaches Resulting Primarily from Distention of Cerebral and Pial Arteries

Headache Associated with Infection and Fever

Septicemia, bacteremia, and fever are commonly associated with headache. It is unlikely, however, that the agent responsible for the fever is identical to that resulting in the headache. The most intense, prolonged headaches associated with infections occurring in this part of the world are those that accompany typhoid fever, typhus fever, and influenza. The headache is dull, deep, aching, generalized, but is often worse, especially at the beginning, in the back of the head. It is increased in intensity by bodily effort. It is often worse in the latter part of the day, especially if the patient is ambulatory, or when the patient is most exhausted or prostrated. The intensity of pain is decreased by manual compression of the common carotid artery. It is not modified appreciably by ergotamine tartrate, except possibly toward the end of the period of the headache.

A 19-year-old laboratory technician, who daily manipulated both murine and scrub typhus virus at her work, entered the hospital complaining of severe headache with occasional fever. Six days before admission she developed a moderately severe occipital headache. During the intervening 5 days this headache was of increasing intensity, recurred daily, was worse in the late afternoon and evening, and persisted through the night. It was usually absent the following morning. At the time of the headache her face was flushed. The headache was of a throbbing, aching quality, made worse by turning the head, by bending over, or by bodily effort. It became generalized, and was often most intense in the frontal region, especially during the 3 days before admission. The headache was not affected by acetylsalicylic acid, 0.6 g, but was appreciably diminished by codeine phosphate, 60 mg. The patient had no stiff neck, nausea, or vomiting. She was able to work until the day of hospitalization, and the fierce headache was out of all proportion to the general constitutional symptoms and signs. She had a moderate leukopenia and a temperature of 38.5°C. Two rose-colored macules were found under each breast.

Seven months before this illness the patient had been inoculated with both murine and scrub typhus vaccine. Three days after her hospital admission, or 9 days after onset, the headache spontaneously ended, and she became symptom free. Tests of antibody titer established the diagnosis of murine typhus fever.

It was possible to observe in experimental animals, prepared so that the pial vessels could be visualized through a skull window, that the intravenous injection of foreign protein (typhoid vaccine) was followed by cerebral vasodilatation. Such vasodilatation was sometimes, but not always, associated with fever. Because of the use of barbiturates in inducing anesthesia, which was necessary to the experiment, fever was inconstantly obtained. No change in the pressure of the cerebrospinal fluid was observed, though sometimes the pressure became slightly higher. The vaşodilatation was usually extreme, and it was suggested that headache would probably follow such a state.

Since it has been observed that the fever induced by the intravenous administration of typhoid vaccine is frequently associated with headache or with sensations of fullness in the head, the relation of the cranial arteries to the headache was experimentally investigated in observations of patients who were undergoing fever therapy for chorea or rheumatoid arthritis.

Method. A tambour was placed on the temporal artery, a needle introduced into the lumbar sac, and the pulsations simultaneously recorded as heretofore described. After a suitable control period, during which records were made, an appropriate amount (25,000,000 to 1,000,000,000 bacteria per cubic centimeter) of typhoid vaccine was administered intravenously. If no chill or rise in temperature took place within 60 or 90 minutes, a second and smaller amount was given. Estimates of the state of the headache, determinations of the blood pressure, and records of the pulsations of the cerebrospinal fluid and the temporal artery were made at frequent intervals throughout the procedure.

Results. Twelve such experiments were performed. Because of the many hours of immobilization necessary for a complete record of the beginning and the end of the cycle of fever and the consequent discomfort to patients with arthritis, experiments completely satisfactory from a technical point of view were not obtained. However, the observations were adequate and consistent and permitted inferences (Figure 9-7).

Onset of a headache or a sensation of fullness in the head was found in all instances to follow increased amplitude of pulsations of the cerebrospinal fluid and of the temporal artery. Spontaneous lessening of the headache closely paralleled the decrease in amplitude of these pulsations, and as the amplitude of the pulsations again increased, the headache became more severe. With the ultimate decline in amplitude of the pulsations the headache ended. The pressure of the cerebrospinal fluid was at all times within the usual physiologic limits.

Observations of the temporal artery and the cerebrospinal fluid showed that here, too, the spontaneous increase and decrease of the headache paralleled the amplitude of pulsations.

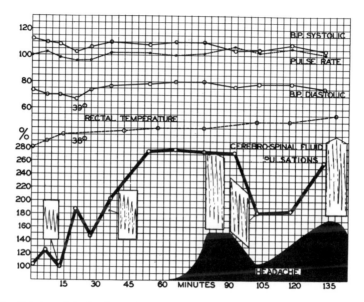

Figure 9-7. Relation of the headache associated with intravenous injection of typhoid vaccine to the amplitude of pulsations of the cerebrospinal fluid. The onset, increase, and decrease in intensity of the headache paralleled the amplitude of pulsations of the cerebrospinal fluid. A spontaneous remission in the severity of the headache paralleled the decrease in the amplitude of pulsations of the cerebrospinal fluid.

The similarity between the pyrexial headache and those induced by histamine was previously noted. The amplitude of pulsations of the cerebrospinal fluid in headache induced by fever and by histamine was greatly increased, in contrast with that in migraine headache, in which there was no increase in amplitude. Pickering and Hess (1933) added the observation that increasing the cerebrospinal fluid pressure by means of a manometer attached to a needle in the lumbar subarachnoid space reduced fever headache.

The fact that increasing the intracranial pressure decreased the intensity of the headache indicates that the mechanism of the headache in fever and that of the headache following injection of histamine are similar and that in both the intracranial arteries are the chief contributors to the pain. It is likely that the headache associated with acute infections, fever, sepsis, and bacteremia has such an explanation.

Although any fever or infection may be associated with headache, some of the common fevers and infectious diseases that have been linked with severe headache as initiating or accompanying symptom, but that in themselves have no special identifying characteristics, are as follows:

Those of bacterial origin include: pneumonia, septicemia, tonsillitis and adenoiditis, scarlet fever, chorea, typhoid fever, paratyphoid fever, undulant fever (brucellosis), tularemia, bubonic plague, Haverhill fever.

Those of probable viral origin include acute coryza, influenza, herpes simplex, measles, mumps, smallpox, poliomyelitis, yellow fever, dengue, rabies, rubella, infectious mononucleosis.

Those of rickettsial origin include: typhus fever, trench fever, oroya fever.

Headache with the attack of malarial fever may be intense.

Accessory evidence that dilatation of intracranial vessels accompanies some acute systemic infections is provided by observations of changes in the force required to produce headache by rapid head movement during the illness. It has been noted, for example, that during a 3-week period of recurrent chills and fever induced by therapeutic tertian malaria, the threshold to jolt headache (expressed in g units) fell from a control level of 6.9 to values as low as 1.6 g. This depression of threshold was not entirely dependent upon the presence of high body temperature, for it varied independently of the height of the fever.

Similarly, in another patient, a lowered threshold to jolt headache could be demonstrated during the first stage of an acute nasopharyngitis accompanied by malaise and lethargy, and during an attack of acute gastroenteritis, also with systemic symptoms, and presumably of the winter viral type.

"Hangover" Headache

As mentioned earlier, there is a good deal of evidence that hangover headache due to excessive alcohol ingestion belong in the category under discussion. Although cerebral blood flow is increased in acute alcoholic intoxication, the mechanism of headache that follows, usually in the morning after alcohol intoxication, is complicated. So-called impurities in alcoholic beverages may also have significant pharmacodynamic effects, but their relevance to hangover headache is difficult to define. Although ethyl alcohol causes cerebral vessels to dilate and CBF to increase, the period of maximum alcohol concentration in the blood does not necessarily correlate with the severity of headache. The headache is usually most severe when the alcohol concentration in the blood is reduced or minimal. However, alcohol is well known as a precipitator of migraine and cluster headache, possibly because of increased prostacyclin synthesis, and aspirin and indomethacin, which are potent cerebral vasoconstrictors, usually lessen hangover headaches. Repeated trials with the experimental administration of 60 to 90 ml of 95% ethyl alcohol have not been followed by headache, even in those who suffer from frequent vascular headaches.

Intake of alcohol under laboratory conditions, however, is quite different from social drinking. The discipline imposed by experimental situations precludes the excitement that accompanies its use in a party setting. It appears, therefore, as though the action of the alcohol in inducing headache is indirect, although it is likely that the headache results from cranial vasodilatation. The throbbing quality, the increase in intensity with elevation of blood pressure or sudden head movement, the decline in intensity on carotid artery compression, which sometimes follows the administration of vasoconstrictor agents, such as caffeine by mouth or ergotamine tartrate by intravenous injection, support this view. It is unlikely that edema of the brain is relevant to the headache.

The common observation that hangover headache is readily aggravated by head movement offers suggestive evidence for dilatation of intracranial vessels as a factor in this type of headache. Accelerometer measurements in one patient revealed that jolts of 4.0 to 4.2 g would intensify his usual right temporal hangover headache, whereas on symptom-free days jolts of 5.5 g or much higher would be required to induce headache.

It is suggested that the vasodilator type of headache results not only from the pharmacodynamic action of alcohol and impurities on cranial vessels, but also from the effects on the subject of late hours, loss of sleep, excitement of social intercourse (talking, singing, and laughing), sustained effort and exhaustion, loss of restraint, and perhaps some remorse. In short, it is associated with psychobiologic factors akin to those operating in certain other types of vascular headaches.

However, since hangover headache is by no means a rare phenomenon and can be produced for experimental purposes so readily, it presents an inviting problem for further study.

It has been demonstrated that oral fructose increases the rate of alcohol metabolism in the healthy human (Pawan, 1968). Mean blood alcohol levels are lower after the ingestion of fructose, using the subject as his own control. Thirty grams of fructose will increase the rate of metabolism of alcohol by 15 to 30 %. No other sugars have this effect on alcohol metabolism, including glucose, galactose, and sucrose. Large amounts of vitamins including the B-complex vitamins, ascorbic acid, vitamin E, and the like do not effect the rate of alcohol metabolism in the healthy human. This being the case, it is possible to reduce the intensity and frequency of hangover headache by employing fructose, either therapeutically or prophylactically.

The mechanism of action of fructose is uncertain. However, alcohol dehydrogenase is the rate-limiting enzyme in the degradation of alcohol and this is dependent, to a considerable extent, on the availability of the hydrogen acceptor, nicotinamide-adenine-dinucleotide (NAD). It is suggested that fructose stimulates the conversion of NADH to NAD, which allows the rate of alcohol metabolism to be partially accelerated.

Postseizure Headache

The headache that follows an epileptic attack with loss of consciousness, with or without convulsive movements, is a generalized, moderately intense, throbbing pain, usually of several hours' duration. It is noted when the patient regains consciousness, is often associated with a desire to sleep, and may be absent when the patient awakes.

The human brain has been repeatedly observed during the convulsive seizure. An initial pallor may be noted just preceding and during the first part of the fit. However, whether or not initial pallor is noted, the latter part of the fit and the postfit stage are always accompanied by widespread vasodilatation of cerebral vessels. The dilated vessels are first cyanotic, and then bright red. Because this bright red dilated phase persists for several hours, it is suggested that this cerebral artery dilatation is the basis of the postepileptic headache.

Measurements of CBF in humans, as well as in experimental animals, support the view that cerebral congestion is responsible for postseizure headaches (Meyer et al., 1966). During the seizures cerebral metabolism and blood flow are generally increased, cerebral autoregulation is lost, and marked acidosis and hyperemia of the brain result.

Headache Associated with Hypoxia

Experimentally induced cerebral hypoxemia (Wolff & Lennox, 1930), especially when coupled with an increase in carbon dioxide tension in the blood, results in extreme dilatation of cerebral vessels, notably of the arteries and arterioles. This observation is probably related to the fact that some persons at high altitudes (Monge, 1942; Barcroft et al., 1922) complain of headache that persists for hours or days until physiologic adjustments have been achieved, or until the individual returns to a lower altitude. Associated with the intense throbbing headache is a sensation of fullness of the head, hot flushes of the face, photophobia, injection of the ocular mucosa, and deep cyanosis. It is likely that such headaches are due to cerebral vascular distention.

An intense, throbbing headache of hours' or days' duration is a striking feature in persons exposed for a shorter or longer period to carbon monoxide. That the headache is due to distention of pial and cerebral vessels is extremely likely. Thus, hypoxemia resulting from inhalation of carbon monoxide has a dilator effect on the cerebral vessels. When, for experimental purposes, dilute mixtures of carbon monoxide and air were given to animals, and the cerebral blood vessels observed through cranial windows, cerebral vasodilatation, and increased cerebrospinal fluid pressure were noted. An increased cerebrospinal fluid pressure in man as well as in animals has also been demonstrated, the result, probably, of vasodilation and a change in permeability of the blood vessel walls.

It has also been shown in humans that during brief hypoxia cerebral blood flow increases remarkably (Meyer et al., 1969) so that vascular headache is a predictable outcome of more prolonged hypoxia.

Headache Associated with Ischemic Hypoxia

It has been demonstrated in animals that after sudden localized or generalized cerebral ischemia, when collateral or general circulation was reestablished, extreme cerebral vasodilatation and increased cerebral blood flow comparable to the so-called reactive hypermia of muscle and skin. This situation has also been called "luxury perfusion" because cerebral perfusion is in excess of tissue demand (Lassen, 1966). Reactive hyperemia of the brain has also been demonstrated to occur in humans after cerebral ischemic hypoxia due to temporary vascular occlusion, and these patients frequently complain of headache (Fisher, 1968).

Headache Associated with High Altitude

Appenzeller (1972) pointed out that headache may be associated with acute mountain sickness, acute pulmonary edema of altitude, and chronic mountain sickness in well-acclimatized subjects. Altitude headache is uncommon below 8000 feet, appears with increasing frequency at higher elevations, and above 12,000 feet is more or less universal in persons not acclimatized to altitude.

Altitude headache often appears hours after exposure to low oxygen tension and is not relieved by administration of oxygen. The headache is assumed to be related to vasodilatation and/or brain edema and is aggravated by maneuvers that increase intracranial pressure such as coughing, straining at stool, head jolting, and particularly exertion. Persons with altitude headache are uncomfortable when lying down. Papilledema and retinal hemorrhages have been observed in some patients with acute mountain sickness. Lumbar punctures in 34 subjects exposed to high altitude demonstrated a significant increase in cerebrospinal fluid pressure, and in one patient a biopsy of the brain revealed brain edema (Singh et al., 1960).

Table 9-1 Headache and hypoxia: neurologic signs and symptoms

Altitude, in meters (feet)	Symptoms	Alveolar PO_2 (mm Hg)	Headache
3,048 (10,000)	Impairment of recent memory, judgment, and ability to perform complex calculations; increased heart rate and pulmonary ventilation	60	Frequent in unacclimatized subjects
3,658 (12,000)	Dyspnea, impaired ability to perform complex tasks, headache, nausea, decreased visual acuity	52	Frequent in all
4,573 (15,000)	Decrease in auditory acuity, constriction of visual fields, impaired judgment, irritability; exercise can lead to unconsciousness	46	Frequent in all
5,486 (18,000)	Decrements in personality and intellect; threshold for loss of consciousness in resting unacclimatized individuals after several hours' exposure	40	Universally present
6,096 (20,000)	Handwriting illegible in conscious subjects	33	Universally present
6,706 (22,000)	Almost all individuals unconscious after sufficient exposure time	30	Universally present

Experimentally induced cerebral hypoxemia, especially when coupled with an increase in carbon dioxide tension in the blood, results in extreme dilatation of cerebral vessels, notably of the arteries and arterioles. This observation is probably related to the fact that some persons at high altitudes complain of headache that persists for hours or days until physiologic adjustments have been achieved, or until the individual returns to a lower altitude (Bancroft et al., 1922, 1925; Houston, 1976; Leufaut & Sullivan, 1971). Associated with the intense throbbing headache is a sensation of fullness of the head, hot flushes of the face, photophobia, injection of the ocular mucosa, and deep cyanosis. It is likely that such headaches are due in part to cerebral vascular distention.

Appenzeller (1972) has pointed out that altitude headache may be associated with either acute mountain sickness, acute pulmonary edema of altitude, or chronic mountain sickness in well-acclimatized subjects. Altitude headache is uncommon below 8000 feet and appears with increasing frequency at higher elevations such as 12,000 feet. Above 16,000 feet, altitude headache is more or less universal (Table 9-1).

Altitude headache often appears hours after exposure to low oxygen tension and is not relieved by administration of oxygen. The headache is assumed to be related to vasodilation and/or brain edema and is aggravated by maneuvers that increase intracranial pressure such as coughing, straining at stool, head jolting, and particularly exertion. Persons with altitude headache are uncomfortable when lying down. Papilledema and retinal hemorrhages have been observed in some patients with acute mountain sickness.

Singh et al. (1960) have investigated headache associated with acute mountain sickness. Lumbar punctures in 34 subjects exposed to high altitude demonstrated a significant increase in cerebrospinal fluid pressure, and in one patient a biopsy of the brain revealed brain edema. Manifestations usually develop in 8 to 24 hours after arrival at the high altitude and remit over 4 to 8 days. The syndrome is thus distinguished from hypoxia per se, or from chronic mountain sickness, by virtue of its time of onset, duration, and course.

Mental symptoms are frequently associated with altitude headache. If the ascent is slow, sensations of exhilaration and well-being are often described. As altitude increases, more serious mental problems develop. Mental tasks become difficult, and irritability and depression are common. To quote Barcroft: (1922)

> Alcohol affects different persons in different ways; so on my journeying in high altitudes I have seen most of the symptoms of alcoholism reproduced. I have seen men vomit, I have seen them quarrel, I have seen them become reckless, I have seen them become morose. I have seen one of the most disciplined of men fling his arms about on the ledge of a crevasse to the great embarrassment of the guide. I have seen the most loyal companion become ill-tempered and abusive to the point at which I feared international complications would arise.

These symptoms can be relieved to some degree by careful and gradual ascent, to allow acclimatization. Acetazolamide, given 250 mg every 8 hours, before and during exposure to altitude, may reduce manifestations of acute mountain sickness. Furosemide, 80 mg every 12 hours, has also been suggested. For some, the symptoms are unrelieved and descent to a lower altitude is necessary.

DECOMPRESSION HEADACHE

Arterial hypoxia, not contaminated by hypercapnea, occurs in those exposed to high altitudes and in those in decompression chambers. Decompression sickness appears when a sudden change in the pressure of ambient gases, to which the subject has become equilibrated, occurs. A sudden reduction in pressure of 45% is usually sufficient to cause symptoms.

The symptoms produced by rapid decompression are caused primarily by the formation of nitrogen gas bubbles in blood and fatty tissues. Nitrogen does not diffuse readily and is not used in body metabolism. Thus, when body fluids and tissues, saturated with N_2, are suddenly exposed to a lower pressure, bubbles of N_2 form, which lodge in small blood vessels and fatty tissues, since N_2 is five times more soluble in oil than in water (Behnke, 1965).

Similar problems occur in aviators in rapid ascent, at about 30,000 feet. This phenomenon is altered by breathing 100% O_2, or an oxygen–helium mixture, before flight, to wash N_2 out of the body, in part. When this is done, rapid ascent to 40,000 feet can be accomplished. In a pressurized cabin, of course, these problems are minimized.

Most decompression sickness now occurs in sports divers, and all patients seen by the author have been in this category. The neurologic complications can be striking (Erde & Edmonds, 1975; Kidd & Elliott, 1975). As shown in Table 9-2, both spinal cord and the brain are affected. Bilateral throbbing headache occurs frequently and

Table 9-2 Neurologic manifestations of decompression

Site	Manifestations
Central (brain)	Blurred vision, scintillating scotomata, visual field defects, bilateral throbbing headache, vertigo, speech disturbance, confusion, hemiparesis, hemisensory defects, focal or generalized seizures
Spinal cord	Low-back, radicular pain, often bilateral, and girdling, commonly in upper lumbar region; paraparesis, loss of bladder and sphincter control, hypoesthesias, sensory levels; paraplegia may occur

at times may be the only symptom of decompression sickness. The headache is often indistinguishable from classic migraine. A migraine attack after decompression may require recompression therapy, because it may be indistinguishable from arterial gas embolism to the brain.

Treatments for both high-altitude and decompression sickness are generally preventive. Descent from altitude will abolish some manifestations but may only retard others. Thus, aviators who have experienced decompression sickness should not be reexposed to even low altitudes of flight for 72-96 hours, since reexpansion of nitrogen bubbles already present in fatty tissues may exacerbate their signs and symptoms.

Adequate recompression therapy is the only specific treatment for decompression sickness. At times this may require prolonged recompression, for more than several days. All other measures can be considered as ancillary, including the use of 100% O_2, and methods to retard or prevent brain edema (dexamethasone, 8–10 mg every 4–6 hours, and intravenous injection of mannitol or dextran).

Headache Associated with Anemia

Anemia associated with hypoxemia induces headache by causing dilatation of the intracranial vessels. According to J.R. Graham (1959), anemia from sudden loss of blood is more likely to be followed by headache than that due to slow loss; but even in chronic states of anemia when the hemoglobin falls below 7.0 g, headache may follow. Nevertheless, except in the case of acute blood loss or hemolysis, anemia, with levels of hemoglobin above 11 g, is rarely in itself the cause of headache.

Hemolytic crises, whether due to congenital or acquired hemolytic anemia, transfusion reactions, sickle cell disease, Mediterranean anemia, paroxysmal hemoglobinemia, and favus bean poisoning; polycythemia vera and polycythemia secondary to hypoxia experienced with chronic pulmonary disease, congenital heart lesions, high altitude, and chronic exposure to carbon monoxide, may, because of the vasodilatation they induce, result in headache.

In addition to the cerebral oxygen deficit caused by the various anemias, similar deprivation occurs in the course of circulatory collapse, impaired pulmonary ventilation, pulmonary infiltration, pulmonary artery obstruction, and shunting cardiovascular anomalies.

Nitrite Headache

The headache experimentally induced by amyl nitrite was studied in five subjects (Wolff, 1929). The inhalation of amyl nitrite produced a prompt fall in both systolic and diastolic blood pressure. Headache was experienced when the blood pressure had returned toward the previous level, with increase in the amplitude of pulsations of the cranial arteries. The headache subsequently disappeared, with return of the pulsations to the initial level.

Some individuals exposed to nitrites, either as medicament, in food, or in industry, complain of headache (Evans, 1912; Laws, 1910). Such headaches are of a dull aching quality and are usually accompanied by a flushed face (Henderson & Raskin, 1972). The gradually increasing tolerance to the nitrites of those exposed to them usually results after a time in the spontaneous reduction or elimination of headache. A too-sudden increase in the amount of nitrites absorbed, beyond the tolerance of the subject, is commonly followed by a recrudescence of the headache. Reduction in amount, or withdrawal of the agent, is then followed by recession of the headache. It is reported that the use of vasoconstrictors such as ephedrine and benzedrine has been followed by elimination of nitrite headaches or a reduction in their intensity. This statement is difficult to accept without suitable evidence, because, as shown above, even the powerful constrictor effect of ergotamine tartrate is nullified by the nitrite dilator action. Moreover, no control series of subjects with such headaches who received only placebos has been studied.

Headache Caused by Chemical Agents, with and without Anemic Cerebral Vasodilatation

Chief among these headaches are those caused by carbon monoxide. Acetanilid, when used in excess, may cause headache by converting hemoglobin to methemoglobin, with resultant hypoxemia. In addition to the methemoglobinemia and sulfhemoglobinemia such as follows the ingestion of nitrates, sulfonamides, aniline compounds, acetanilid, and phenacetin, are those headaches that occur in the acute stage of poisoning from ethyl alcohol, carbon tetrachloride, benzene, arsenic, lead, anticholinesterase, insecticides, and the nitrates including nitroglycerin. Apresoline, thorazine, and calcium channel blockers, by virtue of their vasodilating action, may produce headache in some patients. Withdrawal of cerebral vasoconstrictive agents such as ergotamin, amphetamine, and methysergide from those who have been using them in excess for long periods, may precipitate severe headache. A common situation in patients with chronic cluster and migraine headaches is habitual use of ergotamine with resulting ergotamine-withdrawal headaches when the drug is discontinued. This results in a vicious circle of daily headaches, which is best treated by total withdrawal of ergotamine.

Headache with Electrolyte Disturbance due to Ill-Defined Factors

Headache may also be associated with states of dehydration and disturbed electrolyte balance, that is, excess loss of fluid and electrolytes in the course of diarrhea, vomiting, postoperative fistulas, heat exhaustion, diuresis, and removal of ascitic fluid.

Caffeine-Withdrawal Headache

Pharmacologically, caffeine is a cerebral vasoconstrictor, and withdrawal presumably results in excessive cerebral vasodilatation and vascular congestion. In studies of two subjects, caffeine-withdrawal headache has been shown to have many features suggesting that the pain arises from distention of intracranial, and possibly of extracranial, arteries. Like the headache induced by histamine given intravenously caffeine-withdrawal headache is reduced in intensity by sustained straining or jugular compression, is readily accentuated by "jolt' movements of the head, and is eliminated during exposure to centrifugal force of 2.0 g in the head-to-seat direction.

"Hunger" Headache

When a meal is missed or postponed, the subsequent hypoglycemia in persons subject to vascular headache may induce headache. Headache may also occur as a symptom of impending insulin shock in diabetics and patients with islet cell tumor of the pancreas. Headache as a manifestation of hypoglycemia may be a feature in patients suffering from hypopituitarism, adrenocortical insufficiency, hypothyroidism, and liver disease. Von Brauch (1957) called attention to the fact that headache may occur with hypoglycemic states. An important implication from this and other papers on the subject is that a serious change in the internal environment of the organism, such as occurs with low oxygen, high carbon dioxide, low sugar, or acidosis that threatens survival of the neuron, evokes extreme cerebral vasodilatation. This then becomes the essential element in inducing the headache.

In a small series of subjects, Kunkle and Barker of the New York Hospital demonstrated that there is a relation between headache, food deprivation, the blood-sugar level, and threshold of jolt headache. Food deprivation, either with or without a fall of blood-sugar level, may be associated with lowering of the pain threshold. Thus, in one subject after 8 hours of fasting, the jolt headache threshold dropped from 7.0 to 5.1 g. In another subject, after insulin injected intravenously, when the blood-sugar level fell from 85 to 24 mg/100 cc, the threshold of jolt headache fell from 5.9 to 3.3 g. And inversely, after ingestion of 50 g of glucose, when the blood-sugar rose to normal (95 mg/100 cc) the threshold of jolt headache also rose to 6.3 g. These data further support the view that hunger headaches stem from pain-sensitive intracranial vessels.

Salzer (1960), who has examined and treated many patients with functional hyperinsulinism, describes a patient who had had resection of the right temporal artery for what was assumed to be a temporal arteritis of 2 years' duration. She also had had a laminectomy for removal of bony spurs impinging on the second cervical root—all without beneficial effect. A 6-hour glucose tolerance test revealed a blood-sugar fall to levels of 25 mg/100 ml at the fourth hour. The author, unfortunately, does not state if headache was precipitated during these periods of low glucose level! The patient was free of headache after a few weeks on a modified diet.

It is freely conceded that vascular headache may result during some episodes of hyperinsulinism and during the hunger that results from missing a meal. Sometimes under these circumstances there is fatigue, tension, irritability, and mood changes. It is in such a setting that headache of the vascular type or of the muscle-contraction variety may develop. On the other hand, low blood sugar, so-called functional hyperinsulinism, may be but one aspect of a patient's reaction to his or her difficult situation and not necessarily the direct mediator of the headache.

Thus granting that some persons with headache probably do develop a headache with low blood-sugar levels, functional hyperinsulinism still cannot be considered a common primary cause of headache.

Clinical Application. The headaches associated with fever, sepsis, bacteremia, anoxia, nitrites, and convulsions are modified by acetylsalicylic acid in 0.3-to 0.6 g amounts, and by codeine phosphate in 60-mg amounts; which agent should be used depends on the intensity of the pain. It is obvious, however, that the eradication of the underlying infection is most pertinent.

An increase in the oxygen content of the blood is followed by narrowing of cerebral and pial arteries (Wolff & Lennox, 1930). Hence, the breathing of high concentrations of oxygen may sufficiently oxygenate the blood that headache due to dilated intracranial arteries is diminished in intensity or eliminated. The headaches associated with carbon monoxide poisoning and other anoxemias, and the postseizure headache, may be modified by the inhalation of high concentrations of oxygen. For the same reason, patients with cluster headache who appear to have an unusually marked cerebral vasoconstrictive response to inhalation of 100% oxygen often report temporary but effective symptomatic relief of cluster headache during inhalation of 100% oxygen for 15 minutes (Sakai & Meyer, 1979).

"Ice Cream" Headache

Raskin and Knittle (1976) have noted the tendency for "ice-cream headache" and orthostatic symptoms to occur in patients with migraine. This occurs provided the stimulus is cold enough, prolonged, and applied to the pharynx. Application of similar cold materials in the esophagus or stomach does not cause headache. The pain may be situated at the vertex, is often felt behind the eyes or in the frontal areas; it is almost always associated with the ingestion of ice cream, hence the name. Raskin and Knittle suggest that patients with migraine are particularly susceptible to ice cream headache; they imply that this phenomenon is a biological marker for migraine.

Postendarterectomy Hemicrania

Leviton et al. (1975) have described postendarterectomy hemicranial headache, a benign and self-limited condition occurring in patients 3 to 4 days after the operative procedure has been performed. The pain is hemicranial, throbbing, and indistinguishable from the usual migraine episode. It occurs primarily in those who have had migraine attacks prior to the carotid surgery. This disorder is perhaps due to a sudden increase in blood flow through a vascular system conditioned to low flow because of atherosclerosis.

Orgasmic Headache

A particular variety of exertional headache is associated with the physical activity of sexual intercourse, and hence the term orgasmic headache. In 1974 Paulson and Klawans called attention to this variety of severe headache that appeared to occur in association with orgasm. They described 14 patients seen over the course of several years who had severe head pain, either during or immediately after orgasm. The headache was often behind the eyes, bilateral or occipital, and of varying intensity, though usually rather short-lived. The pain was almost always throbbing. Paulson and Klawans divided the patients into two groups on the basis of the presumed pathophysiology of the headache. Three patients were thought to have low spinal fluid pressure, which was documented in two patients, perhaps as a result of a tear in the subarachnoid membranes that occurred or was widened during the physiologic stress of coitus. The relationship of posture to pain in these patients was identical to that seen in patients with headache following lumbar puncture. In 11 other patients, Paulson and Klawans suggested that vascular factors were of pathophysiologic significance. The point of their paper was that the benign course of 14 patients differed from the usual impression that headaches associated with intercourse result from rupture or expansion of a vascular malformation or aneurysm.

In reply to this report, Lundberg and Osterman (1974) presented a brief report on the benign and malignant forms of headache associated with orgasm. They agreed with Paulson and Klawans that there is a benign but sometimes very troublesome and usually recurring type of vascular headache starting at the climax of sexual intercourse, and mentioned a number of such cases that had been followed for several years at the University of Uppsala. They pointed out, however, that bleeding associated with subarachnoid hemorrhage may occur at the time of intercourse; they described six patients in whom this had happened. Lundberg and Osterman emphasized that the occurrence of vomiting, disturbance of consciousness, stiff neck, and residual pain the day after the incident characterized the headache caused by subarachnoid hemorrhage and distinguished it from that of benign orgasmic cephalgia. Fisher (1968) reviewed his experience with 66 representative cases of subarachnoid hemorrhage caused by the rupture of saccular aneurysms; in 3 of these, the hemorrhage was associated with intercourse.

Levy (1981) has described a 24-year-old male who suffered a stroke in the setting of sexual intercourse and orgasm. This patient developed a hemiparesis, without aphasia, and gradually recovered over the next month. He had a prior history of migraine. Levy suggests that this case represents an example of complicated migraine occurring in association with coitus.

We have examined four men with orgasmic headache. In all, the pain was bilateral, bioccipital, and throbbing in character. It generally occurred at climax, lasted approximately 1 hour, and was not associated with nausea, vomiting, photophobia, or speech and movement defects. Three of our four subjects had multiple episodes of this type. None had serious sequelae (Table 9-3).

Thus, it seems evident that there are benign and malignant forms of headache associated with intercourse or, in formal terms, orgasmic cephalgia. In most cases this is a benign syndrome. However, the alert clinician will be aware that a severe and disabling headache may result from bleeding at the time of intercourse due to rupture of a saccular aneurysm. The subsequent course of patients should differentiate the benign from the malignant forms of head pain. where there is doubt, however, further neurologic studies are certainly indicated, particularly spinal puncture, computerized tomographic (CT) scan of the head, and/or contrast studies.

The etiology of effort headache is multifactorial. Many effort headaches are obviously those of classic migraine, particularly the headaches occurring after prolonged exertion, as in long distance races. In most effort headaches, hypoxia does not play a role, although hypoxia is capable of extending and increasing the vascular headache produced by effort. Headache is a common complaint of the individual who exerts at high altitude, and it may be made worse by exposure to cold, breath-

Table 9-3 Benign orgasmic headache

Researcher	Date	No. of patients	Manifestations	Sequelae
Paulson & Klawans	1974	14	Bilateral throbbing low CSF in 3	No serious sequelae
Lundberg & Osterman	1974	50	Bilateral throbbing at climax	SAH in 6
Fisher	1968	60 with SAH	3 had onset at intercourse	
Levy	1981	1	Climax onset	Right hemiparesis slow recovery
Dalessio	1974	4 (all male)	Bilateral brief throbbing at climax	No serious sequelae

lessness, dyspnea, and fatigue. This leads naturally to considerations of the next topic.

Effort (Exertional) Headache and Migraine

Exertional headache is an uncommon disorder in which head pain appears to be related to exertion or straining (Rooke, 1968). It commonly affects men in a broad age range from 10 to 70 years. Almost always, exertional headache is a benign, though disconcerting, symptom. Approximately 30% of patients are improved or free of this symptom within 5 years, and over 70% are free of headache within 10 years. Diamond (1977) has suggested that indomethacin, 75 mg per day, may be helpful in patients with this disorder.

Jokl (1965) was perhaps the first to note migraine occurring after exercise. His own description of this problem is graphic:

> During my freshman year in medical school I ran as an anchor man in the mile relay team of my university and the German track championships of Jena, Thuringia. We won by the smallest possible margin. I was then 17 years old and this was the first time I had been clocked in under fifty seconds. A few minutes after the race my happiness over the victory was interrupted by an attack of nausea, headache, prolonged weakness and vomiting. It lasted fifteen minutes whereupon it quickly subsided. None of my professors were able to explain this episode, not could I find appropriate reference in any textbooks of physiology or medicine.

Jokl and Jokl (1977) noted several profound cases of effort migraine during the Olympic games in Mexico City and described these to one of the authors (Dalessio, 1974). The high altitude was an obvious predisposing factor, as was heat, humidity, and perhaps lack of training. Migraine after effort tended to occur with prolonged running rather than sprints. These highly conditioned athletes developed scotomata, unilateral retro-orbital pain, nausea, vomiting, and in some cases a striking prostration occurred.

Rooke's (1968) series of benign exertional headache, encompassing 103 cases, includes some in which no significant exertion is described. Nonetheless, he finds

Table 9-4 Effort migraine in runners

Age	Sex	History of migraine	Family history of migraine	Scotomata/ field defects	Paresis/ sensory defects	Permanent neurologic defects
26	M	Yes	Yes	Yes	Transient left paresis	No
19	M	Yes	Yes	Yes	Transient left paresis	No
50	M	No	Yes	Yes	Left sensory defect	No
18	M	No	Yes	Yes	Expressive aphasia Right hemiparesis, transient	No
32	M	Yes	Yes	Yes	Right hemiparesis, 1 hour	No

only 10% in whom an organic disease was finally diagnosed. The majority of these persons were found to have a structural disorder at the base of the brain. None had aneurysm as the primary lesion.

Headache with effort implies that adequate physical activity has produced the requisite cephalgia. Mental effort, no matter how onerous, is not included here. Nor should one include positional or movement headache (paraxysmal headache) in this category. Thus, for example, cough headache is omitted; in the latter case, the headache is almost always associated with the head movement that is a part of the cough.

How much effort, then causes headache? Arbitrarily, enough to double the resting pulse and sustained for at least 10 seconds, but ordinarily for minutes or hours. With this definition, a clear group of headache syndromes associated with physical activity emerge.

The personal experience of the authors with effort headache is limited to five lay distance runners. All had either a history of migraine or a family history of migraine. Classic migraine occurred during or after prolonged running at sea level in all cases. Two runners experienced episodic hemiparesis, but none had any permanent defects (Table 9-4). Other patients with migraine report that exercise during a migraine attack makes the headache worse, and this has also been our experience in interviewing many patients with migraine. This is accounted for by the fact that the normal ability of the brain to maintain a constant blood flow, a property called "autoregulation," is lost during a migraine attack (Sakai & Meyer, 1978). Hence, if blood pressure and cardiac output are increased by exercise during a migraine attack, cerebral blood flow increases and the pounding headache is intensified.

SUMMARY

The intravenous injection of histamine results in dilatation of the intracranial arteries, which, with normal systemic arterial pressure, causes increased cerebral blood flow, cerebral vasodilatation, and increased amplitude of intracranial pulsations. The intense headache associated with these changes has been studied as a means of analyzing other, nonexperimental headaches. The following conclusions were drawn:

- The intensity of the headache experimentally induced by histamine is proportional to the degree of dilatation and stretch of the pial and dural vessels and the perivascular tissue.
- Headache does not result from vascular dilatation unless the intracranial vessels are sufficiently distorted. Carbon dioxide, when used as a vasodilator, is less effective than histamine in increasing the amplitude of intracranial pulsations and does not commonly produce headache.
- Headache experimentally induced by histamine does not depend on the integrity of sensation from the superficial tissues.
- The extracranial arteries play a minor role in contributing to the pain of headache experimentally induced by histamine.
- Cerebral arteries, principally the large arteries at the base of the brain, including the internal carotid, the vertebral, and the basilar artery and the proximal segments of their main branches, are chiefly responsible for the quality and intensity of headache experimentally induced by histamine.
- Although there may be other less important afferent pathways for the conduction of impulses interpreted as headache following injection of histamine, (a) the fifth cranial nerve on each side is the principal afferent pathway for headache resulting from dilatation of the supratentorial cerebral arteries and felt in the frontotemporoparietal region of the head, and (b) the ninth and tenth cranial nerves and the upper cervical nerves are the most important afferent pathways for headache resulting from dilatation of arteries of the posterior fossa and felt in the occipital region of the head.
- Headaches that result primarily from distention of cerebral and pial arteries and resemble in mechanism the headache that follows the intravenous injection of histamine include the following: headaches associated with fever, bacteremia, as a side effect of drugs, and sepsis; headaches resulting from carbon-monoxide poisoning; headaches that follow the industrial and therapeutic use of nitrites; headaches associated with polycythemia vera, chronic mountain sickness, and other hypoxemias; probably the so-called hangover headache; and the postseizure headache.

REFERENCES

Amano, T., J.S. Meyer (1982). Prostaglandin inhibition and cerebrovascular control in patients with headache. *Headache 27*:52–59.

Amano, T., J.S. Meyer (1982). Cerebrovascular changes in patients with headache during antiserotoninergic treatment. *Headache 22*:249–255.

Appenzeller, O. (1972). Altitude headache. *Headache 12*:126–130.

Barcroft, J. (1925). The Respiratory Functions of the Blood. Part II. Lessons from High Altitudes. Cambridge University Press, London.

Barcroft, J.C., C.A. Binger, A.V. Bock et al. (1922). Observations upon the effects of high altitude on the physiological process of the human body, carried out in the Peruvian Andes, chiefly at Cerro de Pasco. *Phil. Trans. Roy. Soc. (London) Ser. B. 211*:351.

Behnke, A.R. (1965). Problems in the treatment of decompression sickness (and traumatic air embolism). *Ann. N.Y. Acad. Sci. 117*:843–859.

Bronk, D.W. (1935). The nervous mechanism of cardiac-vascular control. *Harvey Lectures,* p. 245

Clark, D., H.B. Hough, and H.G. Wolff (1936a). Experimental studies on headache: Observations on histamine headache. *Assoc. Res. Nerv. Dis. Proc. 15*:417.

Clark, D., H.B. Hough, and H.G. Wolff (1936b). Experimental studies on headache: Observations on headache produced by histamine. *Arch. Neurol. Psychiatry 35*:1054.

Dalessio, D.J. (1974). Effort migraines. *Headache 14*:53.

Dandy, W.E. (1931). Treatment of hemicrania (migraine) by removal of the inferior cervical and first thoracic sympathetic ganglion. *Bull. Johns Hopkins Hosp. 48*:357.

Diamond, S. (1977). Recurrent exertional headache. *JAMA 237*:580.

Engel, G.L., J.P. Webb, E.B. Ferris et al. (1944). A migraine-like syndrome complicating decompression sickness. *War Med. 5*:304–314.

Erde, A.E. and C. Edmonds. (1975). Decompression sickness: A clinical series. *J. Occup. Med. 17*:324.

Evans, E.S. (1912). A case of nitroglycerine poisoning. *JAMA 58*:550.

Fisher, M. (1968). Headache and cerebral vascular disease. In *Handbook of Clinical Neurology, Vol. 124.* North Holland, Amsterdam.

Forbes, H.S., S. Cobb, and F. Fremont-Smith (1924). Cerebral edema and headache following carbon monoxide asphyxia. *Arch. Neurol. Psychiatry 11*:264.

Forward, S.A., M. Landowne, J.N. Follansbee, and J.E. Hansen (1968). Effect of acetazolamide on acute mountain sickness. *N. Engl. J. Med. 279*:839.

Graham, J.R. (1959). Headache in systemic disease. In *Headache: Diagnosis and Treatment* (A.P. Friedman, and H.H. Merritt, eds.), Chap. 7. F.A. Davis, Philadelphia.

Hardy, J.D., H.G. Wolff, and H. Goodell (1940). Studies on pain. A new method for measuring pain threshold: Observations on spatial summation of pain. *J. Clin. Invest. 19*:649.

Heiss W.D., B. Kufferle, I. Dewel et al. (1976). Cerebral blood flow and severity of mental dysfunction in chronic alcoholism. In *Cerebral Vascular Disease, 7th International Salzburg Conference*, pp. 89–93. George Thieme, Stutgart.

Henderson, W.R. and N. Raskin (1972). Hot dog headache: Individual susceptibility to nitrite. *Lancet 2*:1162–1163.

Heyman, A., J.L. Patterson, Jr., F.T. Nichols, Jr. (1950). The effects of induced fever on cerebral functions in neurosyphillis. *J. Clin. Invest. 29*:1335.

Houston, C.S. (1976). High altitude illness. *JAMA 236*:2193–2195.

Jokl, E. (1965). Indisposition after running. *Med. Dello Sport 5*:363.

Jokl, E. and P. Jokl (1977). Der Beltrag der Sportmedizin zur Klinischen Kardiologic—das Sporterz. In *Altern Leistungsfahigkeit Rehabilitation*, pp. 47–56. F.K. Schattauer Verlag, Munchen.

Kidd D.J. and D.H. Elliott. (1975) Decompression disorders in divers. In *The Physiology of Medicine of Diving and Compressed Air Work* P.B. Bennett and O.H. Elliott (eds.), Williams & Wilkins pp. 471–495. Baltimore.

Lassen, N.A. (1966). The luxury perfusion syndrome and its possible relation to acute metabolic audosis localized within the brain. *Lancet ii*:1113–1115.

Laws, C.E. (1910). The nitroglycerine head. *JAMA 54*:793.

Leufaut C. and K. Sullivan (1970). Adaptation to high altitude. *N. Engl. J. Med. 284*:1298.

Levine, M. and H.G. Wolff (1932). Afferent impulses from the blood vessels of the pia. *Arch. Neurol. Psychiatry 28*:140.

Leviton, A., L. Capland, and E. Salznan (1975). Severe headache after carotid endarterectomy. *Headache 15*:207–210.

Levy, D.K. (1981). Stroke and orgasmic cephalogia. *Headache 21*:12–14.

Lundberg, P.D. and P. Osterman (1974). The benign and malignant forms of orgasmic headache. *Headache 14*:164.

Meyer J.S., F. Gotoh, E. Favole (1965). Effects of carotid compression on cerebral metabolism and electroencephalogram. *EEG Clin. Neurophysiol. 19*:362-376.

Meyer, J.S., F. Gotoh, and E. Favole (1966). Cerebral metabolism during epileptic seizures in man. *EEG Clin. Neurophysiol. 21*:10–22.

Meyer, J.S., F. Gotoh, and M. Tomita (1966). Acute respiratory acidemia. *Neurology 16*:463–474

Meyer J.S., and J. Handa. (1967). Cerebral blood flow and metabolism during experimental hyperthermia (fever). *Minn. Med. 50*:37–44.

Meyer, J.S., T. Ryu, M. Toyoda, et al. (1969). Evidence for a Pasteur effect regulatory cerebral oxygen and carbohydrate metabolism in man. *Neurology 19*:954-962.

Monge, C. (1942). Life in the Andes and chronic mountain sickness. *Science 95*:79.

Northfield, D.W.C. (1938). Some observations on headache. *Brain 61*:133.

Paulson, G.W. and H.L. Klawans (1974). Benign orgasmic headache. *Headache 13*:181.

Pawan, G.L.S. (1968). Vitamins, sugars, and ethanol metabolism in man. *Nature 220*:374.

Pickering, G.W. (1939). Experimental observations on headache. *Br. Med. J. 1*:4087.

Pickering, G.W. and W. Hess (1933). Observations on the mechanism of headache produced by histamine. *Clin. Sci. 1*:77.

Raskin, N.H. and S.C. Knittle (1976). Ice cream headache and orthostatic symptoms in patients with migraine. *Headache 16*:222–225.

Ray, B.S. (1954). The surgical treatment of headache and atypical neuralgia. *J. Neurosurg. 2*:596.

Rooke, E.D. (1968). Benign exertional headache. *Med. Clin. North Am. 52*:801–808.

Sakai, F. and J.S. Meyer (1978). Regional cerebral hemodynamics curing migraine and cluster headaches measured by the ^{133}Xe inhalation method. *Headache 18*:122–132.

Sakai F. and Meyer J.S. (1979). Abnormal cerebrovascular reactivity in patients with migraine and cluster headache. *Headache 19*:257–266.

Salzer, H.M. (1960). Cephalgia; questions and answers. *JAMA 173*:146.

Schumacher, G.A., B.S. Ray, and H.G. Wolff (1940). Experimental studies on headache. Further analysis of histamine headache and its pain pathways. *Arch. Neurol. Psychiatry 44*:701.

Singh, L, P. Khanna, and M.G. Srivastava (1960). Acute mountain sickness. *N. Engl. J. Med. 280*:175–184.

Strauss, R.H. (1978). Diving medicine. *Am. Rev. Respir. Dis. 119*:1001–1023.

Szczcklik A. and R.J. Gryglewski (1979). Actions of prostracyclin in man. In *Prostacyclin*. J.R. Vane and S. Bengstrom (eds.), Raven Press, New York. pp. 383–408.

von Brauch, F. (1957). Hypoglycemic headache. *Dtsch. Med. Wochenschr. 76*:828.

Weiss, S., G.P. Robb, and L.B. Ellis (1932). The systemic effects of histamine in man, with special reference to the responses of the cardiovascular system. *Arch. Intern Med. 49*:360.

Wolff, H.G. (1929). The cerebral circulation: 11a. The action of acetylcholine. 11b. The action of the extract of the posterior lobe of the pituitary gland. 11c. The action of amylnitrite. *Arch. Neurol. Psychiatry 22*:686.

Wolff, H.G. (1938). Headache and cranial arteries. *Trans. Assoc. A.m. Physicians 53*:193.

Wolff, H.G. and W.G. Lennox (1930). Cerebral circulation: 12. The effect on pial vessels of variation in the oxygen and carbon dioxide content of the blood. *Arch. Neurol. Psychiatry 23*:1097.

10

Muscle Contraction Headache

SEYMOUR DIAMOND

Of all the headache patients seen by either the family physician or the generalist, 80% suffer from muscle contraction or tension headaches. There are two types of muscle contraction headaches, episodic or chronic.

Persons with episodic tension headaches usually seek relief with over-the-counter analgesics. They will consult a physician only when the headaches do not respond to these simple analgesics or when they occur with an increased frequency and severity, causing diminished functioning in either an occupational or social setting. Muscle contraction headache can manifest itself in relationship to stress, depression, anxiety, emotional conflicts, fatigue, repressed hostility, or simply creating an environment too great for the patient to handle.

Muscle contraction headaches can occur at any age but are more common in adulthood, when life's frustrations tend too dominate. Friedman and his colleagues (1964), in their review of 2000 cases, noted that most of the patients with muscle contraction headaches were female, and only about 40% reported a family history of headaches in contrast with 70% of migraine sufferers. Most of their patients indicated the onset of headache occurred between the age of 20 and 40 years. Many had daily pain, and 20% had persistent pain occurring at least four times weekly.

Patients with muscle contraction headaches generally describe the pain as a steady, nonpulsatile ache. Other descriptions include viselike pressure, drawing, soreness, bitemporal or occipital tightness, and bandlike sensations about the head that may be termed a "hatband" effect. Patients may also complain of distinct cramping sensations, as if the neck and upper back were in a cast.

The site of the headache varies, frequently occurring at the forehead and temples or at the back of the head and neck. Patients may describe the pain as unilateral or bilateral, involving the frontal, temporal, occipital, or parietal regions, or any combination of these sites. They often complain of soreness on combing or brushing the hair or when putting on a hat. Although this headache may undergo frequent changes in severity and site, the pain, localized in one region, may continue with varying intensity for weeks, months, or even years. The pain's duration may be short and relieved by the patient changing position. By limiting the movement of the neck, jaws, and head, the patient may be able to reduce the severity of the headache. Relief may be obtained by resting or supporting the head in the hands. Sharply localized "nodules" may be demonstrated when the tender areas of the neck, head, and upper back are palpated.

During physical examination, pressure on contracted, tender muscles may increase the intensity of the headache. Tinnitus, vertigo, and lacrimation may also be elicited by this procedure. The pain may radiate to other parts of the head if pressure is placed on tender areas. Shivering from exposure to the cold may aggravate the headache.

Emotional factors are of primary significance in causing muscle contraction headaches. Martin and his associates (1967) reviewed the psychiatric evaluations of 25 patients with muscle contraction headaches. They found no single psychological factor to be a provocateur of these headaches. Most of their patients demonstrated multiple conflicts, such as repressed hostility, sexual conflicts, and unresolved dependency needs. This study suggests that, in cases of muscle contraction headaches, either somatization of anxiety in the form of increased skeletal muscle tension or psychophysiologic expression is occurring. Family members may be performing an unconscious role in fostering the pain, because secondary gain is often present.

Chronic muscle contraction headaches may conceal a serious emotional disorder, such as depression. The patient will present with a persistent and vague headache, for which no organic cause can be determined. For the patient, the physical symptoms are more socially acceptable than the anxiety or depressive symptoms; many patients are certain there is a somatic basis for their pain. The physician must be cognizant of other signs of depression, such as early morning fatigue, irritability, loss of energy or spontaneity, lack of interest, insomnia, or early morning awakening. The patient may have considered suicide.

It is known that the excitatory effect of noxious stimulation of the soft structures of the head radiates centrally, causing the pain to be experienced at a site distant from the noxious stimulation. For example, when the condylar or basal region is stimulated by the injection of a hypertonic saline solution or by manual pressure in the region, the patient may experience orbital or frontal ache. The stimulation of the nuchal tissues may cause occipital headache. The pain caused by sustained contraction of skeletal muscle is triggered promptly by noxious stimulation and ends abruptly when the source of the stimulation is blocked by procaine.

MECHANISM OF MUSCLE CONTRACTION HEADACHE

The mechanism of this type of headache is similar to that of chronic muscle contraction in any other part of the body. Local pathologic processes and their central influences are related to muscle spasm. This involves three independent reflex arcs and four consecutive steps:

1. Muscle spasm is usually initiated by a multisynaptic reflex of withdrawal. The stimulation of nerve fibers is caused by a local pathologic process, with the impulse transmitted directly to the spinal cord and then to the ventral roots. The stimulus then passes over the efferent nerves to the neuromuscular

junction, which in turn causes the muscle to contract acutely and to spread the painful stimulus.

2. Via the polysynaptic spinal pathways and the lemniscal system, which are also stimulated, the initial impulse is conducted up the spinal cord to the thalamic and central levels. At these areas, the stimulus is perceived as painful.

3. At this point, the brain will transmit impulses through the reticulospinal system to activate the gamma-efferent neurons that contract the muscle spindle.

4. During the contraction of the muscle spindle, a monosynaptic stimulus is evoked, which travels directly to the ventral horn. The discharge in the efferent peripheral nerve is augmented and, more important, muscle contraction is augmented.

It should be noted that the contraction of the muscle spindle itself (the third reflex arc) is a monosynaptic pathway and is related to the simple tendon stretch reflexes demonstrated in neurologic examination. Normally, the contracting muscle inhibits firing of the muscle spindle and terminates the third arc stretch reflex, providing relaxation of the muscle. The state of activity of the gamma motor system determines the degree of muscle tone. If cortical influences or local or systemic disease causes the gamma-efferent system to continue to fire, the muscle spindle will remain tight. The muscle continually contracts until the contraction itself becomes painful. The cycle of pain evolves as spasm, anxiety, and pain, or a muscle contraction headache.

Many modern researchers (Lance et al., 1983) have observed that chronic muscle contraction headache may not be a result of disorders of the blood vessels and muscles. Instead, they maybe affected by a chronic or intermittent disturbance of the monoaminergic, serotonergic, and endorphin function, involving the hypothalmus, brain stem, and spinal cord. This occurrence may be due to referral or a central pain phenomenon from the intermingling of major circuits of the brain and spinal cord.

The headache is due to anxiety, stress, tension, or psychogenic determinants. As part of the medical history, a carefully detailed psychiatric inventory should be obtained. This should include details of the patient's marital relations, occupation, social relationships, life stresses, personality traits, habits, methods of coping with stressful situations, and sexual difficulties.

For the episodic muscle contraction headache, treatment is limited to abortive therapy, including over-the-counter analgesics or prescribed simple analgesics. These agents are usually helpful in relieving the pain. However, the importance of biofeedback training and counseling should be stressed if the headaches occur frequently.

DEPRESSION AND CHRONIC MUSCLE CONTRACTION HEADACHE

It has been estimated that, in family practice in the United Kingdom (Hodgkins, 1976), depression is the fourth most frequently diagnosed disorder. In the United States, it ranks twelfth (Marsland et al., 1976). The presence of depression is often subtle and the diagnosis is frequently missed. Most physicians are probably able to recognize the classically depressed patient. This is the patient who walks into the

Table 10-1   Physical complaints

Complaint	Percentage of patients
Sleep disturbances	97
Early awakening	87
Headache	84
Dyspnea	76
Loss of weight	74
Trouble getting to sleep	73
Weakness and fatigue	70
Urinary frequency	70
"Spells"—dizziness	70
Appetite disturbances	70
Decreased libido	63
Cardiovascular disturbances	60
Sexual disturbances	60
Palpitations	59
Paresthesias	53
Nausea	48
Menstrual changes	41

office with a sad look, as well as slow speech and movement. This depressed person exhibits little interest in anything and sighs frequently (Emergency Medicine, 1971). However, the depressed patient often presents with a wide variety of complaints that can be categorized as physical, emotional, and psychic. The physical complaints include chronic pain and headaches, sleep disturbances, severe insomnia and early awakening, appetite changes, anorexia and rapid weight loss, and a decrease in sexual activity, ranging at times to impotence in males and amenorrhea or frigidity in females. Emotional complaints include feeling "blue," anxiety, and rumination over the past, present, and future. Finally, psychic complaints may include such statements as "morning is the worst time of the day," suicidal thoughts, and death wishes (Table 10-1, 10-2, and 10-3).

A headache secondary to depression is usually considered a muscle contraction headache. This headache consists of a steady, nonpulsatile ache, often distributed in

Table 10-2   Emotional complaints

Complaint	Percentage of patients
Blue; low spirits; sadness	90
Crying	80
Feelings of guilt, hopelessness, unworthiness, unreality	65
Anxiousness or irritability	65
Anxiety	60
Fear of insanity, physical disease, death; rumination over past, present, future	50

Table 10-3 Psychic complaints

Complaint	Percentage of patients
"Morning is the worst time of day"	95
Poor concentration	91
No interest; no ambition	75
Indecisiveness	75
Poor memory	71
Suicidal thoughts; death wishes	35

a bandlike pattern around the head. It may be described as viselike, a steady pressure, a weight, a soreness, or a distinct cramplike sensation. They are capricious, bizarre, and follow no definite pattern as to location, although the occipital portion of the skull is frequently affected. Their duration is a distinguishing feature. A depressed person will describe his headache as lasting for years or throughout his life. A depressive headache is usually dull and generalized, characteristically worse in the morning and in the evening. This diurnal variation is the most distinctive characteristic of the headache and has provided a correct diagnosis of severe depression when other features have been inconspicuous.

Certain details about the headache may indicate an underlying depression. These headaches usually appear at regular intervals in relation to daily life, occurring on weekends, Sundays, or holidays, and on the first days of vacation or after exams. The greatest incidence of "nervous-type" headache occurs from 4:00 P.M. to 8:00 P.M. and from 4:00 A.M. to 8:00 A.M. These are usually the periods of the greatest and sometimes the most silent family crises.

These headaches may occur early in the morning, when the depressed patients awakens and his or her fantasies of conflict with family members or at work are manifested. In discussion with the depressed patient, we find that the headaches often occur when the patient leaves the relatively quiet atmosphere of the office for a weekend at home. The headache often coincides with interpersonal situations in which the sufferer feels compelled to appear comfortable, relaxed, and agreeable although he or she is struggling to repress resentment toward someone he or she is expected to love and respect.

People with depressive illness may develop bodily symptoms, and conversely people with painful organic diseases tend to become depressed. It should be noted that too little attention is given to the depressive aspects of chronic pain and its treatment. The physical complaints dominate the situation so that the underlying depression tends to be overlooked.

Two basic factors often provide insight for a possible depression. First, the physician should determine if there is a prior history of depression in the patient or family. The patient should be questioned about similar symptoms in relatives, friends, or self. Many will indicate previous occurrences of these symptoms. The patient may relate obscure symptoms that are actually depressive equivalents. Second, the patient may relate the onset of the symptoms to a particular event. The depressive attacks may follow a wide variety of events the patient perceives as traumatic or feels as a personal loss. The event may be out of proportion to the severity of the resultant depression. A patient may relate the symptoms to some form of bodily injury, an illness, an injection, surgery, or a diagnostic examination. Also, the patient may emphasize that each of his or her symptoms results from this event. The incident that precipitated the headache or other depressive equivalents would not be compatible with the illness or as overwhelming as perceived. The patient usually feels weakened or maimed by the event.

If not subsequent to an illness or accident, depression may follow some change in personal role, position, or socioeconomic status. Loss of a loved one often triggers normal depressed states. It can also initiate a malignant depression beyond the scope of the loss. The patient's history will reveal the loss to be very important, but it must be considered within the personal scope of the individual, for whom it may have a peculiar significance.

Statistically, we have found that 84% of depressed patients indicated that headache was one of their complaints or their only complaint. In Table 10-1 the most frequently listed complaint with depression is sleep disturbance (Diamond, 1964). Of the patients that I or my colleagues examined, 97% presented with this complaint. In younger patients, there is less variation in sleep. The older individual experiences more difficulty with sleep. Sleep disturbances may manifest themselves as hypersomnia, insomnia, early awakening, or disturbing dreams. Early awakening is one of the most common sleep disturbances with depression.

The emotional complaints characteristic of depression may vary, as reviewed in Table 10-2 (Diamond, 1964). The clue to depression is the introversion of the patient. Emotionally, the patient focuses on self and illness, repeatedly reviewing mistakes and misdeeds, and deprecating himself or herself. Feelings of inadequacy and incompetence are common and persist in these people, and they look to the future with despair. Phobias and fears of a variable nature are common, such as fear of insanity, being alone in the house, changing jobs, or moving, all of these are indicative of depression. Irritability and hostility are common emotional symptoms.

In Table 10-3, a multitude of psychic complaints are presented (Diamond, 1964). An impairment in concentration or memory, loss of interest, difficulty in making decisions, and despondency occur frequently in depression. These produce thoughts of suicide, ideas of reference, and delusions. A few patients will hallucinate.

To the depressed patient, everything is an effort. Some people experience complete psychomotor retardations, and they have difficulty eating, sleeping, thinking, and dressing themselves. Daily tasks become major chores. Older people have serious memory defects and may have delusions of cancer or other incurable illnesses.

The biochemical determinants of depression have been researched heavily for the past 30 years. Much of our present knowledge comes from work completed in the mid-1950s (Maas, 1973). During that time, it was observed that tubercular patients treated with iproniazid developed euphoric states. It was later learned that iproniazid is a monoamine oxidase inhibitor and produces increasing levels of norepinephrine and serotonin in the brain and body tissue. About this time it was observed that a small percentage of patients being treated for hypertension with the rauwolfian alkaloids, such as reserpine, developed severe depression indistinguishable from endogenous depressions. These alkaloids were noted to deplete the brain of both biogenic amines. These observations evolved in our present theory of depression, which may be considered an illness involving multiple defects of neurotransmitters. However, these biogenic amines have not been fully explained.

The importance of antidepressant drugs in pain control results from their effects on the synthesis and metabolism of serotonin (5-hydroxtryptamine) and norepinephrine. It has been found that neurons containing serotonin and norepinephrine are part of the brain's analgesia system (Diamond, 1983; Messing et al., 1975). A descending serotonin pathway in the dorsal spinal cord, originating in the raphe nucleus, and an interlacing of norepinephrine and opioid neurons in the locus ceruleus, are of particular interest to pain researchers (Diamond, 1983). Drugs that alter the synthesis or uptake of serotonin and/or norepinephrine, which includes virtually all antidepressant agents, would be expected to play a role in the brain's regulation of pain. Serotonin antagonists have been known to influence both opiate- and stimulation-induced analgesia (Messing & Lytle, 1977). In animals, tricyclics produce analgesia directly (Saarnivaara & Mattila, 1974) or through potentiation of opiates (Malseed & Goldstein, 1979).

The most popular biologic theories of depression hold that the disorder is associated with depletion of brain monoamine neurotransmitters such as serotonin and norepinephrine. Determining the most important substance in depression is controversial. Evidence is available to support both the norepinephrine and serotonin hypotheses (Feighner, 1982). Other neurotransmitters, such as dopamine and endorphin, may also be involved in depression (Fawcett, 1980). The discovery of endogenous, opiatelike substances in the brain, the endorphins and enkephalins, has significantly advanced our understanding of pain. Recent findings suggest that pain transmission in the central nervous system is controlled by an endorphin-mediated analgesia system that can be activated by several exogenous actions, including opioid substances, electrical stimulation, acupuncture, and even placebo (Fields, 1981; Basbaum & Fields, 1978; Mayer & Price, 1976; Snyder & Childers, 1979).

Several tests have been developed to evaluate depression and select the therapeutic agent to be used. The dexamethasone suppression test (DST) (Cobbin et al., 1979) basically involves administering a small amount of dexamethasone to the patient at midnight and measuring serum cortisol levels the following day. It has been found that a subgroup of patients with an endogenous depression also exhibit nonsuppression. Most of these patients show normal suppression in the morning and nonsuppression later in the day.

Approximately 45% of endogenously depressed individuals have an abnormal DST. Because the test is 96% specific for endogenous depression an abnormal DST will occur in only 4 to 7% of patients with other psychiatric disorders including schizophrenia, mania, personality disorders, and minor or neurotic depression. If a patient has an abnormal response to the test, the physician must rule out organic illnesses that may cause an abnormal result. These include Cushing's syndrome, pregnancy, and uncontrolled diabetes. The physician must also review the patient's current medications because many drugs alter the results. Currently, the DST is most valuable in monitoring the patient's response to therapy. Normalization of the DST seems to correlate with an improved clinical picture. Patients with an abnormal DST appear more likely to suffer from recurrent depressions than those patients who exhibit normal suppression. Studies are under way to determine if a patient's response to the

DST can be used as a guide for drug therapy. Preliminary work indicates that the nonsuppressors have a better response to treatment. The relationship between the pituitary–adrenal axis and depression is unknown at the present time. The limbic system and cholinergic pathways have been implicated, but further research is required.

Another diagnostic test is the thyroid stimulation hormone (TSH) response to thyrotropin-releasing hormone (TRH). It has been noted that a large percentage of endogenously depressed patients have a blunted TSH response to the administration of TRH. The mechanism for this blunted response is unknown, and the clinical value of this test has yet to be demonstrated.

The 3-methoxy-4-hydroxyphenylethylenglycol (MHPG) urine test is used to evaluate the main metabolite of norepinephrine in the central nervous system. The urinary levels may demonstrate the norepinephrine metabolism (Maas, 1975; Cobbin et al., 1979; Blackwell, 1979). It has been noted that subgroups of depressed patients have decreased MHPG in the urine and other groups of depressed patients have normal or increased levels of MHPG.

It has been suggested that perhaps two groups of depression exist, one in which norepinephrine metabolism is disrupted and serotonin and dopamine systems are normal, and the second with a disorder of serotonin but not norepinephrine or dopamine. Studies revealed that low-MHPG depressives have a higher response to imipramine and desipramine as opposed to amitriptyline and nortriptyline. High-MHPG patients responded more effectively to amitriptyline or nortriptyline. Maas (1975) argued that low-MHPG patients had low norepinephrine but normal serotonin and high-MHPG patients had a low serotonin but normal norepinephrine repression. The possibility of three distinct subgroups of depressive disorders has been suggested. The groups would be differentiated on the basis of low, intermediate, and high MHPG levels (Schatzberg et al., 1980, 1981, 1982). The patients with low MHPG demonstrated a clear response to imipramine or maprotiline, which may have decreased norepinephrine synthesis or release. Normal norepinephrine metabolism may occur in patients with intermediate MHPG levels (poor responders to maprotiline or imipramine). However, they may manifest some other neurochemical abnormality in patients with high MHPG who have intermediate subsensitive postsynaptic receptors and/or increased acetylcholine activity. To explain the disparate results from other studies, a three-group paradigm should be formulated. Low-MHPG patients have demonstrated relatively low levels of cerebrospinal fluid 5HIAA in other recent studies. A low-norepinephrine versus low-serotonin hypothesis would be disputed with these observations (Maas et al., 1982).

The treatment of depression-associated muscle contraction headaches includes the use of the antidepressant agents. Tricyclics are usually the drugs of choice. This group includes amitriptyline, imipramine, desipramine, nortriptyline, doxepin, and protriptyline. The efficacy of these drugs has been shown in numerous studies (Ayd, 1980; Diamond & Baltes, 1969; Diamond, 1963; Diamond, 1966; Ayd, 1971). The tricyclics are considered more effective in endogenous depression and less beneficial when the depressed patient has many accompanying neurotic traits. The choice of tricyclic is not simple because each drug has unique characteristics, as reviewed in Table 10-4 (Diamond, 1977).

Monoamine Oxidase inhibitors (MAOI) are generally considered to be the second

Table 10-4   Effects of tricyclic antidepressants

Drug	Serotonin inhibition	Norepinephrine inhibition	Dopamine inhibition	Sedative effects	Anticholinergic effects
Amitriptyline	Moderate	Weak	Inactive	Strong	Strong
Desipramine	Weak	Potent	Inactive	Mild	Moderate
Doxepin	Moderate	Moderate	Inactive	Strong	Strong
Imipramine	Fairly potent	Moderate	Inactive	Moderate	Strong
Nortriptyline	Weak	Fairly potent	Inactive	Mild	Moderate
Protriptyline	Weak	Fairly potent	Inactive	None	Strong

line of drugs for depression. They are not considered as efficacious as the tricyclics and are known to have more drug interactions. A patient on an MAOI must follow a special diet and avoid foods with tyramine (Table 10-5). The most commonly used MAOI is phenelzine sulfate (Nardil) (Robinson et al., 1973). MAOIs block the oxidative deamination of numerous monoamines, including epinephrine, norepinephrine, serotonin, and dopamine. According to prevailing theories, the amounts of these substances are increased in the brain and other tissues, and the depression created by their deficiency is ameliorated or cured. Despite the precautions and fears with MAOIs,

Table 10-5   Diet for the headache patient on MAO inhibitors[a]

Food group	Foods allowed	Foods to avoid
Beverages	Decaffeinated coffee, colas containing no caffeine. Caffeine sources to be limited to 2 cups daily include coffee, tea, colas	Alcoholic beverages, wines, ale, beer
Milk	Homogenized, skim, 2%	Chocolate, buttermilk
Dairy products	Cottage cheese, cream cheese, American cheese, Velveeta or synthetic cheese. Yogurt in ½ cup portions or less	Aged and processed cheese: includes cheddar, Swiss, Mozzarella, Parmesan, Romano, brick, Brie, Camembert, Gouda, Gruyere, Emmentaler, Stilton, Provolone, Roquefort, blue, and cheese-containing foods (pizza, macaroni and cheese), yogurt and sour cream
Meat and meat substitutes	Freshly prepared meats, eggs	Aged, canned, cured, or processed meats, those containing nitrates or nitrites, commercial meat extracts, pickled or dried herring, chicken livers, sausage, salami, pepperoni, bologna, frankfurters, patés, peanuts and peanut butter, marinated meats, meat prepared with tenderizers, soy sauce or yeast extracts

Food group	Foods allowed	Foods to avoid
Bread and bread substitutes	All except those on the avoid list. Commercial bread	Homemade yeast breads, fresh coffee cake, doughnuts, yeast and yeast extracts, sourdough breads, breads and crackers containing cheese, breads containing chocolate or nuts
Fruits	All except those to avoid. Citrus fruits (oranges, grapefruit, pineapple, lemon, lime) are limited to $\frac{1}{2}$ cup serving per day	Canned figs, raisins, papaya, passion fruit, avocado, red plum, $\frac{1}{2}$ banana allowed per day
Vegetables	All except those on avoid list	Italian broad beans, Fava beans, lima beans, navy beans, pea pods, sauerkraut, onions except for flavoring
Desserts	All except fresh-yeast-raised desserts or those containing chocolate	Any with chocolate
Miscellaneous	White vinegar, commercial salad dressing in small amounts	Brewer's yeast, chocolate, soy sauce, monosodium glutamate, meat tenderizers, papaya products, Accent, Lawry's and other seasoned salts, soup cubes, canned soups, frozen TV dinners. Some snack items and instant foods contain items to be avoided. Read all labels

[a] Tyramine content may vary among brand names available in the market because of preparation, processing, or storage. It is best to eat only freshly prepared foods to avoid the risk of eating foods that may have been aged, fermented, pickled, or marinated. Tenderizers, monosodium glutamate, nitrate, or nitrite compounds are likely to be provoking agents. It is important to read labels carefully when shopping and ask question when eating out.

they are often found effective when the tricyclics fail. In studies comparing tricyclics and MAOIs (Ravaris et al., 1980), the MAOIs tended to exert a stronger antianxiety action whereas the tricyclics were more effective in reversing weight loss and improving sleep.

Combination therapy of a tricyclic and MAOI simultaneously was previously verboten in practice. There had been isolated reports of hypertensive, hyperpyretic crises leading to death due to combination therapy. Standard practice was to initiate therapy with a tricyclic. If no improvement was noted within 4 to 6 weeks, the drug was discontinued, and after waiting 10 days to 2 weeks the MAOI was started. The two drugs were never given in combination. In 1971, Schuckit and his associates reviewed 25 reported cases of morbidity secondary to the combination therapy. The results of that study indicated that the risks of combination therapy had been greatly exaggerated. Many of the complications reported could be attributed to drug overdose and others could be related to the concomitant use of other drugs that act on the central nervous system. In the remaining cases, the tricyclic involved was imipramine and the MAOIs included iproniazid, tranylcypromine, isocarboxazid, pargyline, and phenelzine.

MIXED HEADACHE SYNDROME

A discussion of muscle contraction headaches would be incomplete without a review of the diagnosis and treatment of the mixed headache syndrome. The mixed headache patient is the case most frequently seen by the neurologist or headache specialist. This type of headache is comprised of the following symptomatology: (1) daily, continuous headache; (2) a hard or sick headache (migraine) occurring 1 to 10 times monthly; and (3) easy susceptibility to habituation to over-the-counter or prescribed analgesics and/or ergotamine tartrate (Mathew, 1981).

When the diagnosis of mixed headache syndrome has been determined, the physician should avoid the use of sedation, tranquilizers, habituating analgesics, and narcotics, to prevent addiction which thereby perpetuates the problem. To prevent the rebound phenomenon, the use of ergotamine should be restricted to relief of the hard or sick headache, and never be prescribed on a daily basis.

The tricyclic antidepressants or the MAOIs are the drugs of choice in the prophylactic treatment of the mixed headache syndrome. For refractive cases, combination therapy consisting of a tricyclic antidepressant and an MAOI may be indicated. However, this treatment should be cautiously selected with regard to patients and pharmaceutical agents. The cautious addition of propranolol (Inderal) in the long-acting form may be considered in doses of 80, 120, and 160 mg on a daily basis. Occasionally, adding a nonsteroidal anti-inflammatory agent to the therapeutic regimen may be helpful.

The patient with the mixed headache syndrome may require a copharmacy approach with several agents. To ensure the successful treatment of chronic muscle contraction headaches and mixed headache syndrome, the patient must receive continuity of care, and habituating analgesics must be avoided.

CERVICAL SPINE DISEASE AND MUSCLE CONTRACTION HEADACHES

Headache is not limited to the head. Head pain may also be referred to and include the neck as a component of the pain syndrome. The patient may complain of pain in the upper cervical spine as part of both migraine and cluster headache syndromes. Disorders of the cervical spine may create localized pain but may also produce referred pain to the head. Migraine and cluster headaches as a cause of pain at the cervical spine have been described previously in this text. The following discussion will focus on disorders of the cervical spine as a cause of pain.

Structures and Mechanisms in Cervical Pain

There are multiple etiologies for pain involving the cervical spine. The mechanisms for such pain are numerous and, frequently, obscure. A review of the involved structures should enhance an understanding of the complexity of this problem.

Cervical nerves and roots, the vertebral arteries, ligaments, periosteum, the annulus fibrosus of the disks, and synovial joints are capable of producing pain. The second cervical nerve's sensory root produces the fibers that become the greater occipital nerve. This nerve provides the major sensory input from the posterior half of the head (Chouret, 1967; Edmeads, 1978). Irritation of the greater occipital nerve can produce headache. A variety of mechanisms can produce this condition, including inflammation (Dalessio, 1972), entrapment (Cameron, 1964), direct trauma, and compression between the atlas and the axis (Hunter, 1949). In addition, irritation of the sensory fibers of C1 through C2 may result in pain at both the neck and head. The role of C3 and C4 nerve root compression as a cause of head pain is not as well established (Braag & Rosner, 1975; Brain, 1963).

Occipital neuralgia may be present when there is an intermittent, jabbing quality to the pain, in the distribution of the greater or lesser occipital nerves. Tenderness may be present over the point where the occipital nerve crosses the superior nuchal line. Diminished sensation or dyesthesias are usually present over the affected area.

The distinction between occipital neuralgia and referred pain from the atlantoaxial or C3 zygapophyseal joints must be established. At the latter site, there is usually more continuous pain with no sensory loss. To isolate this distinction, the second cervical ganglion may be blocked (Bogduk, 1981), or the tender area may be infiltrated locally with xylocaine and corticosteroids.

As in other forms of neuralgic pain, carbamazepine is the drug of choice for treatment of this syndrome. The initial dose of carbamazepine is usually 100 mg per day; this is gradually increased up to 800 mg per day, in divided doses. In some cases, immobilization of the area with a cervical collar may be indicated. Transcutaneous stimulator (TENS) units have reportedly benefited some patients (Hammond & Danta, 1978). Neurosurgical procedures, including decompression of the greater occipital nerve through the muscular channel percutaneous radio frequency neurotomy and peripheral or intradural nerve root section, may be considered for refractive cases.

Cervicogenic headache (Sjaastad et al., 1983) may be triggered by mechanical factors involving the cervical spine. The pain is unilateral and may be associated with blurred vision, tinnitus, lacrimation, tingling, and arm pain. In more severe and protracted cases, symptoms associated with migraine, such as nausea and anorexia, may occur. Moving the neck in various positions or palpation of the cervical spine may induce an attack. The duration of a cervicogenic headache may continue from minutes to days. Diagnosis of the condition is enhanced by a cervical nerve block of C2 and C3 ipsilateral to the headache. Recent work presented by Pfaffenrath, Mayer, and their associates (1984) have demonstrated a computerized technology utilizing tomography of the cervical spine in two positions, flexion–extension and lateral flexion, which may provide evidence of abnormality of joint motion of the C2–C3 articulations. Indomethacin may provide relief in this condition, although in refractive cases surgical treatment may be required.

Occlusion of the vertebral arterial system in the neck has long been suspected to be a source for occipital headache (Yates & Hutchinson, 1961). Headache is a common complaint in patients with vertebrobasilar insufficiency (Grindal & Toole, 1974). The vertebral arteries are closely associated with the first six cervical vertebrae rendering them susceptible to compression. Direct blows to the neck, attempted strangulation, aggressive cervical manipulation, or other neck trauma (Schneider & Crosby, 1959) may occasionally cause small tears in the intimal lining of the vertebral arteries, with subsequent development of thrombus formation. The embolization that may ensue will produce various brain-stem stroke syndromes, with the site dependent on the location of the emboli. In these cases, anticoagulant therapy must be started immediately. Compression of the vertebral arteries may occur with advanced osteophyte formation. However, how this mechanism causes headache has not been fully explained. The sympathetic nerve supply that surrounds the vertebral arteries possibly affects the cerebral blood flow and thus may induce headache (Bartschi-Rochaix, 1968; Harper, et al., 1972).

Bony anomalies of the craniovertebral junction may induce neck pain in 13 to 26% of those affected cases (McRae, 1960, 1966, 1969). Anomalies such as occipitalization of the atlas, congenital atlantoaxial dislocation, and basilar invagination, may produce pain. In many of these cases, flexion of the neck will trigger pain. The pain, which is localized to the suboccipital and occipital areas, is aggravated by the supine position (Edmeads, 1978). Congenital conditions, such as Dandy-Walker syndrome or Arnold-Chiari malformation, may cause cervical pain (Watkins, 1969) or exertional headache (Rooke, 1968).

Headache Associated with Cervical Spondylosis

Degenerative changes begin with the disk. The process may involve herniation of the disk through the annulus fibrosis, or the development of osteophytic changes of the articulated surfaces of the vertebrae as well as the anterior longitudinal wall. While the process is usually asymptomatic, the patients may describe pain that encompasses the head and neck (Petersen, et al., 1975). When the degenerative changes are severe, nerve root entrapment by osteophytes may occur. Compression of the cervical cord and nerve root fiber may occur with herniation of a cervical disk. Pain in the cervical spine may occur through local inflammatory changes or through reflex spasm of the paraspinal muscles (Brain, 1963; Graham, 1964). This is the mechanism responsible for the headache associated with cervical spondylosis.

Spondylotic head pain begins as an ache in the morning and may progress to a more constant and nagging pain. The physical examination of the patient with moderate to advanced spondylosis will frequently reveal muscle spasm as well as suboccipital tenderness. Movement of the neck may be somewhat limited. Early in the course of therapy, an anti-inflammatory agent and immobilization through a soft cervical collar is indicated. Cervical traction may enhance pain relief. However, surgery may be considered if the following are observed: spinal cord compression, significant root involvement, long tract signs such as motor weakness or reflex changes, or numbness.

Rheumatoid arthritis and ankylosing spondylitis are also associated with symptomatic involvement of the cervical spine. The major problem that occurs is atlantoaxial subluxation; contributing factors are inflammation, atlantoaxial bony dissolution, and stretching. Pain frequently occurs with subluxation. The patient often complains of a deep occipital ache, which increases in intensity as the head is flexed forward. A sharp pain may also occur. The pain may radiate to encompass the head in a hatband distribution, or the ache may localize to the temple or eye. Compression of the lower medulla and upper cervical cord may occur secondary to the increased mobility that is present, with the odontoid process being displaced backwards into the spinal canal or foramen magnum. The headache may present with signs of cord compression, including paresthesias, long tract signs, or numbness. Pain secondary to inflammation may also occur with rheumatoid arthritis, presenting at the occiput and neck. Immobilization of the head or extension of the neck may temporarily relieve the condition. In refractive cases, surgery may be considered. Neck exercises and traction are not indicated.

Trauma to the Cervical Spine

Trauma to the neck may produce a variety of pain syndromes, ranging from a mild and self-limited condition to a prolonged pain problem involving the head and neck.

Acceleration injury, whiplash, and cervical sprain or strain are common terms for soft tissue injuries of the cervical region. Motor vehicle accidents are the major cause of the more serious injuries. Following the typical rear-end auto collision, the unsupported head and neck hyperextend. This hyperextension occurs within the first quarter second. The muscle reflexes, which are the major protective mechanism for the neck, are unable to respond adequately in this short period. If head supports are properly fitted and correctly positioned in autos, there is a significant decrease in the incidence of hyperextension and the ensuing injuries.

In addition to hyperextension, hyperflexion or lateral flexion may occur following auto accidents or other traumas to the neck. The injuries incurred are not usually as extensive or serious as those precipitated by hyperextension because of the limited amount of flexion through which the head can progress.

The physical examination is usually normal during the initial 2 to 3 hours following neck trauma. However, after this initial period, anterior neck swelling and tenderness may be observed, particularly in acceleration–extension injuries, thus restricting neck movement. Trapezius spasm may also appear. The stiffness and decreased cervical range of motion will usually continue from days to weeks, with a gradual improvement. Headache is a common symptom in these injuries, along with tinnitus, pain in the cervical area, dizziness, vertigo, and visual disturbances. The patient may experience pain radiating down one or both arms, which results from nerve root pressure or spasm of the scalene muscles.

General treatment measures for soft tissue neck injuries include rest and protection of the neck. A soft cervical collar may offer relief. However, this treatment should be used on a limited basis and not continued after the healing period. Heat applied locally to the neck will relieve the muscle spasm. Physical therapy in its various forms may be employed and will usually enhance the comfort of the patient. It should be noted that traction is contraindicated, as injured and inflamed muscles and ligaments would be stretched during this particular therapy. The cautious use of muscle relaxants may help (Hohl, 1983). After the spasm and tenderness regress, isometric exercises have been used successfully.

For many unfortunate patients, the symptoms will persist for a long period after the injury. Headache as well as neck pain and stiffness are the major continuing complaints. The physical examination on follow-up is usually normal. There is evidence that the initial injury to the neck may initiate the prolonged process of disk degeneration, demonstrated on follow-up cervical radiographic studies performed many years later. After studying 179 consecutive patients with soft tissue injuries, Greenfield and Ilfeld (1977) concluded that progress was much slower in those patients who presented initially with shoulder, arm, or back pain, in addition to the usual symptoms.

Reviewing follow-up reports of soft tissue neck injuries revealed that litigation is not a predictor of prolonged disability. Hohl and Hopp (1978) and Hohl (1974), indicated that injuries independent of the neck region, appear to heal faster with less persisting symptoms. If litigation were the solitary reason for the symptomatology, these other injuries would also persist as long as the soft tissue neck injuries. Of Hohl's 266 patients, 45% continued to suffer significant symptoms 2 years following final settlement of their litigation.

Injury to the soft tissue of the anterior neck may produce headache. Traumatic dysautonomic cephalalgia has been described by Vijayan (1977). Symptoms include a unilateral vascular headache associated with pupillary dilation and facial swelling ipsilateral to the side of the injury. Vijayan proposed that the syndrome was caused by a stretching injury to the carotid arteries. Propranolol has been used successfully in the prophylaxis of this condition.

Thoracic outlet syndrome following neck trauma may present with obvious symptoms of subclavian artery aneurysm, gangrene, and brachial or subclavian artery thrombosis. In less distinct cases (Jamieson & Mersky, 1985), the clinical history and examination may be ambiguous and suggest a psychoneurotic disorder. Almost invariably, a triad of findings is present. These consist of neck, shoulder, and arm pain, postural discomfort of the arm, and paresthesias of the hand and finger. Only one fourth of the cases have postural effects or vascular changes. Although Adson's sign may be present, tenderness over the brachial plexus or the margin of trapezius, along with provocation of symptoms by military bracing of the arms or hyperabduction and extension of the arms, may enable confirmation of the diagnosis.

ACKNOWLEDGMENT

Frederick G. Freitag, D.O., and Larry D. Robbins, M.D., of the Diamond Headache Clinic, Chicago, Illinois, assisted in the preparation of this chapter.

REFERENCES

Ayd, F.J. (1971). Recognizing and treating depressed patients. *Mod. Med. 39*:80–86.
Ayd, F.J. (1980). Amitriptyline (Elavil) therapy for depressive reactions. *Psychosomatics 21*:November–December.
Bartschi-Rochaix, W. (1968). Headache of cervical origin. In *Clinical Neurology,* Vol. 5 (Vinken and Bruyn, eds.), pp. 192–201. North Holland Publishing, Amsterdam.
Basbaum, A.I. and H.L. Fields (1978). Endogenous pain control mechanisms: Review and hypothesis. *Ann. Neurol. 4,* 451–462.

Blackwell, B. (1979). MHPG in depression. *Psychiat. Opinion*, July–August.

Bogduk, N. (1981). Local anesthetic block of the second cervical ganglion; a technique with application to cervical headache. *Cephalgia 1*:41.

Braag, M.M. and S. Rosner (1975). Trauma of cervical spine as cause of chronic headache. *J. Trauma 15*:441–446.

Brain, W.R. (1963). Some unsolved problems of cervical spondylosis. *Brit. Med. J. 1*:771–777.

Cameron, B.M. (1964). Cervical spine sprain headache. *Am. J. Orthop. 6*:9.

Chouret, E.E. (1967). The greater occipital neuralgia headache. *Headache 7*:33–34.

Cobbin, D., Requin-Blow, B. Williams R.L. et al. (1979). Urinary MHPG levels and tricyclic antidepressant drug selection. *Arch. Gen. Psychiatry 36*:1111–1115.

Dalessio, D.J. (1972). *Wolff's Headache and Other Head Pain*, 3rd ed., pp. 552–555. Oxford University Press, New York.

Diamond, S. (1963). The use of amitriptyline hydrochloride in general practice. *Il Med. J. 123*:347–348.

Diamond, S. (1964). Depressive headaches. *Headache 4*:255–259.

Diamond, S. (1966). Double-blind controlled study of amitriptyline-perphenazine combination in medical office patients with depression and anxiety. *Psychosomatics 7*: 371–375.

Diamond, S. (1977). Nine experts review a FP's depression regimen. *Patient Care 11*:42–77.

Diamond, S. (1983). Depression and headache. *Headache 23*:122–126.

Diamond, S. and B.J. Baltes (1969). The office treatment of mixed anxiety and depression with combination therapy. *Psychosomatics 10*:360–365.

Editorial (1971). The great pretender. *Emergency Med. 3*:21–27.

Edmeads, J.R. (1978). Headaches and head pains associated with diseases of the cervical spine. *Med. Clin. North Am. 62*:533–544.

Fawcett, J. (1980). Depression at the biochemical level. *Psych Ann 109* (Suppl):362–368.

Feighner, J.P. (1982). Pharmacological management of depression. *Fam. Pract. Recert. 4 (suppl 1)*:13–24.

Fields, H.L. (1981). Pain II: New approaches to management. *Ann. Neurol. 9*:101–106.

Friedman, A.P., T.J.C. Von Storch, and H.H. Merritt (1964). Migraine and tension headaches. A clinical study: 2000 cases. *Neurology 4*:773.

Graham, J.R. (1964). Treatment of muscle contraction headache. *Mod. Treatment 1*:1399–1403.

Greenfield, J. and F.W. Ilfeld (1977). Acute cervical strain. Evaluation and short-term prognostic factors. *Clin. Orthop. 122*:196.

Grindal, A.B. and J.F. Toole (1975) Headaches and transient ischemic attacks. *Stroke 5*:603–606.

Hammond, S.R. and G. Danta (1978). Occipital neuralgia. *Clin. Exp. Neurol. 15*:258.

Harper, A.M., V.P. Deshmuth, O.V. Ronan et al. (1972). The influence of sympathetic nervous activity on cerebral blood flow. *Arch. Neurol. 27*:1–6.

Hodgkins, K. (1976) Educational implications of the Virginia study. *J. Fam. Pract. 3*:1.

Hohl, M. (1974). Soft tissue injuries of the neck in automobile accidents; factors influencing prognosis. *J. Bone Joint Surg. 56A*:1675.

Hohl, M. (1983). Soft tissue neck injuries. In *The Cervical Spine* (R.W. Bailey, ed.), pp. 282–287. J.B. Lippincott, Philadelphia.

Hohl, M. and E. Hopp (1978). Soft tissue injuries of the neck II. Factors influencing prognosis. *Orthop. Trans. 2*:29.

Hunter, C.R., and F.H. Mayfield (1949). Role of the upper cervical nerve roots in the production of pain in the head. *Am J Surg 78*:743–749.

Jamieson, W.G. and H. Mersky (1985). Representation of the thoracic outlet syndrome as a problem in chronic and psychiatric management. *Pain 22*:195–200.

Lance, J.W., G.A. Lambert, P.J. Goadsby, and J.W. Duckworth (1983). Brainstem influences on the cephalic circulation: Experimental data from cat and monkey of relevance to the mechanism of migraine. *Headache* 23:258–265.

McRae, D.L. (1960). The significance of abnormalities of the cervical spine. Caldwell Lecture. *Am. J. Roentgen. 84*:1–25.

McRae, D.L. (1966). The cervical spine and neurologic disease. *Radiol. Clin. North Am.* 4:145–158.

McRae, D.L. (1969). Bony abnormalities at the craniospinal junction. *Clin. Neurosurg. 16*:356–375.

Maas, J. (1973). The biology of depression: Where we stand. *Psychiatry 1973 5*:67–69.

Maas, J. (1975). Biogenic amines and depression. *Arch. Gen. Psychiatry 32*:1357–1361.

Maas, J.W., J.H. Kocsis, C.D. Bowden et al. (1982). Pretreatment neurotransmitter metabolites and response to imipramine or amitriptyline treatment. *Psychol. Med. 12*:37–43.

Malseed, R.T. and F.J. Goldstein (1979). Enhancement of morphine analgesia by tricyclic antidepressants. *Neuropharmacology 18*:827–829.

Marsland, D.W., M. Wood, and F. Mayo (1976). Content of family practice. *J. Fam. Pract.* 3:1.

Martin, M.J., H.P. Rome, and W.M. Swenson (1967). Muscle contraction headache. A psychiatric review. *Res. Clin. Stud. Headache. 1*:184.

Mathew, N.T. (1981). Prophylaxis of migraine and mixed headache. A randomized controlled study. *Headache 21*:105–109.

Mayer, D.J. and D.D. Price (1976). Central nervous system mechanisms of analgesia. *Pain* 2:379-404.

Mayer, E., G. Herrmann, V. Pfaffenrath et al. (1985). Functional radiographs of the craniocervical region and cervical spine. A new computer aided technique. *Cephalgia 5*:237–243.

Messing, R.B., L. Phebus, L.A. Fisher et al. (1975). Analgesic effect of fluoxetine HC1 (Lilly 110140), a specific uptake inhibitor for serotonergic neurons. *Psychopharmacol. Comm. 1*:511–521.

Messing, R.B. and L.D. Lytle (1977). Serotonin-containing neurons: Their possible role in pain and analgesia. *Pain 4*:1–21.

Peterson, P.F., G.M. Austin, and L.A. Dayes (1975). Headaches associated with discogenic diseases of the cervical spine. *Bull. Los Angeles Neurol. Soc. 40*:96–100.

Pfaffenrath, V., E.T. Mayer, W. Pollman et al. (1984). The cervicogenic headache—correlation of the symptomatology with results of a computer aided evaluation of radiographs of the cervical spine, with attention to the atlantoaxial articulations. In *Proceedings of the Fifth International Migraine Symposium,* pp. 19–20, London.

Ravaris, C., C.L. Ravaris, D.S. Robinson, and J.O. Ives et al. (1980). Phenelzine and amitriptyline in treatment of depression. A comparison of present and past studies. *Arch. Gen. Psychiatry 37*:1057–1080.

Robinson, D.S., A. Nies, and C.L. Ravaris, et al. (1973). The monoamine oxidase inhibitor, phenelzine, in the treatment of depressive-anxiety states. A controlled clinic trial. *Arch. Gen. Psychiatry 29*:407–413.

Rooke, E.D. (1968). Exertional headache. *Med. Clin. North Am. 52*:801–808.

Saarnivaara, L., and M.J. Mattila (1974). Comparison of tricyclic antidepressants in rabbits: Antinociception and potentiation of the noradrenalin pressor responses. *Psychopharmacologia 35*:221–236.

Schatzberg, A.F., A.H. Rosenbaum P.J. Orsulak, et al. (1980). Toward a biochemical classification of depressive disorders IV: Pretreatment urinary MHPG levels as predictors of ˂ntidepressant response to imipramine. *Comm. Psychopharmacology 4*:441–445.

Schatzberg, A.F., A.H. Rosenbaum, P.J. Orsulak et al. (1981). Toward a biochemical classification of depressive disorders III: Pretreatment urinary MHPG levels as predictors of response to treatment with maprotiline. *Psychopharmacology 75*:34–38.

Schatzberg, A.F., P.J. Orsulak, and A.H. Rosenbaum et al. (1982). Toward a biochemical classification of depressive disorders V: Heterogeneity of unipolar depressions. *Am. J. Psychiatry 139*:471–475.

Schneider, R.C. and E.C. Crosby (1959). Vascular insufficiency of brain stem and spinal cord in spinal trauma. *Neurology 9*:643–656.

Schuckit, M., E. Robins, J. Feighner et al. (1971). Tricyclic antidepressants and monoamine oxidase inhibitors. *Arch. Gen. Psychiatry 24*:509–514.

Sjaastad, O., C. Saumte, H. Hovdahl et al. (1983). Cervicogenic headache, an hypothesis. *Cephalalgia 3*:249–256.

Snyder, S.H. and S.R. Childers (1979). Opiate receptors and opioid peptides. *Annu. Rev. Neurosci. 2*:35–64.

Vijayan, N. (1977). A new post—traumatic headache syndrome: Clinical and therapeutic observations. *Headache 17*:19.

Watkins, W.S. (1969). Paroxysmal headache due to the Chiari malformation. *Dis. Nerv. Syst. 30*:693–695.

Yates, P.O. and E.C. Hutchinson (1961). Cerebral infarction: The role of stenosis of the extracranial cerebral arteries. In *Medical Research Council Special Reports,* No. 30. H.M. Stationery Office, London.

11

Cranial Arteritis and Polymyalgia Rheumatica

DONALD J. DALESSIO
GARY W. WILLIAMS

Cranial arteritis (CA) is a febrile, often self-limiting disease that affects the aged of both sexes and is characterized by painful inflammation of the temporal and other cranial arteries and generalized systemic signs and symptoms including malaise, weakness, weight loss, anorexia, fever, and sweating (Huston et al., 1978).

Other names for this arterial disease include temporal arteritis, granulomatous arteritis, and giant-cell arteritis. Of these several terms, the most descriptive is giant-cell arteritis, which is probably employed least. Temporal arteritis is actually misleading, because it implies localization of the inflammatory process to the superficial temporal arteries, whereas in the usual case the disease is widespread. We will use the term cranial arteritis in this chapter.

A related disease is polymyalgia rheumatica (PMR), characterized by complaints of pain and stiffness of the limbs and trunk, often associated with systemic signs of a nature similar to those of CA described above.

A significant number of patients with PMR, ranging from 30 to 50 %, will eventually develop CA during the course of their illness. This suggests that the two diseases are in fact one; the myalgias and synovitis of polymyalgia rheumatia may represent a developmental stage of cranial arteritis.

LABORATORY FINDINGS

The laboratory data in CA and PMR are similar. The principal findings are those associated with inflammation. Marked elevation of the erythrocyte sedimentation rate is characteristic of these two diseases, and the absence of such an elevation makes the diagnosis suspect. Rare cases of ''normal'' sedimentation rates in patients with biopsy-proven CA occur, but it must be emphasized that these occur infrequently. The authors have never personally examined a patient with CA with a ''normal'' sedimentation rate; however, it is not unusual to confirm the diagnosis in patients with mild elevations, especially if the patient has been treated with nonsteroidal anti-inflammatory agents. Normal values for sedimentation rates are age-dependent but, in general, rates above 35 to 40 mm/hour can be accepted as abnormal in patients of any age. Values of 100 mm/hour or greater are common in these diseases. When possible, the Westergren method should be used. Variations in results occur when blood is allowed to stand, and therefore the test should be set up within 1 hour of drawing the sample.

In addition to elevated sedimentation rates, a mild to moderate normochromic anemia is often seen along with mild leukocytosis. Nonspecific changes in plasma proteins are common, including elevation of plasma fibrinogen levels, alpha-2-globulins, complement, and gamma globulins with slight depression of the serum albumin. Liver function tests are frequently abnormal; especially common are mild elevations of the alkaline phosphatases with elevations of serum transaminases. In several cases percutaneous liver biopsies were performed. Most often, fine bile ducts with intracellular deposition of bile pigment characteristic of cholestasis has been reported. In one personally observed case, in addition to cholestasis, a granuloma was present in the biopsy specimen. In spite of the prominent proximal muscle pain in patients with polymyalgia, the tests for muscle inflammation are normal. An elevated creatine kinase or aldolase level suggests the diagnosis of an inflammatory myopathy of another sort.

Interest has been increasing in markers of vessel inflammation that might be helpful in distinguishing the subgroup of patients with polymyalgia rheumatica who also have cranial arteritis. Elevated levels of von Willebrand factor antigen have been found in the blood of patients with CA and other forms of vasculitis (Nusinow et al., 1984). Studies currently in progress should further our understanding of the factors released by endothelial cells in response to injury and the ways in which such factors can be used to identify patients at risk for serious complications of vessel inflammation.

Should the temporal artery be biopsied when a diagnosis of CA is suspected? In most cases, yes. In an emergency, for example, in which vision is threatened, the biopsy can be done after corticosteroid therapy has been started. When consigning patients to long-term therapy with corticosteroids, however, we prefer to have a tissue diagnosis whenever possible. In patients with a diagnosis of PMR in whom there is no clinical or historical evidence of CA, we do not proceed to biopsy.

BIOPSY FINDINGS

In cranial arteritis the involved arteries are grossly seen as tortuous, swollen, nodular vessels with or without pulsation, with cellulitis of contiguous tissue. Biopsies of temporal arteries have been performed in more than half of the cases reported, and some patients have come to autopsy. Microscopic examination reveals a panarteritis. The typical section reveals hypertrophy of the intima, medial necrosis associated with the formation of granulomatous tissue and the presence of foreign body giant cells, periarterial cellular infiltration, and thrombus formation (Figs. 11-1, 11-2). Eosino-

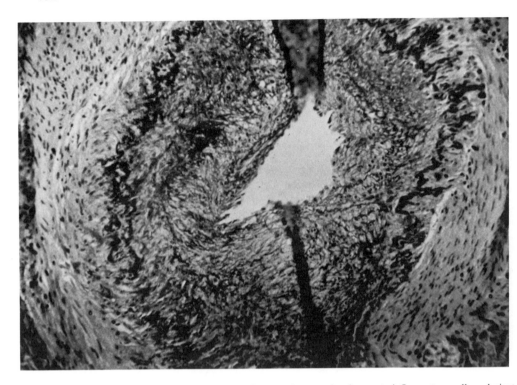

Figure 11-1. Cranial arteritis. Section of a biopsy of temporal artery showing acute inflammatory cells and giant cells (H&E stain).

philic invasion of the artery in cranial arteritis is rare. The presence of giant cells has suggested a tuberculous etiology, but no tubercules have been seen, and no acid-fast bacilli have been demonstrated.

Consecutive biopsies on three cranial arteritis patients were studied by electron microscopy by Kuwabara and Reinecke (1970). All biopsies showed a combination of pathologic changes of various stages of the disease with information of the smooth muscle cell involvement. Biopsies obtained in the clinically acute periods showed predominantly inflammatory elements. Later biopsies from the same patients showed granulomatous reactions and muscular regeneration.

Klein et al. (1976) called attention to the intermittency of pathologic changes (skip lesions) that may occur in cranial arteritis. They identified skip lesions in 17 of 60 patients with temporal arteritis, based on a retrospective and prospective examination of temporal artery biopsy specimens. Examining more than 6000 serial sections of arteries from patients with skip lesions, they found foci of arteritis as short as 330 mm in length in an otherwise normal biopsy specimen. Their study suggests the need to biopsy long segments of the artery, to examine multiple histologic sections, and perhaps to consider performing a contralateral temporal artery biopsy when frozen section examination of the first side is normal.

Lie, Brown, and Carter (1970) made a study of 150 temporal arteries from cadavers and described senile changes in these arteries occurring with advancing age. Pro-

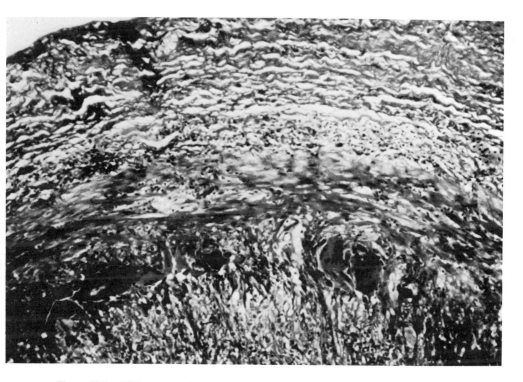

Figure 11-2.   Higher-power view of Figure 11-1, graphically demonstrating the giant cells.

gressive intimal thickening and alteration of the internal elastic lamina occurred from infancy to senility without development of atheroma.

Senile changes in temporal arteries are not associated with giant-cell reaction and should not be confused with the active phase of cranial arteritis. The residual changes of cranial arteritis that may persist for many years are sufficiently different from the ordinary changes of senescence to enable one to distinguish between the senescent arteries and the arteries previously involved with the inflammatory reaction characteristic of temporal arteritis.

IMMUNOLOGIC STUDIES

Liang et al. (1974) performed immunofluorescent studies on 15 consecutive temporal artery biopsy specimens and on control specimens obtained from 10 patients with unrelated diseases. They found four different patterns of immunoglobulin deposition. Immunoglobulins (Ig) were prominent in nuclei outlined by cytoplasmic staining and were also at the disrupted internal elastic membrane in 7 of 15 patients. These patterns were not present in the 10 control temporal artery specimens obtained at autopsy. The authors suggest that the cytoplasmic staining for IgG, IgM, IgA, and the third component of complement resulted from phagocytosis of antibodies, complexed with antigen and complement within the vessel wall. They suggest, further, that the elastic pattern is consistent with two mechanisms: (1) elastic tissues may bind anti-body specific to the tissue or (2) immune complexes may penetrate the endothelium and then lodge passively against the internal elastic membrane. These findings par-allel those for other forms of vasculitis and suggest that antibodies participate in the pathogenesis of cranial arteritis. The immunoglobulins in these vessels may be anti-bodies to a component of the arterial wall, presumably elastin, or they may result from the deposition of circulating immune complexes.

Reyes et al. (1976) described a 67-year-old woman with a 5-month history of progressive, multiple neurologic deficits; an autopsy revealed viruslike particles as-sociated with granulomatous angitis of the central nervous system. The small paren-chymal and leptomeningeal blood vessels of the brain and spinal cord were particu-larly affected. Electron microscopic studies of formalin-fixed brain disclosed intranuclear particles resembling herpes virus. Although definitive proof cannot be established, Reyes and his collaborators suggest that some cases of granulomatous angitis of the central nervous system may result from virus infection.

Malmvall and associates (1976) studied immunoglobulin levels in the serum of 36 patients (25 women and 11 men) with a mean age of 70 years. Twenty-four (15 women and 9 men) had histologic findings of cranial arteritis in temporal biopsy specimens. Complement levels were determined in 30 of the patients. A control group consisted of 39 hospitalized patients with a mean age of 74 years, none of whom had fever or elevated sedimentation rate, and in whom there was no evidence of immunologic, malignant, or infectious diseases. In the group with giant-cell arteritis, the mean values of IgE, total complement, and complement factors C_3 and C_4 were statistically significantly higher than those in the control group. There was no in-crease of IgM concentration. The concentration of IgA was higher in men with giant-cell arteritis than in men in the control group, but no difference was seen among the women.

We have surveyed 36 temporal artery biopsies obtained from 1975 through 1978. All were examined with standard pathologic techniques, hematoxylin and eosin stain-ing (H&E), and with immunofluorescent methods (IF). Of the 36 patients, 21 were women and 15 were men. In some selected cases, elastic stains were done. IF in-cluded IgG, IgA, IgM, C_{1q}, C_3, and fibrinogen. The results from nine representative patients with giant-cell arteritis are presented in Table 11-1.

In addition, only H&E and IF studies were done in eight other cases. Of these, half showed fibrinogen within the lumen and IgG on the internal elastic membrane.

These data suggest that giant-cell arteritis probably represents a disorder of im-munologic vasculitis associated with the deposition of immune complexes within the walls of affected blood vessels. This would lead to localized vascular injury and inflammation, producing the systemic signs of the disease.

CLINICAL ASPECTS

The symptomatology of the disease may be divided into the nonspecific complaints of a generalized systemic nature and specific complaints directly attributable to in-

Table 11-1 Hematoxylin/eosin and immunofluorescence findings in nine patients with cranial arteritis

Age (years)	H/E stain diagnosis (Dx)	IF					
		IgG	IgA	IgM	C1q	C3	Fib
74	Temporal arteritis	Luminal	—	Luminal	—	—	Luminal
68	Giant-cell arteritis	Internal elastic membrane	—	—	—	—	Diffuse
71	Consistent with temporal arteritis	Linear in smooth muscle	Minimum amount in smooth muscle	Minimum amount in smooth muscle	Linear in smooth muscle	—	Linear in smooth muscle
74	Giant-cell arteritis	—	—	—	—	—	—
68	Giant-cell arteritis	—	—	—	—	—	Luminal
69	Giant-cell arteritis	—	—	—	—	—	—
62	Giant-cell arteritis	—	—	—	—	—	—
78	Arteritis with intact elastica "not temporal"	Scattered in intima/media	—	Fine granular deposits at elastica	—	—	Deposits in all parts
76	Temporal arteritis	In media and intima	—	—	In media	In media	In media

Key to abbreviations:
H/E = hematoxylin and eosin.
IgA, IgG, IgM = immunoglobulins A, G, M.
C1q, C3 = complement components.
Fib = fibrinogen.

flammation and distension of the temporal and other arteries (Table 11-2) (William-son & Russell, 1972).

Not all patients with CA have headache, but when present, the headache is of high intensity, of a deep aching quality, throbbing in nature, and persistent. In addition to the aching and throbbing, there is often a burning component, unlike most other vascular headaches. The headache is slightly worse when the patient lies flat in bed, and is diminished in intensity by the upright or half-upright position. It is somewhat reduced in intensity by digital pressure on the common carotid artery on the affected side and is made worse by stooping over. Hyperalgesia of the scalp is present; be-cause the distended arteries are extremely tender, any pressure greatly increases the pain.

Some patients may suffer pain on mastication, and in some this may be the initial symptom. Facial swelling and redness of the skin overlying the temporal arteries, with the addition of the burning component of pain, are usually noted after the onset of headache. Immediate relief from burning pain and headache may follow biopsy of the inflamed temporal artery, and it is assumed that this follows the interruption of the afferents for pain about the vessel.

Before the onset of full-blown CA, pain often occurs in the teeth, ear, jaw, zyg-oma and nuchal region, and the occiput. The distribution of these symptoms suggests primary involvement of other branches of the external carotid artery, notably the external and internal maxillary arteries.

OCULAR SYMPTOMS

The presenting complaint may be of ocular origin. It has become evident that more than a third of patients with CA are threatened with partial or even complete loss of vision. Diplopia and photophobia have been noted, ophthalmoscopic evidence of oc-clusion of the central retinal artery has been apparent in some cases, and some cases with complete loss of vision have been reported.

CEREBRAL SYMPTOMS

Some patients have presented signs suggestive of cerebral damage and encephalitis during the acute stage of the illness. Mental sluggishness, dizziness, vomiting, dy-sarthria, delirium, and even coma have been described.

Cases of CA with involvement of intracranial arteries may occur. In addition to the usual constitutional symptoms of weight loss, anorexia, low-grade fever, and headache, these patients also demonstrate lethargy, depression, and cranial nerve palsies. Major stroke may occur.

Table 11-2 Numerical incidence of involvement of the various arteries (from Wilkinson & Russell)

Artery	No. of arteries described (i.e., their state was definitely ascertained at the time of autopsy) in the 12 patients	No. of arteries severely involved in the 12 patients	No. of arteries mildly involved in the 12 patients	"Incidence" of severe involvement (%)	"Incidence" of mild involvement (%)
Superficial temporal	22	22		100	
Vertebral	13	13		100	
Ophthalmic	17	13		76	
Posterior ciliary	12	9		75	
External carotid	15	7	4	47	27
Petrous and cavernous segments or internal carotid	8	3	5	38	62
Proximal central retinal	10	6	3	60	30
Distal central retinal	11	3	4	26	36
Cervical segment of internal carotid	8		2		25
Common carotid	14		2		14
Large arteries at base of brain	10		2		20
Small intracranial	10		1		20

Table 11-3 Presenting symptoms in 50 patients with GCA

Symptoms[a]	Patients (No.)	Percentage
Headache	45	90
Jaw pain	20	40
Generalized aching, stiffness	19	38
Visual complaints	17	34
Cerebral symptoms	15	30
Tender aching temporal arteries	12	24
Fatigue, malaise, insomnia	14	28
Neck and back pain	10	20

[a]Not mutually exclusive.

OTHER SYMPTOMS

In every case, signs and symptoms have been present that cannot be plausibly related to the sterile inflammation of the temporal arteries alone, and are more suggestive of systemic arteritis.

Prevalent symptoms and signs are weight loss, anorexia, general malaise, fever, sweating, and weakness. The weight loss may be profound, and the patient may be emaciated. This condition is probably secondary to anorexia, which, though in certain cases is a concomitant of the excruciating pain and headache, may antedate the onset of pain. Sweating is a common symptom.

Inconstant low-grade fever not associated with shaking chills is recorded in 70% of the cases. The average temperature is 37.8°C, although recordings as high as 39.5° have been made.

Other complaints of a nonspecific nature are weakness, lassitude, malaise and "grippy feelings," and fatigue (occasionally to the point of prostration) (see Table 11-3).

PAINFUL OPHTHALMOPLEGIA (TOLOSA–HUNT SYNDROME)

Six cases of retro-orbital pain and involvement of the structures lying within the cavernous sinus and its wall were studied by Hunt et al. (1961). Pain may precede the ophthalmoplegia by several days, or may not occur until some time later. It is not a throbbing hemicrania occurring in paroxysms, but a steady pain behind the eye that is often described as "gnawing" or "boring." The defects are not confined to the third cranial nerve; the fourth, sixth, and first division of the fifth cranial nerves are also implicated. Periarterial sympathetic fibers and the optic nerve may be involved. The symptoms last for days or weeks. Spontaneous remissions occur, sometimes with residual motor or sensory deficit. Attacks recur at intervals of months or years. No systemic reaction occurs. The syndrome is presumably caused by an inflammatory lesion of the cavernous sinus. Tolosa (1954) of the Neurological Institute of Barcelona, published the report of a single case that met the preceding criteria. His patient expired after an exploratory operation, and autopsy showed an inflammatory lesion of the cavernous sinus. The syndrome, also called pseudotumor of the orbit, has been carefully considered, reviewed, and discussed by Ingalls (1953) and as a "syndrome of the superior orbital fissure," it has been studied by Lakke (1962), who supplies an additional bibliography.

Occasional cases of Tolosa–Hunt syndrome still appear in the medical literature. Smith and Taxdal (1966) have emphasized the dramatic response of the syndrome to systemic corticosteroid therapy. Takeoka et al. (1978) have described angiographic findings in a patient with the Tolosa–Hunt syndrome. During the acute episode, at a time when a right third nerve paresis was present, there was evidence of irregular narrowing in the carotid siphon and incomplete opacification of the anterior cerebral artery when angiography was repeated. Ten days later, after treatment with corticosteroids, a remarkable improvement in the prior stenosis had occurred.

A few observations on the Tolosa–Hunt syndrome deserve emphasis. There is a close relationship between the oculomotor paresis that occurs and the angiographic abnormalities. In most patients pupillary function remains normal, with only 20% showing some pupillary involvement. The onset of the third-nerve paresis is rather rapid, but recovery is almost always complete when appropriate therapy is provided.

POLYMYALGIA RHEUMATICA (PMR)

Polymyalgia rheumatica (PMR) does not have an "official" set of criteria for its diagnosis. It may represent a group of related disorders; however, it is generally recognized as a clinical syndrome characterized by the following:

1. Marked stiffness and pain in the muscles of the shoulder and pelvic girdles at night and especially in the morning. Improvement occurs throughout the day with activity.
2. Patients generally over age 50.
3. Absence of prominent symmetrical synovitis.
4. Negative latex fixation test for rheumatoid arthritis.
5. Elevation of the erythrocyte sedimentation rate (ESR) to 50 mm/hour (Westergren).
6. Prompt (usually within 48 hours) response to 15 mg/day of prednisone.

The etiologies of CA and PMR are unknown and although they are often found together, their precise relationship is controversial. They may represent stages in a common inflammatory process, and the clinical picture may reflect certain host responses to an inciting agent. PMR is a more commonly recognized clinical entity, and although it may precede the development of CA it also exists as a stable clinical syndrome for long periods without the development of clinically recognized vessel inflammation. Whether or not all PMR patients are at risk for the development of vessel inflammation is not clear; however, if one biopsies the temporal arteries of patients with PMR in the absence of any signs or symptoms of vessel inflammation, evidence of arteritis will be found in 10 to 15%. The significance of determining the presence or absence of vessel inflammation—that is, PMR versus PMR with CA— has great prognostic and risk significance in the untreated patient; however, in the patient who is about to be started on therapy, the difference is more a matter of levels of steroid use than choices between therapeutic agents. The inability to detect occult vessel inflammation in a certain subgroup of patients with a clinical diagnosis of polymyalgia rheumatica does raise questions regarding the use of nonsteroidal anti-inflammatory agents in this disease, since such agents do not eliminate the possibility of blindness or stroke.

TREATMENT OF CA AND PMR

Short-Term and Long-Term Goals

CA can be considered as a semiacute inflammatory disease that demands rapid treatment. On occasion, if vision is threatened, treatment should be considered as a medical emergency. In the short term the goal is to relieve the patient's complaints. Longer term goals are to suppress the disease sufficiently using the least amount of medication, presuming that the illness will eventually prove self-limiting and will "burn out."

Indications for hospitalization include rapid progression of complaints, especially if vision is threatened. Usually patients with giant-cell arteritis are easily managed on an outpatient basis. The temporal artery biopsies are well suited to an outpatient surgical procedure. Long-term management is almost always in the outpatient department.

Nonpharmacologic Measures

A graduated physical therapy program should be instituted for patients with PMR, particularly emphasizing range of motion, exercise, heat, and hot packs. After the diagnosis has been made and corticosteroids have been begun, similar programs may be useful for patients with CA.

Drug Therapy

Corticosteroids should be used promptly in the therapy of CA and PMR. They should be begun as soon as the diagnosis is made—if necessary, before a temporal artery biopsy. The corticosteroids control the progress of the arteritis, reducing symptoms and preventing the development of ocular complications. Blindness or defects in vision do not always correlate with the severity of the cranial arteritis; thus, all patients should be treated promptly. In CA the treatment is usually initiated with 40 to 60 mg of prednisone daily. Thereafter, this does may be rapidly tapered to a maintenance level, depending on the relief of symptoms and the decline in the sedimentation rate toward normal. In PMR, prednisone may be started at a dosage of 15 mg given as a single dose in the morning. The duration of therapy is uncertain. It may be necessary to continue corticosteroids for months or even years, although eventually it is possible to discontinue treatment in almost all patients.

Absence of response to prednisone within 5 to 7 days is unusual and indicates a more comprehensive evaluation of the presenting complaints. In PMR the response usually, but not invariably, occurs within the first 24 to 72 hours.

Alternate-day corticosteroid therapy is not advisable in CA, at least initially, because systemic symptoms will not be controlled by the drug when used in this manner (Hunder et al., 1975). It is advisable to use a single morning dose of prednisone to minimize the additional side effects associated with split-dose regimens, although the latter may be useful in the initial treatment program when the maximum effect of the drug is desired.

If treatment is stopped in less than 2 years, about 20% of patients with CA will relapse. As the dose of steroids is being tapered in patients with CA, mild to moderate symptoms of PMR sometimes become evident. Generally, this does not constitute an indication to increase the prednisone levels unless there is significant elevation of the sedimentation rate. The sedimentation rate should be checked for several months after the cessation of therapy and the physician should be aware of possible relapses at extended intervals. We recently observed a relapse of PMR after a 2-year asymptomatic steroid-free interval and the development of a vasculitic lesion in another patient previously treated for PMR for 18 months, again, with a 2-year drug-free interval. These examples illustrate the continued risk of patients with this disease and point out the problems in considering any individual patient as "cured."

In long-term treatment of PMR, it may be possible to manage the patient on a low maintenance steroid dose, in the range of 1 to 5 mg/day. If this is done, the clinician should be alert to the appearance of CA despite the low-dose steroid therapy; involvement of the ophthalmic artery producing blindness is a particular concern in this situation.

It is known that other anti-inflammatory drugs, such as the nonsteroidals, are capable of lowering the sedimentation rate and relieving some of the constitutional symptoms of PMR. There are those who argue for their use in PMR patients without signs or symptoms of CA. One of the authors had such a patient referred to him who developed sudden, irreversible monocular blindness while on nonsteroidal anti-inflammatory agents for PMR. Clearly, these agents do *not* protect patients from such serious complications and we do not advocate their use in the initial management of PMR or CA. They may have a role in the later therapy of patients when corticosteroids have been tapered to a low level and the patient experiences symptoms of a musculoskeletal nature associated with the steroid discontinuation. In all cases the physician must be aware of the potential for relapse and the use of the nonsteroidal anti-inflammatory agent in this group of patients may mask the sedimentation rate elevation that accompanies a relapse of either CA or PMR.

Finally, it is important to realize that in every series of patients there are those who, in the process of tapering of corticosteroids, eventually develop a polyarthritis which develops into classic rheumatoid arthritis. Such patients may or may not have positive latex fixation tests. We have observed several patients who have had biopsy-proven CA and subsequently developed seropositive rheumatoid disease.

Complications of Treatment

The complications are those of treatment with corticosteroids. In a personal series of patients with CA, about 40% developed a moonface—Cushingoid appearance; 15% had symptomatic vertebral compression fractures; and 10% had demonstrable proximal muscle weakness.

Some diabetic patients will note increased insulin requirements. The physician needs to be alert to rapid development of cataracts, exacerbation of peptic ulcers, avascular necrosis of bone, reappearance of pulmonary infection, especially tuberculosis, which may occur in treating patients with CA with prednisone.

SUMMARY

- Cranial arteritis and polymyalgia rheumatica may represent different phases of the same disease.
- Most patients will present with signs and symptoms generally associated with inflammation, namely, anorexia, prostration, fever, sweats, weight loss, and leukocytosis; and, in CA, locally, over the artery, heat, swelling, tenderness, redness, and pain.
- Cranial arteritis probably represents an example of immunologic vasculitis associated with the deposition of immune complexes within the walls of the affected blood vessels, thereafter producing localized vascular injury and inflammation.
- Prompt therapy with corticosteroids is indicated in all patients with cranial arteritis and, we believe, in polymyalgia rheumatica.
- Long-term follow-up is indicated in both diseases and the possibility of relapse must be kept in mind, even several years after the discontinuation of corticosteroids.

REFERENCES

Cooke, W.T., P.C.P. Cloake, A.D.T. Govan, and J.C. Colbeck (1946). Temporal arteritis: A generalized vascular disease. *Q. J. Med. 15:*47.

Crompton, M.R. (1959). The visual changes in temporal (giant-celled) arteritis. *Brain 82:*377–390.

Enzmann, D. and W.R. Scott (1977). Intracranial involvement of giant cell arteritis. *Neurology 27:*794–797.

Gocke, D.J., C. Morgan, M. Lockshin, et al. (1970). Association between polyarteritis and Australia antigen. *Lancet 2:*1149–1153.

Heptinstall, R.H., K.A. Porter, and H. Barkely (1954). Giant cell (temporal) arteritis. *J. Pathol. Bacteriol. 67:*507–519.

Hollenhorst, R.W., J.R. Brown, H.P. Wagener, and R.M. Shick (1960). Neurologic aspects of temporal arteritis. *Neurology 10:*490.

Horton, B.T. and T.B. Magath (1937). Arteritis of temporal vessels; report of seven cases. *Proc. Mayo Clin. 12:*548.

Hunder, G.G., S.G. Sheps, G.L. Allen, et al. (1975). Daily and alternate-day corticosteroid regimens in the treatment of giant-cell arteritis: Comparison in a prospective study. *Ann. Intern. Med. 82*:613–618.

Hunt, W.E., J.N. Meagher, H.E. LeFever, and W. Zeman (1961). Painful ophthalmoplegia. Its relation to indolent inflammation of the cavernous sinus. *Neurology 11*:56.

Huston, K.A., G.G. Hunder, J.T. Lie et al. (1978). Temporal arteritis: A 25 year epidemiologic, clinical and pathologic study. *Ann. Intern. Med. 88*:162–167.

Ingalls, R.G. (1953). *Tumors of the Orbit.* C.C. Thomas, Springfield, Ill.

Klein, R.G., R.J. Campbell, G. Hunder, and J. Carney (1976). Skip lesions in temporal arteritis. *Proc. Mayo Clin. 51*:504–510.

Kuwabara, T. and R. Reinecke (1970). Temporal arteritis. *Arch. Ophthalmol. 83*:692–697.

Lakke, J.P.W.F. (1962). The superior orbital fissure syndrome caused by local pachymeningitis, with a case report. *Arch. Neurol. 7*:289.

Liang, G.C., P. Simkin, and M. Mannik (1974). Immunoglobulins in temporal arteritis. *Ann. Intern. Med. 81*:19–23.

Lie, J.T., A.L. Brown, Jr., and E.T. Carter (1970). Spectrum of aging changes in temporal arteries. *Arch. Pathol. 90*:278–285.

Malmvall, B., B. Bengtsson, B. Kaijser et al. (1976) Serum levels of immunoglobulin and complement in giant cell arteritis. *JAMA 236*:1876–1878.

Nusinow, S.R., A.B. Federici, T.S. Zimmerman, J.G. Curd (1984). Increased von Willebrand factor antigen in the plasma of patients with vasculitis. *Arthritis Rheum. 27*:1405–1410.

Reyes, M.G., R. Fresco, S. Chokroverty, and E. Salud (1976). Virus-like particles in granulomatous angiitis of the central nervous system. *Neurology 26*:797–799.

Russell, R.W. (1959). Giant cell arteritis; a review of thirty-five cases. *Q. J. Med. 28*:471–489.

Scott, T. and E.S. Maxwell (1941). Temporal arteritis; a case report. *Intern. Clin. 2*:220–222.

Smith, J.L. and D.J.R. Taxdal (1966). Painful ophthalmoplegia: The Tolosa-Hunt syndrome. *Am. J. Ophthalmol. 61*:1466–1472.

Takeoka T., F. Gotoh, Y. Fukuuchi, and Y. Inagaki (1978). Tolosa, Hunt syndrome. *Arch. Neurol. 35*:219–223.

Tolosa, E. (1954). Periarteritic lesions of carotid siphon with clinical features of carotid infraclinoidal aneurysm. *J. Neurol. Neurosurg. Psychiatry 17*:300.

Wilkinson, I.M. and R.W. Russell (1972). Arteries of the head and neck in giant-cell arteritis. *Arch. Neurol. 27*:378–391.

12

Major Vascular Diseases and Headache

DONALD J. DALESSIO

Headache is a common complaint of patients with cerebrovascular disease. It is consistently associated with acute events characterized by vessel rupture and bleeding. It may not be present when thrombosis is present; for example, even with a major cerebral infarction patients rarely complain of pain, another striking example of the insensitivity of the brain parenchyma to ischemia.

ANATOMIC CONSIDERATIONS

The cerebral arterial tree in humans, unlike that of many organs, has no hilum from which the vessels plunge into the body of the structure. On the contrary, the internal carotid and vertebral arteries are united by the circle of Willis and its six large branches, which encircle the globoid hemispheres at the base of the brain. These six great trunks then divide into branches. A few enter the basal ganglia and choroid plexus, but for the most part they spread themselves like a net in finer and finer branches over the surface of the cortex. Smaller arteries at innumerable points dive deeply into the cortical and subcortical tissues where, through their capillaries, they anastomose with one another and with others coming through the brain substance from the opposite surface of the hemisphere.

The cerebral veins are divided into two groups, the internal and the external, with incomplete anastomoses between them. The internal group drains through the great cerebral vein of Galen, running back directly over the pineal body. The external veins emanate from the region of the insula. Because with growth there is anterior displacement of the frontal lobe and posterior development of the main mass of the hemispheres, the direction of the terminal portion of the great veins is altered; the anterior veins are thus directed posteriorly and the posterior veins course obliquely and anteriorly as they pass to the superior sagittal sinus. The large venous sinuses drain into channels at the base of the skull. The blood then flows from the cranial cavity like fluid from a flask with a gradually tapering neck.

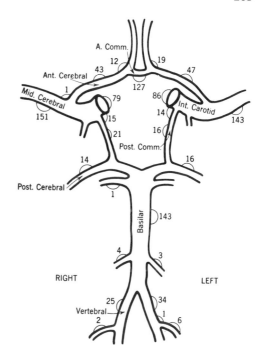

Figure 12-1. Location of intracranial aneurysms in 1023 cases (from McDonald & Korb, 1939).

SUBARACHNOID HEMORRHAGE

The Genesis of Cerebral Aneurysm

The main cerebral blood supply derives from the basilar and internal carotid arteries, meeting in the polygonal arrangement known as the circle of Willis. The internal carotid arteries branch abruptly to give rise to the anterior cerebral and middle cerebral vessels, while a further abrupt branching, the anterior commissure connects two of these, the anterior cerebrals. The paired vertebrals join to form the basilar, which forks at its anterior end into the posterior cerebrals, and these last are connected with the rest of the "circle" by still another abrupt bifurcation, the posterior commissures, which join the internal carotid. A rapidly moving volume of blood is thus forced through a highly angular system of arteries.

The vessels composing the circle of Willis are characterized by a high frequency of aneurysm, particularly at or near the points of bifurcation. A major factor in the occurrence of such aneurysm is congenital weakness of the artery walls, and this appears to be closely related to the angularity of the circle. The relation of the architecture of the circle of Willis to the incidence of aneurysm is shown in Figures 12-1 and 12-2.

Most saccular aneurysms are located on the anterior aspects of the circle of Willis. The most common sites include the following:

1. Adjacent to the anterior communicating artery.
2. At the origin of the posterior communicating artery.

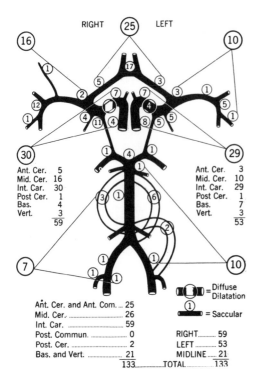

RIGHT (25) LEFT

(16)   (10)

(30)   (29)

Ant. Cer.	5		Ant. Cer.	3
Mid. Cer.	16		Mid. Cer.	10
Int. Car.	30		Int. Car.	29
Post Cer.	1		Post Cer.	1
Bas.	4		Bas.	7
Vert.	3		Vert.	3
	59			53

(7)   (10)

Ant. Cer. and Ant. Com.	25
Mid. Cer.	26
Int. Car.	59
Post. Commun.	0
Post. Cer.	2
Bas. and Vert.	21
	133

= Diffuse Dilatation
① = Saccular

RIGHT	59
LEFT	53
MIDLINE	21
TOTAL	133

Figure 12-2. Arteries involved in 133 aneurysms. There were 108 patients, but in 16 of these the aneurysms were multiple. The total number of aneurysms for each main area is shown in each of the large circles near the outer borders (from Dandy, 1944).

3. At the bifurcation of the internal carotid into the middle and anterior cerebral arteries.
4. At the first bifurcation of the middle cerebral artery.

In 20 to 30% of cases, these may be multiple aneurysms.

Although most aneurysms are saccular, they vary greatly in form. Rarely, giant aneurysms are seen.

The Qualities and Temporal Features of the Headache Associated with Subarachnoid Hemorrhage

Headache is the most common symptom of subarachnoid hemorrhage and occurs in almost every conscious patient. It is usually of very high intensity and of sudden onset. It is often described as "something snapping inside the head," followed by an intense throbbing ache. The ache at the start is commonly located in the occipital region and then radiates down the neck and back. Less commonly, it is located first in the frontal region, bilaterally or unilaterally, in the temporal region, at the vertex, or deep in the eye, but such headache soon radiates into the occipital region. When associated with neck rigidity, the headache is worsened by flexure of the neck.

In more than half of patients, the attack of sudden intense pain is accompanied by vomiting and drowsiness, neck rigidity, and loss of consciousness. Convulsions occur after the onset of headache in approximately 10 to 15% of patients. In 10% there are prodromes lasting a few hours to several days, such as low-intensity frontal or occipital headache, pain in the eye, pain in the back of the neck, backache, or pain in the hamstring muscles. Occasionally the severe headache is preceded by vertigo, photophobia, diplopia, and rarely by vomiting.

The high-intensity headache following subarachnoid hemorrhage persists with little modification for approximately 1 week from its onset, with subsequent complete elimination of pain within 2 months. Sustained, chronic, or recurrent headache persisting longer than 2 months following rupture of intracranial aneurysm with subarachnoid hemorrhage is rare in patients who have not had headaches before the accident.

The initial severe headache associated with sudden hemorrhage into the subarachnoid space about the base of the brain is probably due to traction, displacement, distention, and rupture of pain-sensitive blood vessels and the pia arachnoid. The headache of several days' duration is probably secondary to a sterile inflammatory reaction about the blood vessels and meninges.

Other Presentations of Aneurysms

Full-blown subarachnoid hemorrhages are difficult to miss. Sometimes, however, there are "minibleeds," as only a few cubic centimeters of blood leak from an aneurysm whose point of rupture is partially sealed by thrombus. The occurrence of such aneurysmal leaks is doubted by some physicians; certainly they are uncommon or, at least, uncommonly recognized. The headaches produced by such leaks may be abrupt and severe, though not as prostrating as those from larger hemorrhages. Often they are occipital and, like those from larger hemorrhages, are worsened by movement or jarring. They last a shorter time than the headaches of larger hemorrhages—sometimes for only hours, sometimes for a day or two. If such minibleeds occur in patients who are chronic headache sufferers, they may be dismissed as "an unusually severe migraine."

Fewer than 10% of aneurysms present in ways other than bleeding (Sahs et al., 1969). Most of these aneurysms are at the junction of the internal carotid and posterior communicating arteries. This location affords the aneurysm the opportunity of pressing either on the oculomotor nerve, producing diplopia, squint, ptosis, and/or pupillary dilatation, or on the first division of the trigeminal nerve, producing ipsilateral orbitofrontal pain. Other "prerupture presentations" of aneurysms, even more uncommon, include visual disturbances from involvement of the ophthalmic circulation by aneurysms of the ophthalmic or anterior communicating arteries and hemiparesis or seizures due to pressure on the cerebral cortex from middle cerebral artery aneurysms.

Diagnosis of Aneurysms

If aneurysm rupture is suspect, a CT scan of the head should be done. In the majority of cases, the diagnosis of subarachnoid hemorrhage can be made with the unenhanced scan, which will demonstrate blood in the ventricles and/or basal cisterns.

Acute hydrocephalus is often present as well. One may then decide whether or not to use lumbar puncture, which may not be necessary. If no lesions are seen, contrast medium may be given to complete the CT examination.

Currently arteriography is usually done early in the course, to establish the anatomy and to help plan the surgery. All four vessels should be visualized; it is not enough to demonstrate the aneurysm responsible for the hemorrhage because multiple aneurysms may be present.

Treatment

The modern treatment of subarachnoid hemorrhage is an unsettled and continuously changing issue, since rebleeding may occur throughout the life of the patient. The greatest risk to the patient is in the subsequent month after the initial bleeding episode.

Current therapy of the acute episode is aggressive, emphasizing early operation, management of rebleeding, and amelioration of vasospasm. The prevention of clot lysis using ϵ-aminocaproic acid is controversial. A recent cooperative study of the calcium-channel blocker nimodipine, in preventing ischemia and vasospasm, is promising (Allen et al., 1983). Some suggest employment of hypervolemia and hypertension in vasospasm. If all other forms of therapy fail and the neurologic situation continues to deteriorate, barbiturate coma may be employed. These varied therapeutic maneuvers are controversial, and the matter is far from settled, with treatment regimens varying widely from center to center (Kassell et al., 1981).

Hunt and Kosnick (1974) have developed a classification of patients with aneurysms based on an extensive clinical experience (see Table 12-1). All authors agree that operation should be done rapidly on patients in Grades 0 to II. Many neurosurgeons now believe that the best management of aneurysmal rupture is one that emphasizes early operative intervention in almost all cases (Ljunggren et al., 1982).

Prognosis of Aneurysms

Jane et al. (1977) have studied the natural history of intracranial aneurysms with rebleeding rates during acute and long-term periods of observation. For a patient with an anterior communicating aneurysm seen one day 1, the chance that he or she will rebleed within the first day is approximately 50%. For posterior communicating aneurysms, the expected chance of rebleeding on the first day is 60%. Thereafter, the rate rapidly diminishes for both aneurysms. By day 30, the chance of rebleeding during the first 6 months has dropped to less than 10%. The authors have also followed a group of 213 patients for up to 21 years; of these, 54 had another bleeding episode during the first 10 years, and another 7 patients rebled between the 10th and 20th years. To summarize, the first decade following subarachnoid hemorrhage is characterized by rebleeding episodes at the rate of approximately 3% per year. Subsequent rebleeding occurs at the rate of 2% per year. In 67% of subsequent hemorrhages, death occurs. Jane and his colleagues make the point that subarachnoid hemorrhage

Table 12-1 Classification of patients with intracranial aneurysms according to surgical risk

Grade	Criteria[a]
0	Unruptured aneurysm
I	Asymptomatic, or minimal headache and slight nuchal rigidity
IA	No acute meningeal or brain reaction, but with fixed neurologic deficit
II	Moderate to severe headache, nuchal rigidity, no neurologic deficit other than cranial nerve palsy
III	Drowsiness, confusion, or mild focal deficit
IV	Stupor, moderate to severe hemiparesis, possibly early decerebrate rigidity and vegetative disturbances
V	Deep coma, decerebrate rigidity, moribund appearance

[a]Serious systemic disease, such as hypertension, diabetes, severe atherosclerosis, chronic pulmonary disease, or severe intracranial arterial spasm seen on arteriography results in placement of the patient in the next less favorable grade.

secondary to aneurysms should be considered as a chronic disease with a "relentless rate of rebleeding."

Sahs and his colleagues (1984) have undertaken a long-term follow-up study of patients with subarachnoid hemorrhage seen between 1958 and 1965 and treated "conservatively," or without surgery. Of 568 cases, 378 were dead (66.5%) at the time of the survey in 1981–82. Of the deceased, 40% had expired within 6 months of hemorrhage. Those with multiple aneurysms did not differ significantly from those with a single lesion. Sahs estimates the rebleeding rates, after 6 months from the initial ictus, as follows:

2.2% per year for the first 9½ years.
0.86% per year for the second decade.

PARENCHYMATOUS CEREBRAL HEMORRHAGE

Although it is theoretically possible for hemorrhage in the brain parenchyma to occur without pain, this almost never happens. Cerebral (or cerebellar) hemispheric bleeding of any significant magnitude is accompanied by excruciating headache and, usually, by disturbance of consciousness. The venerable term *apoplexy,* implying sudden paralysis with total or partial loss of consciousness and sensation, is most appropriate in this situation. Usually the intrahemispheric blood distends the brain, producing traction on pain-sensitive structures, and frequently it ruptures into the subarachnoid space, producing typical signs and symptoms associated with subarachnoid bleeding.

Certain signs and symptoms are common to all forms of intracranial bleeding. These include progressive headache, stiffness of the neck, disturbances of consciousness, nausea, and vomiting. Transient or progressive neurologic signs and/or seizures should be anticipated. Severe headaches in hypertensive patients, particularly morning headaches, should be considered a warning symptom of a possible impending cerebral hemorrhage. Hypertension of any etiology is by far the most frequent cause of parenchymatous cerebral hemorrhage. The rupture may occur from an artery or cerebral vein, but the most common source of bleeding is from an arteriole that has degenerated in relation to the hypertensive atherosclerotic process. Persistent elevation of the blood pressure, particularly in acute situations of malignant hypertension, will produce necrosis of the smooth muscle and elastic laminae of the vessel wall, evoking Charcot–Bouchard aneurysms. These frequently rupture and are a common source of parenchymatous hemorrhage and brain destruction. These microaneurysms are distributed particularly in the lenticulostriate branches of the middle cerebral arteries that supply the internal capsule and the basal ganglia. They also occur in the brain stem, especially in the pons. Charcot–Bouchard aneurysms may be identified with arteriographic techniques or a magnified CT scan.

Thus, parenchymatous cerebral hemorrhage usually occurs in the region of the internal capsule or the basal ganglia and pons. Approximately one fifth occur in the brain stem and cerebellum. The remainder are found in the frontal and occipital lobes.

Work-up of the patient with intracranial hemorrhage should proceed rapidly. A CT scan should be done as an emergency procedure. If there is suspicion of increased intracranial pressure, lumbar puncture should be delayed unless infection, such as bacterial meningitis, is a possibility. Spinal puncture may hasten herniation. At times, particularly if anticoagulants are to be used, a careful lumbar puncture is necessary. Emergency arteriography is indicated if a surgical procedure for clot evacuation is contemplated, particularly if acute cerebellar hemorrhage is suspected, in which case surgery may be life-saving.

Most of these patients have preexisting hypertension, and many will have striking elevation of the blood pressure during the cerebral hemorrhage. Because there is evidence that elevated blood pressure will promote further hemorrhage and increasing cerebral edema, the hypertension should be treated.

HEADACHE AND ARTERIOVENOUS MALFORMATIONS (AVMs)

Arteriovenous malformations (AVMs) are uncommon. They account for only about 6% of subarachnoid hemorrhages. At least a third of all diagnosed AVMs do not bleed but present instead as focal or generalized epilepsy or with focal deficits such as hemiparesis. Walker (1956) has found that the incidence of chronic headaches in people with AVMs is not greater than that in the general population. Despite this study, which should deemphasize any relationship between the two, a formidable mythology has grown up to connect AVMs with chronic headaches (Lees, 1962).

It has frequently been stated that the occurrence of migraine headaches persistently localized to the same side of the head should arouse suspicion of an underlying AVM. This has led to the infliction of angiography on many hapless patients who have lacked the versatility to have alternating hemicrania. In the definitive study by Blend and Bull (1967), however, it was found that no patient with migraine alone, even if persistently localized, had an abnormal angiogram; of those patients with migraine and abnormal angiograms, all were found to have persistently abnormal signs on neurologic examination, or bruits, seizures, or a history of subarachnoid hemorrhage. Thus, even the most persistently localized migraine does not warrant angiography unless there are clear-cut neurologic abnormalities.

AVMs may produce small leaks on multiple occasions, and headaches due to these leaks may occur; they are similar to those of leaking aneurysms. Rarely, blood from these multiple leaks organizes within the subarachnoid space of the basal cisterns, leading to a communicating hydrocephalus. The headache produced by the hydrocephalus is that of increased intracranial pressure—a dull, diffuse ache, more likely to be present in the morning, worse in the head-down position, and increasing over weeks and months.

HEADACHE AND OCCLUSIVE DISEASE, INCLUDING TRANSIENT ISCHEMIC ATTACKS

Medina, Diamond, and Rubino (1975) have observed that patients with transient ischemic attacks (TIAs) may describe headache in an incidence ranging from 25 to 40%. Often the head pain occurs in association with neurologic symptoms, or with their resolution. Sometimes headache is appreciated as a harbinger of the TIA. The pain is usually throbbing and brief, and may be accentuated by effort or position. The pain locale is variable, but headache associated with carotid TIAs is generally frontal, and that associated with vertebrobasilar TIAs is often occipital, as one would predict.

Edmeads (1979) has done studies of regional cerebral blood flow during TIAs in patients with and without headaches. No apparent differences that would explain the appearance of headache in some and not in others can be found in these subjects.

Leviton et al. (1975) have described a severe ipsilateral headache following closely upon carotid endarterectomy. This complication may occur in those subject to migraine before surgery. This postendarterectomy hemicranial pain is indistinguishable from migraine. It often appears 36 to 72 hours after surgery and is typically described as intense and pounding. Generally, this is a benign and self-limiting phenomenon, perhaps related previously to sudden increase in blood flow through a system disposed to low-pressure flow.

HEADACHE AND VENOUS OCCLUSION

Thrombosis of the large intracranial venous sinuses, notably the lateral and sigmoid sinuses, may cause increased intracranial pressure with papilledema and no focal signs, mimicking the "pseudotumor cerebri" syndrome. The headache so produced is that of increased intracranial pressure. In the past the common causes were contiguous pyogenic infection, trauma, dehydration, cachexia, and the puerperium; recently, oral contraceptives have been recognized as an important cause.

Thrombosis of the superior sagittal sinus may produce headache from increased intracranial pressure, but this usually also produces hemorrhagic cerebral infarction with focal neurologic deficits, which give a clue to the diagnosis. Fronto-orbital pain may arise from involvement of the fifth nerve in cavernous sinus thrombosis, but the associated chemosis and oculomotor palsies usually make the diagnosis evident.

TRANSIENT MIGRAINE ACCOMPANIMENTS (TMAs)—VASCULAR OR NOT?

We owe interest in this topic particularly to the efforts of Fisher (1968, 1980), whose observations deserve careful review and consideration. His patients presented with episodic transient visual and other neurologic symptoms, but when the conditions were investigated, embolic phenomena and occlusive vascular disease could not be demonstrated. Fisher believes, therefore, that these episodes are migrainous accompaniments of later adult life, occurring without headache—hence the term transient migrainous accompaniments (TMAs).

A reliable sign of migrainous paresthesias is the "march" of numbness as it gradually spreads over the face or fingers and hands and migrates from face to limb or vice versa, or crosses to the face and hand on the opposite side. This evolution may last for 30 minutes, commonly 15 to 25 minutes. This gradual spread is unusual in thrombotic or embolic cerebrovascular disease. Pure sensory stroke due to thalamic ischemia is the only stroke whose evolution may resemble the typical "march" of migraine paresthesias, but this occurs only rarely. Conversely, the march of sensory seizures is much more rapid, being measured in seconds.

The occurrence of two or more episodes, particularly if they closely resemble one another, is important in the diagnosis. This history helps to exclude cerebral embolism, which is a prime diagnostic possibility when there is only one attack. The history of a similar spell as long as 20 to 30 years before is also evidence for migraine. An identical vascular spell or series of spells, occurring years ago, also favors migraine over thrombotic vascular disease. The time between episodes varies widely.

The duration of the episode may also be of importance in the diagnosis. Migrainous episodes classically last 15 to 20 minutes or longer, whereas most transient ischemic attacks last less than 15 minutes.

Other points of value in the diagnosis of transient migraine equivalents are the benign nature of the spell in retrospect and the rarity of permanent sequelae. Repeated good recovery from what appears initially to be a threatening situation is evidence for migraine. In Fisher's series, there were no permanent deficits. Fisher stressed, further, the importance of a normal arteriogram and the absence of a source of emboli as prerequisites for establishing the diagnosis of TMA. Where atherosclerotic plaque and migraine coexist, the diagnosis becomes more difficult and the judgment depends on the experience and expertise of the clinician.

Murphey (1973) has described his own experiences with TIA. He notes that visual

TIAs are usually unilateral and that they may be obliterated by closing the eye and presumably altering retinal arterial flow. This is in contrast with migrainous scotomata, which are often bilateral, sometimes homonymous, are related to occipital cortical ischemia, and persist with eye closure.

SUMMARY

- The headache of subarachnoid hemorrhage is of high intensity and sudden onset, is commonly located in the occipital region, and in almost all patients is associated with neck rigidity.
- The headache of subarachnoid hemorrhage usually persists at a very high intensity for a few days, but seldom for as long as a week, and subsides thereafter, with complete elimination of pain within 2 months. The persistence of headache for longer periods following subarachnoid hemorrhage in patients who have had no previous headaches is rare.
- The initial headache of subarachnoid hemorrhage is probably due to traction, displacement, distention, and rupture of pain-sensitive blood vessels and the pia arachnoid. The headache of several days' duration is probably secondary to a sterile inflammatory reaction about the blood vessels and meninges.
- Ruptured cerebral aneurysm based on a congenital defect with or without arteriosclerotic changes is responsible for the headache, stupor, coma, convulsions, and other disturbances in a high proportion of patients with subarachnoid hemorrhage. However, it is unlikely that periodic headaches of a few hours' duration, recurring over many years, as they do in some patients, could stem from the slowly developing structural changes in an aneurysm.
- Ruptured subarachnoid hemorrhage is an extremely serious disease. Death occurs in approximately 45% of patients with each major bleeding episode and there is a significant risk of recurrence. Approximately one third of those who succumb will do so in the first 48 hours after bleeding, another third within the next month, and the remainder from recurrent bleeding episodes thereafter.
- A precise regimen for every case of subarachnoid hemorrhage cannot be recommended with certainty. Early intervention is justified in many cases of aneurysmal hemorrhage characterized by prompt diagnosis, angiography showing no vasospasm, a favorable location, and the absence of serious neurologic signs.
- Cerebral (or cerebellar) hemispheric bleeding that is of any significant magnitude is accompanied by excruciating headache and usually by disturbance of consciousness. Hypertension is the most frequent cause of parenchymatous cerebral hemorrhage. The hemorrhage usually occurs in the region of the internal capsule or the basal ganglia and pons, but one fifth of such hemorrhages occur in the brain stem and cerebellum.
- Headache may be a manifestation of occlusive vascular disease.
- Transient migrainous accompaniments of later adult life may be confused with recurrent embolic episodes. With attention to the history, however, the former diagnosis can often be established, especially if arterial studies are normal.

REFERENCES

Allen, G.S., H.S. Ahn, T.J. Preziosi et al. (1983). Cerebral arterial spasm: A controlled trial of nimodipine in patients with subarachnoid hemorrhage. *N. Engl. J. Med. 308:*619–624.

Blend, R. and J.W.D. Bull (1967). The radiological investigation of migraine. In *Background to Migraine: First Migraine Symposium,* pp. 1–10. Springer-Verlag, New York.

Dandy, W.E. (1944). *Intracranial Arterial Aneurysms.* Comstock Publishing, Ithaca, N.Y.

Edmeads, J.G. (1979). The headaches of ischemic cerebrovascular disease. *Headache 19:*345–349.

Fisher, C.M. (1968). Migraine accompaniments vs. arteriosclerotic ischemia. *Trans. Am. Neurol. Assoc. 93:*211–213.

Fisher, C.M. (1980). Late life migraine accompaniments as a cause of unexplained transient ischemic attacks. *Can. J. Neurol. Sci. 7:*9–17.

Hunt, W.E., and E.J. Kosnik (1974). Timing and periorbital care in intracranial aneurysm surgery. *Clin. Neurosurg. 21:*79–89.

Jane, J.A., H.R. Winn, and A.E. Richardson (1977). The natural history of intracranial aneurysms: Rebleeding rates during the acute and long-term period and implication for surgical management. *Clin. Neurosurg. 24:*176–184.

Kassell, N.F., H.P. Adams, Jr., J.C. Torner, and A.L. Sahs (1981). Influence of timing on admission after aneurysmal subarachnoid hemorrhage on overall outcome: Report of the Cooperative Aneurysm Study. *Stroke 12:*620–631.

Lees, F. (1962). The migrainous symptoms of cerebral angiomata. *J. Neurol. Neurosurg. Psychiatry 25:*45–50.

Leviton, A., L. Caplan, and E. Salzman (1975). Severe headache after carotid endarterectomy. *Headache 15:*207–210.

Ljunggren, B., L. Brandt, G. Sunbay et al. (1982). Early management of aneurysmal subarachnoid hemorrhage. *Neurosurgery 11:*412–418.

McDonald, C. and M. Korb (1939). Intracranial aneurysms. *Arch. Neurol. Psychiatry 42:*289–307.

Medina, J.L., S. Diamond, and F.A. Rubino (1975). Headaches in patients with transient ischemic attacks. *Headache 15:*194–197.

Murphey, F. (1973). The scotoma of carotid artery disease as I remember them. *J. Neurosurg. 39:*390–393.

Sahs, A.L., H. Nishioka, J.C. Torner, et al. (1984). Cooperative study of intracranial aneurysms and subarachnoid hemorrhage: A long-term prognostic study. *Arch. Neurol. 41:*1140–1151.

Sahs, A.L., G.E. Perret, H.B. Locksley, and H. Nishioka (1969). *Intracranial Aneurysms and Subarachnoid Hemorrhage. A Cooperative Study.* J.B. Lippincott, Philadelphia. Toronto.

Walker, A.E. (1956). Clinical localization of intracranial aneurysms and vascular anomalies. *Neurology 6:*79–90.

13

Allergy, Atopy, Nasal Disease, and Headache

DONALD D. STEVENSON

The term *allergy* was derived by von Pirquet (1906) from the Greek words *allos* (other) and *ergon* (action). Von Pirquet used *allergy* to describe the "changed reactivity" that occurred in a subset of animals after immunization with antigens (allergens). The most striking example of "changed reactivity" is anaphylaxis. A susceptible animal, which has had prior immunization with specific antigens, undergoes a predictable systemic reaction when antigen is reintroduced. This reaction is the consequence of union between specific antigens; specific cell-fixed IgE antibodies; followed by release of chemical mediators and their rapid effects on smooth muscles, vascular beds, and mucous membranes.

Although an antigen-induced, IgE-mediated, anaphylactic reaction is universally accepted as an allergic event, physicians agree less frequently when the term allergy is used to describe other immunologic inflammatory reactions, and agreement disappears when nonimmunologic untoward reactions are included in a classification of "allergic" reactions. Since the 1960s, the classification of Gell and Coombs (1968) has been widely accepted as a reasonable description of directions by which the immune system can respond to the introduction of specific antigens (Figure 13-1).

The atopic state refers to allergic reactions (such as asthma and hay fever), which are familial and in which intracutaneous injection of the offending allergen leads to immediate wheal and erythema in the skin.

TYPE I REACTIONS

When IgE antibodies, fixed to tissue mast cells or circulating basophils, combine with specific antigens, a cascade of intracellular biochemical events is initiated that culminates in the release of chemical mediators into surrounding tissue or fluid (Kaliner & Austen, 1973). These mediators produce the allergic inflammatory response, which in turn produces the pathophysiologic changes of allergic diseases. Figure 13-

	TYPE I	TYPE II	TYPE III	TYPE IV
Immuno-chemical reaction	IgE-mediated chemical mediator release	cytotoxic or cytolytic Ab. (IgM or IgG)	circulating complexes of Ab. Ag and complement	sensitized lymphocytes
Time of reaction	Immediate (15 min)	Immediate to delayed (minutes to hours)	Intermediate (4-24 hr)	Delayed (24-72 hr)
Clinical state	Anaphylaxis Allergic rhinitis	Hemolytic anemia	Vasculitis	Contact dermatitis

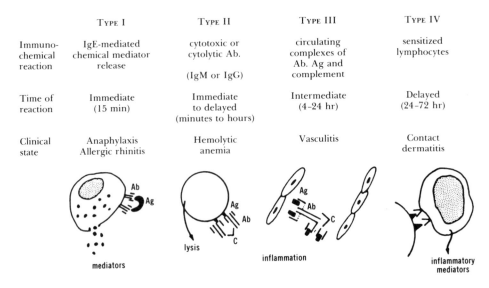

Figure 13-1.   Types of allergic reactions.

2 depicts the interactions between primary effector cells, basophils (circulating in the bloodstream), and mast cells (tissue fixed), releasing primary mediators and their targeted effects to directly stimulate eosinophils, platelets, and neutrophils. These secondary cells also release mediators and participate directly in the late allergic inflammatory reactions. Such events tend to amplify the original inciting stimulus (Austen, 1984).

Although the stimulus to the allergic cascade is frequently an interaction between antigen and IgE antibodies, mast cells and basophils can be activated by nonimmunologic stimuli, such as physical stimuli (trauma, heat, cold, vibration, solar radiation), complement products (C3a, C5a), enzymes (phospholipase A_2, chymotrypsin), polysaccharides (dextran), polypeptides (bradykinin, polymyxin B, eosinophil major basic protein), neuropeptides and hormones (substance P, neurotensin, somatostatin, gastrin, endorphins, enkephalins, acetylcholine), lymphokins from T-cells, and drugs (morphine, tubocurarine, radiocontrast media, codeine) (Plaut & Lichtenstein, 1983).

Described below are the primary mediators of the allergic reaction:

Histamine can combine with receptors in certain tissue cells to produce a variety of special events, depending on the response of the tissue where the receptors reside. For pharmacologic convenience, these receptors are called H_1, which are blocked by standard antihistamines (chlorpheniramine, diphenhydramine, etc.), and H_2, which are blocked by H_2 antihistamines (cimetidine and ranitidine). Table 13-1 summarizes the tissues that contain H_1 or H_2 receptors and the consequences of their stimulation by histamine molecules (Goth, 1978). Important counter mechanisms exist for degrading histamine rapidly. Radiolabeled histamine, injected intravenously, disappears from the circulation in about one minute (Beall & Van Arsdel, 1960).

Eosinophilic chemotactic factor of anaphylaxis (ECF-A) is a glycopeptide with a

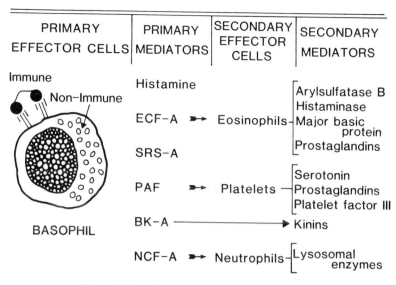

PRIMARY EFFECTOR CELLS	PRIMARY MEDIATORS	SECONDARY EFFECTOR CELLS	SECONDARY MEDIATORS

Figure 13-2. Allergic inflamatory cells and mediators.

molecular weight between 500 and 1000. When released from tissue storage cells, eosinophils are attracted to this site of anaphylactic reaction by ECF-A through countergradient mechanisms (Kay & Austen, 1971). Eosinophils have profound inflammatory effects, releasing major basic protein, leukotrienes, and other products.

Prostaglandins are a group of closely related chemicals that are derived from a common essential fatty acid, arachidonic acid, contained in the wall of many mammalian cells and released by the enzyme phospholipase A_2. Prostaglandin synthetase converts arachidonic acid to hydroperoxide, then into PGH and eventually into PGF and PGE series. For the most part, these mediators appear as a consequence of any inflammation and tend to modulate or amplify other systems. For instance, $PGF_2\alpha$ directly stimulates bronchoconstriction and decreases cyclic AMP levels in mast cells and basophils. PGE_1, on the other hand, stimulates bronchodilatation and increases intracellular cyclic AMP levels in mast cells, diminishing or interrupting mediator release from storage cells (Vane, 1976).

The role of prostaglandins in neurovascular biology is incompletely defined. Some prostaglandins, particularly thromboxanes, can aggregate platelets with disruption and release of stored serotonin, a potent vasodilator. Bergstrom et al. (1959) showed that intravenous injections of prostaglandin E_1 in susceptible individuals was associated with the onset of vascular headaches, whereas all patients experienced burning pain along the vein where PGE_1 was infused.

Leukotrienes C_4, D_4, E_4 (SRS-A), are also newly synthesized molecules, derived from arachidonate in the cell wall. These three powerful lipoxygenase products induce smooth muscle contraction and increased vascular permeability (Wasserman, 1983). Also formed is LTB_4, which is chemotactic for neutrophils and eosinophils.

Platelet-activating factor (PAF) is released from mast cells after antigen challenge. PAF combines with platelet receptors, stimulating release of serotonin and histamine

Table 13-1 Locations and actions of histamine receptors (H$_1$ and H$_2$) in humans

Receptors	Organs	Actions
H$_1$		
Blocked by		
Diphenhydramine	Lacrimal glands	Increased secretions
Chlorpheniramine	Salivary glands	Increased secretions
Cyclizine	Capillary	Vasodilatation and increased permeability
Promethazine	Heart	Tachycardia
Cyproheptadine	Vascular	Vasodilatation (hypotension)
	CNS	Stimulation
	Mast cells	Inhibition of histamine release
	Cutaneous	Pruritus
	Bronchial tree	Bronchoconstriction
H$_2$		
Blocked by	Cutaneous vasculature	Cutaneous vasodilatation
Cimetidine	Larger arteries	Vascular dilatation
Metiamide	Heart	Excitation
	Leukocytes	Inhibit functions
	Gastrointestinal	Secretion HCl and pepsin

from rabbit platelets (Benveniste, 1974). The role of PAF in humans is only partly clarified. Aggregation of platelets has a significant effect on the coagulation and kinin systems. Induction of neutropenia and basopenia, release of platelet amines, and generation of thromboxanes are other effects that have been recently demonstrated (Wasserman, 1983).

Kinin-activating factor is released from IgE-sensitized basophils after antigen challenge, with a time course similar to that of histamine release (Newball et al., 1975). More recently it has been demonstrated that three different proteins are released from basophils after immune or nonimmune challenge. These are basophil kallikrein (molecular weight, 400,000), basophil Hageman factor activator (molecular weight, 13,000), and basophil prekallikrein activator (molecular weight, 80,000) (Wasserman, 1983).

Kinins

A circulating globulin, kininogen is the precursor protein for bradykinin. Kininogen is cleaved by the enzyme kallikrein to produce the active peptide bradykinin (Lewis, 1961). Kallikrein is generated from prekallikrein after interaction with activated Hageman factor (from the coagulation cascade) or released from basophils or mast cells during type I reactions. The generation of the nonapeptide, bradykinin, produces a potent mediator that increases vascular permeability, contracts smooth muscles, and interacts with sensory nerve endings to produce a painful stimulus (Kaplan & Austen, 1975).

For the most part, kinin activation appears to be a secondary system, resulting from release of mediators from basophils, activation of the complement system, or intravascular coagulation. Bradykinin is a potent vasodilator, but is rapidly cleaved in normal plasma to an inactive octapeptide, limiting its systemic effects in normal humans and animals. Because of the liability of bradykinin in normal mammalian circulations, it has been extremely difficult to study its *in vivo* effects and to assign a clear role for the kinin system in disorders such as vascular shock, asthma, pain syndromes, or vascular dilatation of the cerebral circulation (Cochrane & Griffin, 1982).

Neutrophil chemotactic factor (NCF-A) was identified by Wasserman et al. (1977) in the sera of patients with cold urticaria. Partial purification of this material indicates it has a high molecular weight (750,000) and shows a preferential chemotactic activity toward neutrophilic polymorphonuclear leukocytes. Its release into the venous effluent follows a time course identical to that of histamine and low-molecular-weight eosinophil chemotactic factor, suggesting that these mediators are released together during anaphylactic cellular discharge.

> *T-lymphocyte chemotactic factor:* 1400-molecular-weight protein is released from mast cells and attracts T-lymphocytes (Wasserman, 1983).
> *B-lymphocyte chemotactic factor:* 500-molecular-weight protein is released from mast cells and attracts B-lymphocytes (Wasserman, 1983).

Although type I reactions can produce rapid and profound changes in the caliber of circular smooth muscles, vasodilatation, increased vascular permeability, infiltration of eosinophils and neutrophils, aggregation of platelets, and activation of the kinin and coagulation systems; the compensatory and counterregulatory systems that either destroy the circulating mediators or block their effects by activating the sympathomimetic autonomic responses are also well developed. These balances serve to either localize IgE-mediated (type 1) reactions to the site of antigen–antibody interaction or shorten the time of their systemic effects (Austen, 1984).

TYPE II REACTIONS

Cytolytic or cytotoxic reactions occur when the antigens are actually part of the cell wall, as in autoimmune hemolytic anemia or transfusion reactions, or when the antigens adhere to the cell walls. When penicillin or quinidine adhere to red blood cells, they can initiate type II reactions if circulating antibodies of the IgG or IgM classes, which have been synthesized in response to the antigens discussed earlier, combine with these antigens. The union of antibody and adherent antigen or cell wall antigen does not damage the cells. However, antibodies from both IgG and IgM classes activate the complement system through the classic pathway, beginning with the C_1 trimolecular complex, through C_4, C_2, C_3, and $C_{5,6,7}$, C_8, and C_9. With the addition of the terminal complement components, spaces are formed in the lipid membrane of the cell wall, the cellular contents extrude into the extracellular space, and cytolysis occurs (Ruddy et al., 1972). To our knowledge, type II hypersensitivity reactions are not involved in the pathogenesis of headache.

TYPE III REACTIONS

Immune complex reactions occur within the vascular spaces when circulating soluble antigens (drugs, nuclear antigens, virus particles) combine with IgG or IgM antibodies, which fix complement components. This active immune complex of antigen, antibody, and complement adheres to the endothelial surface of blood vessels, greatly aided by certain properties of activated complement. These include release of C_{3a} and C_{5a} anaphylatoxins, which stimulate nonimmunologic release of stored mediators from circulating basophils, activation of the kinin system through C_2, and release of chemotactic complexes of complement cleavage proteins that attract neutrophils to the site of complement activation (Kohler, 1978).

In type III reactions, inflammation occurs in the walls of blood vessels where immune complexes are deposited. The renal endothelial surfaces are common sites of immune complex deposition, presumably because immune complexes leave the plasma when the rate of blood flow diminishes. Biopsy and immunofluorescent staining for antibody or complement show a lumpy, bumpy arrangement of complexes in the subendothelial cell walls with infiltration of inflammatory cells, particularly PMNS. Type III reactions can produce headache if immune complexes are deposited in those arteries that carry blood to both intracranial and extracranial structures.

TYPE IV REACTIONS

Cellular immune reactions occur when thymus-derived T-lymphocytes, previously sensitized to specific antigens arrive at the site of antigen introduction. When the original antigen is either introduced through the skin or arrives with certain lipids (as in *Mycobacterium tuberculosis*), lymphocytes are preferentially sensitized or stimulated. Reintroduction of specific antigens stimulates sensitized lymphocytes to migrate toward the site of antigen entry or concentration. Activated lymphocytes secrete bioactive chemicals or factors (David & David, 1972), which produce inflammation in the area of their release. The tuberculin cutaneous reaction, occurring 24 to 72 hours after introduction of killed *M. tuberculosis* antigens, is the classic example of a delayed cellular reaction. With the exception of tuberculosis and fungal meningitis, cellular immune reactions probably do not produce headaches.

EXPERIMENTAL STUDY OF PAIN FROM THE NASAL AND PARANASAL STRUCTURES

Harold Wolff and his associates studied the distribution and intensity of pain originating from the nasal and paranasal structures. Using a probe, faradic electrical current, and cotton pledgelets soaked in epinephrine (1:1000), they stimulated various sites in the nose and surrounding structures.

Volunteers consisted of 5 normal subjects, 10 subjects who had undergone complete extirpation of a left acoustic neuroma with section of the left facial nerve, 5 subjects with chronic sinusitis, 4 patients with acute sinusitis, and 1 subject with a fistulous opening into the left maxillary sinus.

Subjects covered the tip of their index finger with red wax and were instructed to press the pigment-covered finger against the skin at the place where painful sensation was experienced.

Pain was subjectively classified as 1 (least intense) through 10 (most intense). The degree of faradic current used in these experiments was determined as follows: the level of current that could elicit a 1+ reaction, when the tip of the stimulator was applied to the tongue, was the threshold of electrical current used for that experimental subject.

Sensation from Stimulation of the Pharynx, Nasopharynx, and Eustachian Tube

A 1 to 2 plus aching pain was elicited by pressing against the mucous membrane of the pharynx and posterior nasopharynx. The pain was described as being felt deep within the throat and was marked on the skin as being approximately along the thyroid cartilage of the larynx and at the edge of the hyoid bone, extending to the border of the tragus. Stimulation of the tonsils with faradic current was felt as an uncomfortable tickle at the site of stimulation, but pain was occasionally referred to an area in back of the ear.

Contact of a nasal catheter with the rim of the soft palate and the fossa of Rosenmüller was felt as touch, which was described as unpleasant but not painful. Inflation of the eustachian tube was felt as "air blowing through and striking the eardrum." Section of the fifth or seventh cranial nerve did not disturb sensation in these structures.

In one subject, in whom the fifth and ninth cranial nerves had previously been severed, the pharynx and fossa of Rosenmüller were reported to be insensitive, but blowing air through the eustachian tube produced the usual sensation.

Sensation from Stimulation of the Nasal Floor and the Septum

In all subjects with an intact cranial nerve supply, touch and pressure stimuli were recognized as such on the nasal floor, and local unpleasant sensations were elicited by passage of a nasal catheter. In subjects with complete section of the fifth cranial nerve root, the insertion of a catheter through the nose was not felt until it impinged on the soft palate and the fossa of Rosenmüller. These patients, however, stated that they felt "a pressure from the posterior portion of the nasal floor."

The nasal septum in normal subjects was sensitive throughout to light touch, and both faradic current stimulation and pressure with a probe elicited moderate pain (1 to 2 plus), which was felt locally and was sometimes referred as follows: Stimulation of the middle part of the septum caused pain to be felt along the zygoma and toward the ear. On stimulation of the ethmoid portion, pain was felt in both the outer and the inner canthus of the eye on the homolateral side (Figure 13-3).

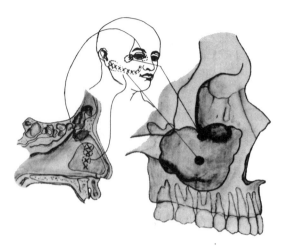

Figure 13-3. The points stimulated on the septum are shown by crosses and on the lateral wall of the maxillary sinus by cross-hatched circles. The areas in which pain of 1 to 2 plus intensity was felt are indicated by crosses within an outline on the small head above. Note that widely separated stimuli cause pain to be felt in the same areas.

Sensation from Stimulation of the Nasal Turbinates

The lower, middle, and upper turbinates, whether stimulated mechanically with a probe, or by faradic current, were considerably more sensitive that the nasal floor or the septum. A sharp, burning pain was felt at the site of stimulation and along the lateral wall of the inside of the nose. A duller, aching pain was referred into the upper teeth when faradic current or pressure was applied to the anterior portion of the lower turbinate. When the middle and posterior portions of the lower turbinate were stimulated, pain was also felt under the eye, along the zygoma, and toward the ear. On stimulation of the middle turbinate, pain was felt along the zygoma, extending back toward the ear and into the temple, and occasionally deep in the ear. On stimulation of the anterior tip of the superior turbinate, pain was felt in the inner canthus of the eye and spread to the forehead and along the lateral wall of the nose (Figure 13-4).

Pain elicited by inserting a cotton pledglet soaked with epinephrine along the turbinates usually reached an intensity of 4 to 5 plus. The intensity of pain elicited by stimulation of these structures, and its extent of spread, varied from subject to subject. It was observed in subjects with engorged mucous membranes of the nose, especially of the turbinates, that experimentally induced pain was more intense, was referred to a larger area, and was longer lasting than when mucous membranes showed no injection or purulent secretion.

In patients with complete section of the fifth cranial nerve root, stimulation of the turbinates by pressure, faradic current, or epinephrine pledglets did not elicit sensation at the site of stimulation, except for a feeling of pressure "deep in." Two such patients also said they felt a pain deep in the ear when the middle turbinate was pressed on with a probe, but they could feel nothing at the site of stimulation, and referred pain was not described.

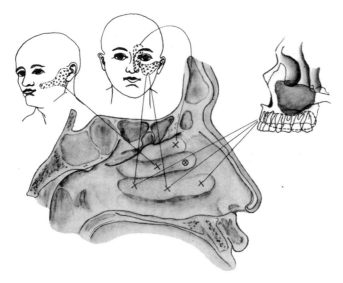

Figure 13-4. The points stimulated on the turbinates are indicated by crosses, from which lines lead to the indicated areas in which pain of 4 to 6 plus intensity was felt.

Sensation from Stimulation of the Ostium of the Maxillary Sinus

The normal ostium in three subjects was stimulated by a probe or faradic electrode. As soon as the probe touched the walls of the ostium there was a sharp, burning pain of 6 plus intensity at the site of stimulation, accompanied by profuse lacrimation and injection of the eye on the side stimulated. When attempts were made to push the probe or electrode through the ostium into the antrum, a 5 to 8 plus sharp, burning pain was felt at the site of stimulation, and an intense 4 plus aching pain was felt in the posterior nasopharynx, in the back teeth, along the zygoma, and back into and well above the temple on the side stimulated. There was a deep aching pain in the pharynx. The skin over the zygoma was flushed and hyperalgesic (Figure 13-5). The skin over the zygoma and the temple remained hyperalgesic, and the upper teeth were ''sore'' for approximately 24 hours following this procedure.

Sensation from Stimulation of the Nasofrontal Duct

The nasofrontal duct and the lower part of the channel leading to the frontal sinus were likewise found to be exceedingly pain sensitive. Figure 13-6 illustrates the areas in which pain was felt when the duct of the frontal sinus was stimulated with faradic current, or merely with the passing of the electrode or a metal probe into the frontal sinus. Pain was felt at the inner canthus of the eye, and in a wide band under the eye along the zygoma and into the temple, on the side stimulated. Pain was also felt at the angle of the jaw and in the last two or three upper teeth. Profuse lacrimation and injection in the eye and photophobia were present.

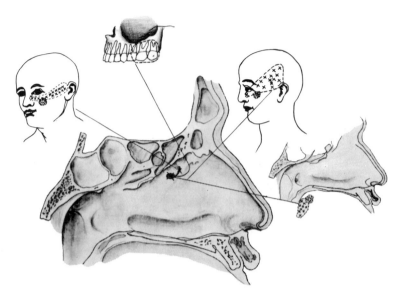

Figure 13-5. Large crosses indicate stimulation of the ostium of the maxillary sinus. Lines lead to the areas indicated by small crosses in which pain of 6 to 9 plus intensity was felt. A dotted circle over the zygoma indicates the area of erythema and hyperalgesia that long outlasted stimulation of the ostium.

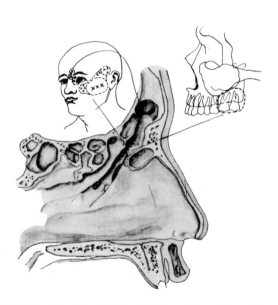

Figure 13-6. Lines lead from the points stimulated in the nasofrontal duct to the areas in which pain of 5 to 7 plus intensity was felt. On stimulation of the inner wall of the frontal sinus minimal pain of no more than ½ plus intensity was felt only in the area indicated directly over the sinus.

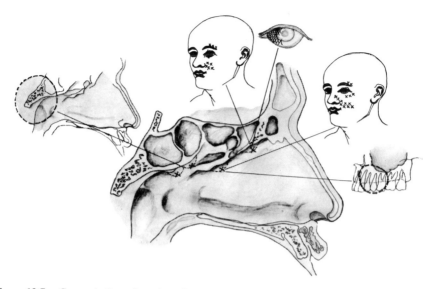

Figure 13-7. Crosses indicate the points of pressure against the walls of the superior nasal cavity in the region of the sphenoid and ethmoid sinuses, with the indicated areas in which pain of 5 to 6 plus intensity was felt.

Sensation from Stimulation of the Sinuses

The Frontal Sinus

When the walls and roof of the frontal sinus were stimulated by pressure with a probe, or by faradic current, minimal pain of no more than a ½ plus intensity was felt directly over the site of stimulation.

The Ethmoid Sinuses

In two of the normal subjects it was possible to investigate the pain sensitivity and sites of pain reference from stimulation in the superior nasal cavity, near the ethmoid sinuses. The sinuses themselves could not be explored. By pressing a probe against the wall of the superior nasal cavity in the general region of the anterior cells of the ethmoid sinuses, pain of 6 plus intensity was felt directly over the eye and deep in the eye at its inner canthus. Pain was also felt in the upper jaw just above the superior nasal cavity over the posterior cells of the ethmoid, the conjunctiva adjacent to the nose became injected, and profuse lacrimation and photophobia were present.

Pressing this region of the superior nasal cavity over the posterior ethmoid cells with a probe produced an intense aching pain of 5 to 6 plus intensity in the upper teeth including the canine, the cuspids, and the first molar; profuse lacrimation in both eyes; and photophobia. The pupils were observed to be dilated. Moderate aching pain occurred just under and over the outer canthus of the homolateral eye. Also, pain extended from the teeth up the side of the nose (Figure 13-7).

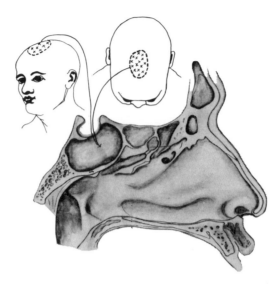

Figure 13-8. The area is indicated in which pain of 1 to 2 plus intensity was felt on faradic stimulation of the mucosal lining of a sphenoid sinus by Dr. Bronson Ray.

The Sphenoid Sinus

When the wall of the superior nasal cavity in the region of the sphenoid sinus was pressed on by a probe, pain of 5 to 6 plus intensity was felt immediately, and most intensely deep in the pharynx, which was described by the subject as seeming to be deep in the head. Pain of lesser intensity was referred over the eye and into the upper teeth on the side stimulated (Figure 13-7).

During an operation on the head for removal of a pituitary tumor, Dr. Bronson Ray stimulated the mucosal lining of the interior of the sphenoid sinus. In this patient, slight pain (1 to 2 plus) was felt at the vertex of the skull (Figure 13-8).

The Maxillary Sinus

The maxillary sinuses, in normal subjects, could not be entered through the ostia. However, in three patients who had completed operative procedures, performed on the nose and paranasal sinuses, the ostia were accessible and so large that a faradic stimulator could be introduced into the antrum with ease, and the walls of the latter could be stimulated by faradic current and by pressure. It was doubtful the mucous membrane linings of these antra were free of inflammation, because all the patients had sinus disease. Stimulation of the upper wall was felt up into the eye. Stimulation of the lower lateral wall was felt in the jaw and the back teeth. The sensation elicited from the walls of the sinus was of the same intensity and quality as that elicited by the same amount of faradic current applied to the tip of the tongue and from the mucous membrane of the septum (see Figure 13-3). When this threshold current was applied to the lower and middle turbinates in the same patient, however, a pain of 3 to 4 plus intensity was elicited. These three patients felt pressure with a probe against the walls of the maxillary sinus as pressure but did not report it as painful.

In two of the patients with complete fifth cranial nerve root section, pressure on the posterior wall of the maxillary sinus was felt as "pressure deep in." Faradic stimuli were not felt on the walls of the sinus, nor was any sensation experienced in the teeth in three of these patients when faradic current was applied to the lateral wall. The ostia on the side of the fifth cranial nerve root section in these patients were also insensitive.

It was possible to explore a normal maxillary sinus in a unique way. A 28-year-old woman, who had a sinus tract into the left maxillary sinus following extraction of the first left molar in the upper jaw, was studied. This fistulous tract was large enough to allow the entrance of a Holmes laryngoscope for visualization of the mucous membrane lining the sinus cavity.

Experiment 1. The mucous membranes of the sinus were seen to be smooth and glistening throughout and were free of inflammation or atrophy. The normal ostium could also be observed as open and without surrounding inflammatory reaction or scar tissue.

When the wall of the maxillary sinus inn this subject was stimulated with faradic current just under the orbital plate, a vibrating sensation was felt at the site of stimulation, and a ½ plus pain up through the eye and over the eye along the supraorbital ridge. On the lateral wall and the posterior wall, faradic stimulation was felt as an electric shock along the upper jaw and in the teeth, but the subject stated that the sensation was not painful. When faradic current was applied to the mucous membrane close to the ostium, however, 2 plus pain was experienced, and pain was felt in the upper teeth, in and over the eye, and along the zygoma toward the left temple.

Experiment 2. This experiment explored the effect of prolonged positive pressure within the maxillary sinus. A thin rubber balloon was attached with adhesive tape binding over the end of a small perforated rubber catheter. This was inserted into the maxillary sinus through the fistulous opening after injection of procaine into the gum around the opening. The catheter was attached to a manometer so that pressure applied inside the sinus could be measured in millimeters of mercury (Figure 13-9).

A positive pressure of 15 to 25 mm Hg elicited a sensation of pressure and fullness in the side of the face but was maintained for 3½ hours without eliciting pain. The pressure in the sinus could be gradually raised to 200 mm Hg before pain was experienced.

Pressure was maintained between 50 and 80 mm Hg for a period of 2¼ hours before the subject experienced a 1 plus pain in and just below the area of the zygoma, and in the upper teeth, radiating back toward the ear. However, quick, forced inhalations of air through the left naris increased the intensity of the pain from 1 to 3 and 4 plus and enlarged the area in which it was felt. Reducing the pressure to 0 mm Hg did not immediately abolish the pain, but its intensity gradually diminished during a 10-minute period.

The state of the turbinates was noted at fixed intervals throughout a 6-hour period of inflation. The left turbinate gradually became swollen during this time, but it was not until this engorgement had occluded the left naris that pain was experienced with a pressure of 50 mm Hg. Moreover, at the beginning of this period, pressure could

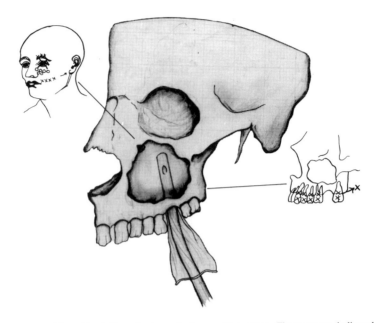

Figure 13-9. The thin rubber balloon is shown in the maxillary sinus. The areas are indicated in which pain was felt when positive pressure was applied to the walls of the sinus for prolonged periods.

be raised to 200 mm Hg before pain was experienced, whereas when the turbinates had become swollen and engorged, pressures over 50 mm Hg caused pain.

This pain, associated with pressure in the maxillary sinus and swollen, engorged turbinates, could be materially reduced in intensity, or almost entirely abolished, by procainization of the engorged turbinates, in spite of continued pressure and a feeling of fullness in the side of the face.

Comment. One might infer from the preceding that sustained, increased intramural pressure within the antrum may be associated with pain. However, such sustained stimulation of the walls of the sinus evokes engorgement of the turbinates. It is the reflex engorgement of these nasal structures that is responsible for most of the pain, since procainization of the inferior and middle turbinates markedly reduces its intensity, even at a time when the pressure within the sinus was maintained and perceived as pressure in the side of the face.

Experiment 3. This experiment investigated the effect of negative pressure within the maxillary sinus. The nasal side of the ostium was occluded by inserting a cotton and petroleum jelly tampon under the middle turbinate well over the ostium. Negative air pressure was then applied to the sinus by inserting a tube through the fistulous opening. A drawing sensation was felt in the face, which the subject described as the feeling that "my face will collapse." This sensation was elicited with a negative pressure of 100 to 150 mm Hg. The experience was accompanied by considerable apprehension on the part of the subject, but in spite of this she maintained that she felt no immediate pain. However, if the negative pressure were subsequently increased to 250 mm Hg, an immediate 4 plus pain was felt in the side of the nose and in the teeth.

Comment. When the cotton pledgelet occluding the ostium was removed at the termination of the experiment, a portion of its surface presented the appearance of having been drawn into the ostium. It is quite likely that the pain, experienced with high negative pressures, resulted from mechanical stimulation of the ostium. Thus, although the effects of negative pressures were not explored as extensively as were those of positive pressure, the available evidence makes it seem likely that most of the pain that resulted was secondary to stimulation of ostium and nasal structures.

Experiment 4. A thin rubber balloon was inserted into the sinus and filled with hot (45°C) and cold (19°C) water. Of these stimuli, the cold was not distinguished immediately and the hot not at all. After 10 minutes, the cold water was recognized as "a slight feeling of coolness." While the balloon was in the antrum, filled, under pressure with a syringe, with either hot or cold water, the teeth in the upper jaw felt sore when pressed on, but these procedures did not elicit any aching pain anywhere in the side of the face.

When the maxillary sinus was irrigated through the fistulous opening with saline, no pain was elicited other than irritation of the fistulous opening itself. When the sinus was irrigated with saline through the nose and the ostium, however, a 4 to 5 plus pain was felt in the nasal wall, along the zygoma into the temple, over the eye, and all through the upper teeth. Similar pain was induced by inserting a cotton tampon soaked with epinephrine under the middle turbinate and over the ostium.

Comment. The feeling of cold after 10 minutes of exposure to cold within the sinus could have resulted from cooling of neighboring structures. The soreness of the teeth probably resulted from direct stimulation of the dental nerves.

"Sinusitis," Headache, and Anesthetization of the Turbinates

The following experiments were from a series of investigations that illustrate the effects of surface anesthetization of nasal mucous membranes in patients with headache associated with disease of the nasal and paranasal structures.

Experiment 1. This patient had pain in the jaws and teeth and on both sides of the face along the zygomas and into the temples. Pain in the frontal region, increased lacrimation, and photophobia were also experienced. The pain was described as a steady ache of a 3 plus intensity except in the forehead, where it was 4 plus.

Roentgenograms showed both maxillary and frontal sinuses to be opaque. The nasal mucous membrane was bright red, and the turbinates were swollen. The inferior turbinate was in contact with the septum. Purulent secretions were present beneath both middle turbinates, in the region of the ostia.

Cotton tampons soaked with 1% procaine hydrochloride were inserted along the inferior turbinates. At the end of 10 minutes the tampons were removed. The subject stated that the pain in the teeth and jaws was nearly gone. Similar tampons were inserted under the middle turbinates approximately 5 mm beneath the ostia for 10 minutes. Within 8 minutes all of the pain in the jaws, teeth, and face was gone, but a 1 plus pain remained in the frontal region. In another 10 minutes the subject stated that all of the pain in the head was gone, and shaking the head vigorously produced no pain.

Experiment 2. On the eighth day of an upper respiratory infection, the patient had pain over the right side of the face, from the side of the nose, under the eye, along the zygoma, into the temple and ear, and in the upper teeth and jaw. The pain was of 1 plus intensity, and of a dull, aching quality. The nasal mucous membranes were injected throughout. The turbinates were swollen and in contact with the septum. The middle turbinate was bright red—redder than the inferior turbinate—and extremely pain sensitive. When it was touched with a probe, pain in the right side of the face was intensified to 3 plus. There were purulent secretions beneath the middle turbinate in the region of the ostium. A procaine-soaked cotton tampon was inserted along the inferior turbinate and left in place for 10 minutes. The pain decreased slightly, especially along the side of the nose. Another tampon was inserted under the middle turbinate, approximately 5 mm below the ostium, for 10 minutes, and when it was removed all pain in the side of the face, temple, ear, and teeth was gone, and only a sense of fullness and stiffness remained. All discomfort was gone within an hour and did not return.

Comment. The effect of placing procaine under the middle turbinate and about 5 mm beneath the ostium cannot be explained as a direct procaine effect on nerves entering the ostium to innervate the walls of the sinus. Such nerves, which penetrate the ostium through the nose, enter mostly posteriorly and along the upper margin of the maxillary bone.

Experiment 3. This experiment involves pressure symptoms associated with a cyst in the left antrum. This patient, with a history of pain for 3 days in the left side of the face and head, was observed to have engorged turbinates that were in septal contact, causing complete occlusion of the nares. A local anesthetic was placed on the mucous membranes of the inferior and middle turbinates. Within 15 minutes the patient was left with a sense of fullness in the left side of the face and beneath the eye, with almost complete alleviation of the pain. The left antrum was entered with a trocar, and straw-colored fluid escaped from the needle under a pressure sufficient to send a stream in a straight line for 10 to 12 inches. Thereafter, the subject had no sensation of head fullness or pain.

Comment. This experiment gives further evidence that increased pressure in the maxillary sinus per se produces sensations of head fullness, and that such pain as the subject experienced had its origin in the inflammation of the turbinates. This experiment further illustrates that increased pressure in the antrum may exist for a long period without symptoms. Only with the onset of an upper respiratory infection and the associated inflammation of the turbinates was pain experienced.

Variations in Venous Pressure and the Size and Appearance of the Turbinates

Experiment 1. This subject had no gross infection of the nose. The jugular outflow on the left side of the neck was occluded for 3 minutes, which caused a gradually increasing engorgement of the turbinates. Ultimately, the inferior turbinate was in contact with an anterior deviation of the septum, so that the air passage was occluded. Toward the end of the 3-minute period there was an increase of watery secretion.

Experiment 2. When the appearance of the nose was again normal, the experiment was repeated so that venous occlusion was produced on the opposite side. The same engorgement occurred, but nasal airway obstruction was not complete because there was no septal deviation on that side.

Experiment 3. The head was tilted to the horizontal in such a way as to avoid pressure on the neck and to minimize venous stasis. No change in the appearance of the turbinates was noted within 3 minutes, although over a 45-minute period some swelling gradually occurred on the dependent side.

Experiment 4. In addition to tilting the head as in Experiment 3, the face and neck were firmly pressed with a pillow or the supporting hand. The turbinates on the dependent side were noted to become swollen to the point of occluding the air passage within 1 to 3 minutes.

The Effect of Vigorously Shaking the Head on Subjects with Engorged Turbinates

The intensity of headache associated with disease of the nasal and paranasal sinuses is increased by shaking the head. The following experiments show that this increased pain results from the sudden displacement of swollen, inflamed structures.

The subject, about 12 days after the onset of an upper respiratory infection, and during a headache-free period when the turbinates in the right naris were moderately engorged, induced further engorgement by occluding venous return in the right jugular vein with pressure of the hand and by lying on the right side for 5 minutes. The air passage in the right side of the nose was completely occluded, and there was a sense of fullness in the right side of the head, but no pain. The turbinates were observed to be swollen, the middle turbinate being especially engorged and in septal contact. At this time, shaking the head vigorously induced pain over the right side of the face from the side of the nose, along the zygoma, into the temple, and in the right upper teeth and jaw. The pain was of a dull, aching quality, of a 1 plus intensity, and persisted for 2 hours. A cotton tampon soaked with a vasoconstrictor (Neo-Synephrine Hydrochloride) was then inserted along the inferior turbinate and in contact with the middle turbinate, and was left in place for 10 minutes. When the pack was removed, the turbinates were observed to be pale and shrunken and all pain in the side of the face was gone. Vigorously shaking the head did not elicit pain.

The Site of Origin of Headache from Disease of the Nasal and Paranasal Structures

It is evident from these studies that the linings of the sinuses are relatively insensitive compared with their extremely sensitive ducts and ostia and the turbinates. Even though with inflammation, the threshold for pain in the sinuses is lowered so that they become more pain sensitive, the situation is altered relatively little, because with generalized inflammation, the ostia, ducts, and turbinates become even more pain sensitive.

Although the term *sinus headache* is commonly assigned to those headaches associated with sinus disease, proof that pain has its source in the mucous lining of the paranasal sinuses is lacking. The issue has been confused by the fact that sinus inflammation rarely if ever occurs without concomitant inflammation of the ostia and nasal structures. The rare exception is sinus infection secondary to periapical abscess, but this type of sinus disease causes minor or no discomfort until the nasal structures are directly or indirectly inflamed as well.

It is inferred, therefore, that the site of the headache is related chiefly to the region of the nose that is most inflamed and engorged. Disease of the superior nasal structures causes headaches primarily in the front and top of the head, and in and between the eyes. Disease of the middle and inferior nasal structures causes headaches primarily over the zygomas and temples and in the teeth and jaws.

THE PATHOPHYSIOLOGY OF HEADACHE FROM DISEASE OF NASAL AND PARANASAL STRUCTURES

Variations in Venous Pressure

Variations in venous pressure modify the intensity of the headache. Unilateral pressure on the jugular veins, both internal and external, increases the turgescence of the turbinates on the homolateral side. When the turbinates are inflamed and engorged, this effect is more striking than when they are normal. When the turbinates are already moderately painful, the pain is augmented by further turgescence, and still further augmented by shaking the head or lowering the head between the knees. When a subject with turgescent turbinates rests in a lying-down position on his or her side, there is a momentary slight increase in pain as the swollen, reddened turbinates are displaced. Gradually the uppermost turbinates shrink slightly, whereas the dependent turbinates become more turgescent and occlude the air passages.

On the other hand, venous pressure is not a factor of first importance in sinus headache, since intensity is usually greatest when the subject is in the erect position, and the cranial venous pressure is lower.

Negative and Positive Air Pressure

The fact that the headache is usually worse in the upright position and better when the patient is lying down has been used as evidence that pain is due to negative or positive air pressure in the sinuses, resulting from the draining out of, or filling up with, purulent secretion. However, because changes in pressure have been demonstrated to be inadequate stimuli for producing serious discomfort in these cavities, other factors must be more important as causes of pain.

Irritants on the Nasal Mucosa

Toxic or noxious chemicals, in either the liquid or gaseous phase, can produce inflammation in the nasal mucosa by direct interaction with the mucous membranes. This is not immunologically mediated, although variations in the degree of sensitivity of dose-effect relationship in certain patients have been observed by careful clinicians. Some individuals with exquisite sensitivity to inhaled cigarette smoke, smog, and chemical fumes are already suffering from other forms of nasal mucosal inflammation (allergic or vasomotor rhinitis). The superimposition of chemical molecules on already inflamed surfaces increases the inflammation and swelling, and this may be enough to exceed pain thresholds and produce a paranasal pain syndrome. In the absence of underlying rhinitis, chemical fumes would not be an adequate stimulus to produce paranasal pain in this subgroup of patients.

Vasomotor Changes in the Nasal Linings

Local vasomotor changes in the erectile tissues of the nose as accompaniments of stress, exhaustion, anxiety, hormonal stimulation, sexual excitement, and various emotional states have been observed. Ordinarily such variations are not associated with nasal symptoms, but sometimes the effects of these changes produce enough congestion of the turbinates to induce obstruction of the nasal passages with or without associated paranasal head pain.

NASAL DYSFUNCTION AND HEADACHE IN PATIENTS HAVING ADAPTIVE DIFFICULTIES

Functional alterations in the structures in the human nose have been studied and correlated with a wide variety of circumstances, including noxious stimulation inside the nose by chemical agents, noxious stimulation of other portions of the head, variations in environmental temperature, interruption of afferent nerve pathways, weeping, and numerous threatening life situations with their accompanying affective states.

In general, two patterns of disturbance of nasal function were recognized. The first involved vasoconstriction in the nose with shrinkage of the membrane and increase in the size of the air passages. Such changes in reaction to threats accompanied feelings of fear, sadness, and other emotions that although strong, involved minimal conflict (Figure 13-10).

The second type of disturbance in the nose appeared to have greater significance with relation to disease. It was characterized by the initial hyperemia associated with

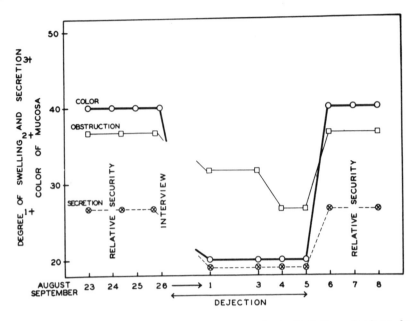

Figure 13-10. Pallor and shrinkage of nasal membranes associated with feelings of sadness, fear, and dejection.

turgescence of the erectile tissues in the turbinates and nasal septum, engorgement of the nasal mucosa, and increased secretion. These changes were accompanied by obstruction to breathing and often by pain. After hyperemia subsided, secondary pallor ensued with the mucous membranes of the nose remaining boggy and edematous. This second type of nasal disturbance, characterized by hyperfunction, occurred in response to a variety of environmental threats against the individual and appeared to constitute part of a defense mechanism for shutting out and washing away a noxious environment at the head of the organism. Such a pattern was found to occur in response to local stimulation by the noxious fumes of ammonium carbonate (Figure 13-11) or by pollens from grasses to which the subject was sensitive (Figure 13-12). It also occurred following noxious stimulation not directed specifically at the nose or respiratory passages—for example, the painful tightening of a metal headband. In fact, this defensive pattern of shutting out occurred even in response to noxious environmental stimuli that did not involve physical contact with the organism, such as situational threats occurring during interpersonal adjustment. Weeping, which followed frustrating or humiliating experiences, was accompanied by swelling, hyperemia, hypersecretion, and obstruction in the nose (Figure 13-13). Such changes also accompanied anger and feelings of frustration without weeping.

One subject, a 25-year-old physician, was studied in detail and continuously over 8 months. He exhibited alterations in nasal function that were observed during naturally occurring day-to-day life stresses. Pallor of nasal membranes with an increase in size of the air channels occurred in a setting of abject fear and dejection following his wife's hemoptysis. In situations of conflict, however, when decisions were required regarding threats to his career or to his position as head of his household,

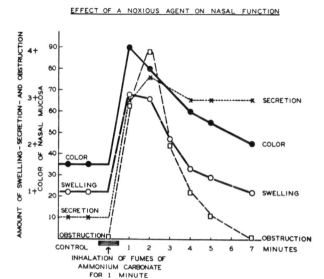

Figure 13-11. Nasal hyperfunction following inhalation of the noxious fumes of ammonium carbonate.

nasal hyperemia with swelling, hypersecretion, and obstruction to breathing occurred. At such times he had frequent colds with sneezing and coughing, postnasal
discharge, and sinus headache.

He approached his problems in an energetic, aggressive, outgoing and self-confident
fashion. Situations within his realm of responsibility were rarely out of his control.
His system of security rested on three props: (1) the approval of his superiors; (2)
his ability to be assertively independent in the economic and social spheres; and (3)
his achievement of a recognized position in a competitive society—that is, "success
in his career."

At the time when the subject's wife was 5-months pregnant, a decision had to be
made to relinquish their own apartment and go to live with the wife's aunt in a
suburb of the city.

During this period, in which the subject was exposed to serious threats to his
independence, he was also subjected to threats to his career and to danger of losing
the approval of his superiors. Working with him under his supervision was an intern
about 4 years' his senior, who found it difficult to perform the menial but essential
chores customarily assigned to an intern, and who was unwilling to accept the responsibility for his patients. The subject hesitated, because of his subordinate's experience and age, to reprimand him openly and frankly. He first tried to cope with
the situation by suggesting a plan to maintain the ward's efficiency. When this failed,
the subject began, in addition to his own work, to perform the intern's neglected
duties himself. He finally confronted the intern frankly with the issue, but the latter
refused to accept criticism from a younger, less-experienced man.

In this setting of threat to his career, with feelings of anger and resentment, and
the fear of loss of the approval of his senior colleagues, as well as the conflict arising
from his being forced to sacrifice those symbols of independence his own home

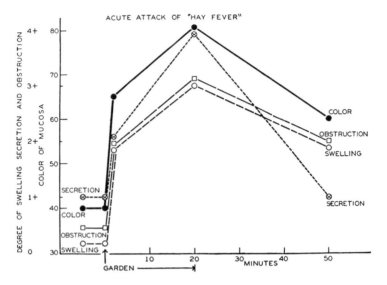

Figure 13-12.   Nasal hyperfunction after exposure to pollens.

represented, the subject was aware of an increase in postnasal accumulations of secretions and the need to "clear his throat" frequently. His nose felt occluded, and there was burning pain in both nostrils. Figure 13-14 demonstrates the increase in redness of the nasal mucosa associated with a significant increase in the amount of secretion, swelling, and obstruction sustained throughout this 12-day period.

During weeping, not only the eyes but also the nose were found to participate in this reaction, and in two individuals in this study, deeper structures including the

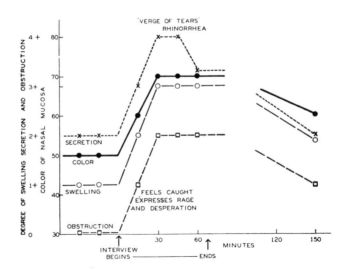

Figure 13-13.   Nasal hyperfunction during an interview in which the subject experienced rage and desperation.

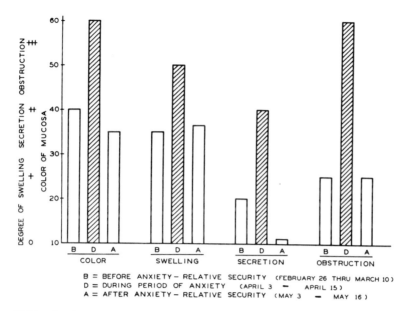

Figure 13-14. Sustained nasal hyperfunction during 12 days of anxiety and resentment compared with control periods before and after.

bronchae constricted during threatening situations, thus participating in the bodily reaction of exclusion. Against local intrusion by dust, for example, or noxious fumes, the reaction of shutting out and washing away proved highly effective. Against situational threats involving interpersonal relations, however, the nasal changes afforded incomplete relief and were often counterproductive.

When the nasal changes in the bodily pattern of shutting out and washing away were unduly sustained, they gave rise to troublesome symptoms including burning pain of low intensity. This was increased by forced inspiration; and a dull, aching pain spread from the bridge of the nose into the orbit and along the zygoma to the ear on each side of the swollen nasal structure. When the swelling shifted to the opposite nostril, the pain correspondingly changed position. The pain, which also involved the teeth, especially those of the upper jaw, alternated with a feeling of fullness, which was worse during the working hours of the day, especially during periods of stress, and was minimal in the early morning and late evening. When pain was relatively intense, local deep tenderness was also noted. Photophobia occurred, especially on the painful side, with injection of the sclerae and the skin of the cheek. Distribution of headache is shown schematically in Figure 13-15.

The data presented indicate that during sustained conflict prolonged nasal hyperfunction may occur, accompanied by obstruction, facial pain, and tenderness. Such symptoms are often attributed to acute sinusitis. In this case no infection of the sinuses was demonstrated, however, and the disturbance with accompanying symptoms subsided completely when the subject's conflicts were resolved.

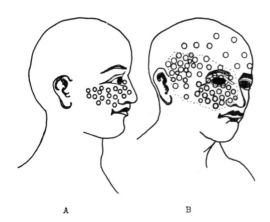

Figure 13-15. Distribution of pain and hyperalgesia during nasal hyperfunction associated with emotional conflict.

A   B

PARANASAL HEAD PAIN AND ALLERGY

It is clear that any stimulus that causes engorgement or inflammation of the nasal turbinates can produce nasal or paranasal head pain. Therefore, the proper perspective to view allergy and headache is within the context of the causes of rhinitis. Because allergic reactions are one of many provoking mechanisms, they are included in the list. However, IgE-mediated reactions do not hold exclusive rights to the pathogenesis of paranasal head pain.

Paranasal Head Pain and Allergic Rhinitis

Paranasal head pain develops in some patients when IgE-mediated reactions occur in nasal mucous membranes. Thus, allergic rhinitis can be responsible for paranasal headache, with or without associated inflammation in the paranasal sinuses. The percentage of patients with allergic rhinitis who also report paranasal head pain is unknown. Many individuals with allergic rhinitis experience mild "pressure" in the paranasal structures, but their individualized definition of pain plays a substantial part in whether or not they report paranasal pain during allergic rhinitis episodes. In our allergy clinic, only 20% of patients with proven IgE-mediated rhinitis report paranasal discomfort as their primary complaint. These patients rarely seek medical attention because of their head pain, but instead volunteer rhinorrhea, nasal congestion, sleep disturbance, or sneezing as their chief complaints.

Other Types of Rhinitis

The term rhinitis is nonspecific. A number of inflammatory mechanisms can induce swelling and congestion of the nasal membranes, and all can lead to paranasal pain. Important variables in the production of paranasal pain include (1) the anatomic arrangements between the nasal septum, turbinates, and sinus ostia; (2) the relative size

Table 13-2 Characteristics of the major forms of rhinitis

	Allergic rhinitis	Infectious rhinitis	Vasomotor rhinitis	Irritant rhinitis
Seasonal incidence	Frequent	Increased in winter	None	Smog
Itching & sneezing	Usual	Rare	Unusual	Unusual
Collateral allergy	Common	Occasional	Occasional	Occasional
Family history allergy	Common	Occasional	Occasional	Occasional
Sore throat	Rare	Common	Rare	Rare
Fever	Rare	Common	Rare	Rare
Conjunctivitis	Itching common	Occasional	Rare	Burning common
Nasal pallor	Usual	Rare	Common	Occasional
Nasal polyps	Occasional	Occasional	Occasional	Occasional
Injection of pharynx	Rare	Common	Rare	Rare
Eosinophil nasal secretions	Usual	Absent	Absent	Absent
Purulent nasal secretions	Rare	Usual	Occasional	Occasional
Positive allergy skin tests	Usual	Rare (coincidental)	Rare	Rare (coincidental)
Paranasal pain	Occasional	Common	Occasional	Occasional

of the nasal passages; and (3) the presence or absence of nasal polyps and their location with respect to sinus ostia.

The characteristics of all forms of rhinitis are compared with those of allergic rhinitis in Table 13-2. *Allergic rhinitis* is the only type that is initiated by IgE and antigen interaction. *Infectious rhinitis* is usually the consequence of a viral agent infecting the nasal membranes and inciting an inflammatory response. A viral infection frequently extends to the sinus ostia, eustachian tubes, pharynx, larynx, and trachea. Primary or secondary bacterial infections, usually *Staphylococcus aureus, Hemophyllis influenza, Pneumococcus pneumonia,* or *Streptococcus hemolyticus,* also occur in the nasal and sinus membranes. Paranasal head pain is more prominent during infectious rhinitis than in any other forms of rhinitis (Solomon, 1967).

Vasomotor rhinitis mimics allergic rhinitis, but antigens and antibodies do not initiate this type of nasal congestion. Instead, a variety of stimuli, including temperature changes, exercise, change in position, change in barometric pressure or humidity, anger, and certain odors, precede the onset of nasal congestion. How these nonallergic stimuli induce nasal congestion is not entirely clear, but most evidence favors dysfunctional control of nasal vascular beds by the autonomic nervous system. Interruption of the cervical sympathetic nerves is followed by unilateral nasal obstruction and hypersecretion. Disruption of the parasympathetic fibers produces dry, crusted atrophic nasal membranes (Millonig et al., 1950). If a cold stimulus is applied to the nasal membranes or to skin of the extremity, there is prompt homolateral engorgement of the nasal turbinates in patients suffering from vasomotor rhinitis (Ralston & Kerr, 1945).

Irritant rhinitis is sometimes subclassified as a form of vasomotor rhinitis. As implied by its name, irritant chemicals activate congestion and inflammation of the nasal membranes through direct contact with these structures. The precise role of the vasomotor autonomic reflexes in the resulting nasal congestion is unclear. Normal individuals who inhale volatile acidic fumes, smoke, or smog invariably develop mild to moderate tearing and nasal congestion. At the other end of the spectrum, selected ''sensitive'' individuals experience severe conjunctival or nasal congestion upon contact with minimal atmospheric concentrations of smog, cigarette smoke, perfumes, or cocaine. Although many of these patients also have vasomotor rhinitis, others experience nasal congestion only when their nasal membranes are in contact with irritant fumes.

Rhinitis medicametosa is the rebound response of the nasal vascular beds to topical application or sympathomimetic drops or sprays. Neo-Synephrine and oxymetazoline HCl are the preparations usually applied to the nasal membranes. Rhinitis medicametosa almost never occurs by itself, and attention to the underlying rhinitis mechanism is necessary, both to wean the patient away from sympathomimetic nasal sprays and also to initiate a treatment plan that will prevent the need for using topical sympathomimetic drugs in the future. By the time these individuals seek medical attention, the syndrome of underlying rhinitis with superimposed rhinitis medicametosa is frequently associated with paranasal head pain. However, despite their discomfort and desire to receive medical assistance, these patients are sometimes reluctant to disclose their use of sympathomimetic sprays. Close questioning and even observation may be necessary to obtain this essential information.

Finally, although the features of rhinitis are presented in Table 13-2 as separate entities, few individuals experience only one type of rhinitis during their lifetime. An individual who develops IgE-mediated rhinitis from inhalating grass pollen in the spring may experience irritant rhinitis in the fall, vasomotor rhinitis while skiing in the winter, and a viral upper respiratory infection with rhinitis in March. This chronology can be further complicated by the simultaneous appearance of two or even more rhinitis mechanisms. Diagnostic and treatment ingenuity can be severely strained when several types of rhinitis occur simultaneously (Tennenbaum, 1972).

In addition, because nasal obstruction leads to sleep deprivation, the disease of rhinitis can cause fatigue and psychosocial disruptions that, through the autonomic nervous system, directly cause further congestion of the nasal turbinates, with paranasal pain, or head pain of either muscle contraction or vascular origin.

Clinical Features of Paranasal Head Pain

The headache associated with frontal sinus disease and the usual inflammation around the sinus ostia are localized diffusely over the frontal region. Antral disease produces headache over the maxillary region. The headache associated with sphenoid and ethmoid sinus disease is experienced between and behind the eyes and over the vertex of the skull. Commonly, when sinus disease is of sufficient duration, pain occurs in the back of the head, neck, and shoulders, in addition to the headache experienced in the front and top of the head.

Headaches are less frequent when the patient has been in the supine position and are less prominent at night than during the day. Moreover, the pain associated with maxillary sinus disease gradually diminishes over about 30 minutes when the patient lies down with the diseased sinus uppermost.

The headache associated with frontal sinus disease commonly begins about 9 A.M., gradually becomes worse, and terminates toward evening, or upon retiring. The pain associated with maxillary sinus disease frequently has its onset in the early afternoon.

In all instances, the pain is of a deep, dull, aching, nonpulsatile quality. It is seldom, if ever, associated with nausea. Chronic sinus disease produces headache pain of lower intensity than that associated with acute sinus disease. In both instances, the intensity of pain is increased by shaking the head or assuming the head-down position. The headache is intensified by procedures that increase the venous pressure, such as "straining," coughing, or wearing a tight collar.

The headache associated with disease of the nasal and paranasal structures is commonly reduced in intensity or abolished by nasal decongestant sprays or pills. Aspirin may reduce the intensity of the pain but usually does not abolish it. Patients frequently report the simultaneous disappearance of nasal congestion and paranasal head pain after appropriate decongestant therapy has been initiated.

NASAL SEPTAL CONTACT HEADACHE

Deviation of the nasal septum can occur in many forms and degrees of obstruction. Because the septum itself is relatively insensitive to pain, the mechanism of pain induction is through pressure of the septum on pain-sensitive structures, such as the nasal turbinates (Ryan & Ryan, 1979).

ANGIOEDEMA AND HEAD PAIN

After release of vasodilating mediators, soft tissue swelling can occur in tissues of the face, tongue, pharynx, or larynx. Antigens such as penicillin, sulfa, horse serum, or insulin can combine with specific IgE antibodies to initiate type I hypersensitivity reactions, manifested by either urticaria, angioedema, or both.

Urticaria—crops of wheals frequently surrounded by erythema and associated with pruritus—occurs in either specific locations or over most of the body's surface. Angioedema, by contrast, is a condition characterized by nonpitting localized edema without associated pruritus (Mathews, 1974). These two forms of abnormal cutaneous or subcutaneous vasodilatation can appear separately or at the same time.

Both urticaria and angioedema are associated with vasodilation and increased permeability of small venules and capillaries; vascular congestion occurs in the upper corium vessels in urticaria and in the subcutaneous vessels in angioedema (Lever, 1961).

Intradermal injection of histamine produces local wheal and flare urticarial lesions, which are indistinguishable from spontaneous urticaria (Lewis, 1961). However, many patients who have urticaria do not respond to antihistamines (H_1 blockers), and the pathogenic mechanisms that produce urticaria and angioedema are now recognized to be heterogeneous with immunologic, nonimmunologic, emotional, neural, and physical inciting events triggering a complicated chain of mechanisms culminating in vasodilatation and increased permeability of cutaneous vessels (Fink, 1972; Kaplan, 1978).

Although most angioedema is painless, in certain forms and/or locations it causes head pain. For the most part, these instances are obvious. Pain is directly related to the area of soft tissue swelling on the scalp or face. Angioedema of the tongue, pharynx, and larynx is almost always manifested by other symptoms, such as obstruction, sensation of a mass, or difficulty with swallowing or speaking. Pain is rarely a manifestation of these latter angioedema locations, and referred pain is even more unusual. Generalized, severe angioedema has been reported in at least one patient with associated headaches, epilepsy, hemiplegia, and coma (Fowler, 1962). We have observed a patient who reacted to parabens (stabilizer chemicals in injectable medications) by developing generalized erythrodermia with tissue edema, including cerebral edema, headache, and semicoma. She was treated with corticosteroids (without parabens) and recovered.

CEREBRAL ARTERITIS SYNDROMES

Systemic lupus erythematosis (SLE) is a disease manifested by deposition of toxic complexes of DNA, antibody, and complement in arterial walls (type III reactions). The resulting inflammation or arteritis can produce systemic symptoms, such as fever, malaise, myalgias, and arthralgias, or localized symptoms that are the consequences of occlusion and perinflammation of specific arteries. When cerebral arteries or the choroid plexus are involved by SLE, the patient can develop head pain adjacent to inflamed superficial arteries, as a consequence of arterial obstruction with ischemic pain or as a generalized cerebritis with a dull, pressure-type pain (Atkins et al., 1972).

Giant-cell arteritis may occur in the cranial arteries. Because the superficial temporal arteries are accessible and can be sacrificed for biopsy, the term *temporal arteritis* has gained popular acceptance. Actually, in this disease, giant-cell arteritis is present in large arteries that supply the skeletal muscles (polymyalgia rheumatic syndrome) (Healey & Wilske, 1977) and viscera (O'Neill et al., 1976); as well as the axillary, brachial, femoral, and coronary arteries (Stanson et al., 1976).

Evolving evidence supports the hypothesis that giant-cell arteritis (temporal arteritis, cranial arteritis, and polymyalgia rheumatica) are diverse manifestations of type III, toxic complex arteritis, appearing in a number of large and medium-sized arteries. Immunofluorescent studies of biopsied arteries (superficial temporal) show deposits of IgG, IgA, sometimes IgM, fibrin, and complement components (Waaler et al., 1976) in a number of biopsy specimens, depending on the stage of disease and the biopsy site (Klein et al., 1976). Hazelman et al. (1975) reported lymphocyte stimulation by arterial wall antigen extracts in polymyalgia rheumatica, suggesting that cellular immune hypersensitivity or type IV reactions may be occurring in this syndrome. If these observations are supported by further studies, the possibility of

Table 13-3 Side effects of drugs used to treat allergic diseases

Drugs	Consequences of drugs	
	Head-pain type	Other side effects and manifestations
Decongestants Antihistamines and sympathomimetics	Vascular, pounding headaches	Somnolence, or excitation
Sympathomimetics Epinephrine Ephedrine Isoproterenol Metaproterenol Albuterol	Vascular, pounding headaches	Tremor, palpitations, tachyarrythmias
Aminophylline or theophylline	Toxic, sick headache, generalized	Nausea, emesis, tremor, excitation, convulsions, tachyarrhythmias
corticosteroids Prednisone Methyl prednisolone	Cervico-occipital headaches Vascular headaches	Hypertension, Cushing's syndrome, osteoporosis

combined hypersensitivity (types III and IV) responses will have been identified. The main deterrent in categorizing giant-cell arteritis as an immune disease, however, has been failure to identify the inciting antigen(s). By contrast, in SLE, a variety of nuclear antigens have been separated and studied by Nutmon et al. (1975).

The relationship between the arteritis syndromes and headaches is described in greater detail in Chapter 11.

HEADACHE REACTIONS TO DRUGS USED TO TREAT ALLERGIC DISEASES

Common and frequently overlooked causes of head pain in patients with allergic diseases are reactions to the drugs used to treat these patients. Individuals with allergic rhinitis receive antihistamine and sympathomimetic decongestants; asthmatics received theophylline, sympathomimetic bronchodilators, and corticosteroids; and patients suffering from systemic arteritis syndromes frequently receive high dosages of corticosteroids. Therefore, when evaluating a patient who has one or more of these diseases and also complains of head pain, physicians are encouraged to assess the consequences of those drugs used to treat the disease, rather than assuming that the disease is responsible for the head pain syndrome.

Table 13-3 lists the major drugs used to treat allergic diseases, along with their side effects.

RELATIONSHIP BETWEEN ALLERGY AND MIGRAINE HEADACHE

Migraine is a common disorder that occurs in 15% of the adult population, twice as frequently in women as in men (Dalsgaard-Nielsen, 1974). Because migraine headaches tend to occur intermittently, it has been tempting to identify provoking factors assumed to be responsible for each migraine attack. Infrequent exposure to allergens or antigens constitutes a hypothetical provoking event for each or even occasional migraine headaches. However, proving that antigens, combining with IgE antibodies, actually cause migraine or vascular headaches has been difficult. Most of the controversy regarding allergy and migraine headaches are the result of differing interpretations of incomplete data.

History of Allergy and Migraine Headaches

Pagniex, Vallery-Radot, and Nast (1919) were among the first to hypothesize an allergic mechanism in migraine. The reports of DeGowin (1932), Rinkel (1933), Balyeat and Brittain (1930), Hahn (1930), Hamburger (1935), Gonzales (1953), Ogden (1951), and others followed. Vaughan's work (1934) is representative of these publications. On the basis of a clinical history of migraine attacks after ingesting certain foods and the presence of positive skin tests to these foods, he concluded that hypersensitivity was a causative factor in 70% of patients with vascular headache of the migraine type. In half of his patients, a reduction in migraine headaches occurred after the diet was modified. The chief food offenders have varied from study to study: wheat, milk, chocolate, and eggs in the opinion of Balyeat and Brittain (1930); celery, peas, and onions in DeGowin's report (1932).

Other physicians have attempted to link migraine headache to allergy by identifying common associations. For example, Neusser (1892) reported eosinophilia during a migraine attack. Von Leeuwen and Zeydner (1922) described an activity in the blood of patients with asthma, urticaria, epilepsy, and migraine that induced smooth muscle contraction *in vitro,* but that was absent from the blood of normal control subjects.

One of the earliest relationships between migraine and allergy was simply based on definitions. In 1873, Trousseau stated that migraine was one of the allergic manifestations of the atopic state. He declared, without evidence, that periodic headache, along with hay fever, urticaria, and eczema were all features of an "asthmatic state." He failed to provide even a shred of data to support his statement. This position was championed in the United States by Vaughan and others (Rowe, 1932; Unger & Unger, 1952). By defining migraine as an allergy, Rinkel, in 1933, was able to show that migraine patients had a family history of "allergy." Although a small number of migraine patients came from families in which true atopic diseases, such as allergic rhinitis, asthma, urticaria, and eczema existed, in the majority of family members interviewed by Rinkel the so-called family history of allergy turned out to be migraine headaches. Another interpretation of the same data is that the majority of migraine patients came from families in which other members also had migraine headaches. Despite the passage of time, the controversy continues. Recent publications by Unger and colleagues (1970, 1974) and Speer (1975) continue to reveal a strong belief that allergy causes spontaneous migraine headaches.

Dietary Migraine

The major arena of controversy with respect to a cause-and-effect relationship between allergic reactions and migraine has been that of food allergy. From the outset, those who favored the allergic migraine hypothesis observed migraine headache attacks after food ingestion in many of their patients. Wolf and Unger (1944) recorded migraine headache attacks in one patient after he consumed food extracts that had given positive skin tests. They then failed to produce headache in the patient after administering harmless extracts presented as the known offending allergen.

Hyslop (1934) reported a patient who suffered migraine after ingesting pork when the patient was under emotional stress.

However, in most of the studies, a critical experimental control was omitted. If the alleged offending food had been administered without the patient's awareness, and headache had always occurred, a direct cause-and-effect relationship between food and headache would be more convincing. When this step was carried out at the New York Hospital, with the administration of chocolate, disguised in capsules for those allegedly sensitive to chocolate, or milk given through a stomach tube to those who were said to be sensitive to milk, the results did not confirm the earlier work. No headache ensued. Moreover, in 1950 Loveless gave milk, corn, arrowroot, and tapioca, as well as placebo preparations, in disguised form, to persons alleged to have had headache attacks precipitated by the ingestion of these foods. She noted, in her well-controlled study, no predictable relationship between the administration of these substances and the occurrence of headache.

In another well-controlled, double-blind food challenge and elimination study, Walker (1960) showed that there was no predictable relationship between disguised offending foods and the occurrence of migraine headache attacks. Many have concluded that the effect of the doctor-and-patients *belief* that the allergen offered would produce a migraine headache could have triggered migraine attacks through fear and psychic anticipation of stress in the earlier, uncontrolled feeding experiments.

Another approach (Grant, 1979) was to eliminate all foods (except lamb, pears, and spring water) for 5 days in a group of 60 migraine patients. All patients had previously been told to avoid cheese, chocolate, citrus fruits, alcohol, cigarette smoke (active or passive), hunger, and excessive stress and yet were still having frequent headaches. At the end of the first 5 days, new foods were tested as follows. Pulse rate and all symptoms were recorded before, 20 minutes after, and 1½ hours after ingestion of each new food. All the patients experienced "reactions' to between 1 and 30 foods/patient, averaging 10 foods for each patient. Patients then eliminated the offending foods from their diet with dramatic improvement in the frequency of migraine headaches. For the group of 60 patients, the number of headaches declined from 402 per month (prediet) to 6 per month (after starting the diet). The author concluded that the elimination of offending food allergens was the cause-and-effect reason for the declining numbers of migraine headaches.

The reduction in frequency and intensity of migraine attacks by the ingestion of so-called elimination diets cannot be relied on as supporting the relevance of ingested allergens to migraine.

This is particularly the case during a "study" in which the investigator must be involved in recording the "results." Her desire to help achieve a positive effect and the patients' motivation to help the results or at least not disappoint the investigator are all variables that contribute to the end result. Wolff (1955) put forth the thesis that the interest and good will of the physician and the expectation of improvement on the part of the patient may effect relief in many patients through neural rather than antiallergic mechanisms.

The presence of positive wheal-and-flare skin test responses to certain foods has been used as evidence for "food allergy" in migraine patients (Vaughan, 1934). Unfortunately, positive skin tests occur in up to 25% of asymptomatic, nonallergic control populations (Smith, 1978).

A variation on food skin testing was provided by Monro et al. (1980), who used RAST to measure serum-specific IgE antibodies. In 47 patients, the authors believed they could predict food allergy from RAST results and after challenge with forbidden foods demonstrated an increase in the serum levels of food specific IgE antibodies. They could "provoke" headaches with open challenges with food and "block" headaches with open ingestion of chromolyn sodium.

Not only are positive food skin tests and elevated titers of serum-specific IgE (RAST) found in asymptomatic individuals, but a cause-and-effect relationship between addition and elimination of foods in known atopic conditions has been difficult to prove. Difficulties of establishing a diagnosis of food hypersensitivity have been outlined by May and Bock (1978). In migraine, the problem is further compounded by a psychological factor—a positive skin test for a food can induce fear or stress in the susceptible patient, which, in turn, can precipitate a migraine headache when that forbidden food is reintroduced.

The many problems in the interpretation of skin tests make it difficult to establish their relevance to migraine. It is noteworthy that although the gastrointestinal tract is more premeable to food allergens in the very young, Vahlquist (1955) has shown that the incidence of migraine in children is at most one third to one half that found in adults. If food allergy, which has a high incidence in children compared with adults, were important in the pathogenesis of migraine, the opposite relationship should exist, with migraine headaches being two to three times more common in children than in adults.

The term *dietary migraine* has been used by Dalessio (1972) to describe the relationship between eating certain foods and the onset of migraine headaches. Despite the controversy as to the existence of food-induced IgE mediated reactions, the observation that certain patients develop headaches after ingesting selected foods remains valid. It is now clear that many of those foods, which appear to produce migraine, have one thing in common. In addition to their food antigens, ingestants also contain vosactive chemicals or substrates for enzyme systems that synthesize vasoconstrictors. These chemicals and substrates have direct or indirect effects on cerebral blood vessel receptors, stimulating vasoconstriction of the susceptible migraine arteries. See Chapter 5 for a list of vasoactive chemicals that all migraine patients should avoid.

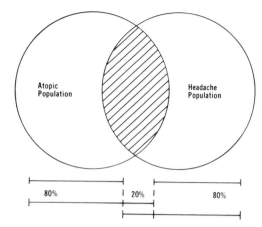

Figure 13-16. Schematic representation of the overlap between the atopic and migraine populations. The hash-marked area between the circles represents those atopic patients who also have migraine headaches.

Epidemiologic Investigations of Migraine and Atopic Populations

Lance and Anthony (1966), in their headache clinic, studied 500 patients with migraine headaches and 100 patients with tension headaches. Of the migraine patients, 17% were found to have allergic disorders, including asthma, hay fever, hives, and eczema; 13% of the patients with tension headaches had similar allergies. There were no statistical differences between the populations, which strongly implied that migraine sufferers had no greater propensity toward allergies than did a control group of patients with muscle contraction headaches. Furthermore, an epidemiologic study of an entire Michigan community (population 11,305) showed that the incidence of asthma and allergic rhinitis was 21.8% for males and 25.3% for females (Broder et al., 1974). Urticaria is extremely common, occurring at least once during the lifetime of at least 20% of the general population (Smith, 1978). Our best available information leads to the conclusion that 20% of the adult population suffers from one or more manifestations of allergy or atopy, an incidence exceeding that found in Lance and Anthony's headache populations.

In a neurology clinic in Chicago, Bassoe (1933) found that only 3% of 270 migraine patients had any historical manifestations of allergy. Ziegler and colleagues (1972) studied 289 migraine patients and also found a very low incidence of associated allergic rhinitis and asthma.

In looking at the allergic population for the incidence of migraine, Schwartz (1952) examined 241 asthmatics and 200 nonallergic controls as well as their 3815 relatives. He found an incidence of approximately 5% for migraine headache among the asthmatics, normal controls, and their relatives. This figure is actually lower than the 15% incidence of migraine in the general population reported by Dalsgaard-Nielsen (1974). In another study by Kallos and Kallos-Deffner (1955), the incidence of migraine in their allergic population was 15%.

Therefore, since migraine and allergy are frequently found in the total population, it is not surprising that nonrandom studies identified some patients with both conditions. It appears that approximately 20% of migraine patients have allergy and 15% of allergy patients have migraine headaches. Figure 13–16 illustrates this point.

Because of the difficulty in identifying some patients with allergic disease even by allergy specialists, a potential criticism of studies that attempted to identify allergies in a migraine population has been that the nonallergist investigators failed to identify allergic patients accurately. Medina and Diamond (1976) measured total serum IgE levels in 89 unselected patients with migraine headaches aned 27 control patients with muscle contraction headaches. Elevated levels of serum IgE were found in 5.7% of patients with migraine and in 3.7% of patients with muscle contraction headaches, incidences not significantly different from each other or from that in the general population. By contrast, elevated levels of serum IgE were found in 41% of patients with both exzema and respiratory allergy and in 79% of patients with atopic dermatitis and respiratory allergy (Smith, 1978).

Although there is no universal test to identify atopy and one must rely on the history to identify migraine patients, no data link these two conditions into a monogenetic or even polygenetic defect. No evidence that classic or common migraine or other forms of vascular headache, such as cluster headache, are truly allergic in origin has been found. However, since both allergy and migraine are common conditions, the presence of one does not appear to protect against the other. Some patients have both. In these individuals, it is important to deal realistically with both disorders.

Migraine Headaches in Allergic Patients

Patients who have allergic disease may also have other disease processes that are not *caused* by their allergy but under certain circumstances may be worsened by the allergy itself, drugs used to treat the allergy, or the psychological consequences of having a chronic disease.

Allergic patients may develop paranasal sinus headaches, muscle contraction headaches from tension and worry over their diseases, and (in susceptible individuals) typical or classic migraine headaches. Is there any evidence that type I IgE-mediated reactions precipitate migraine headaches in the allergic subgroup of migraine patients?

Kallos and Kallos-Deffner's (1955) experiments are particularly interesting. They selected a small group of 28 patients who had both migraine headaches and urticaria, rhinitis, or asthma. They injected extracts of specific allergens into these patients, using concentrations great enough to produce typical IgE-mediated reactions of rhinitis, asthma, or urticaria. In most patients, a vascular headache followed the parenteral injections of large dosages of allergenic extracts. However, two important clarifying observations were made. Headache always appeared in association with rhinitis, asthma, or urticaria and never as the only manifestation of an allergen-induced systemic reaction. Second, the migraine aura (phase 1 or the vasoconstrictive component) was universally absent. The nasopulmonary reaction could then be prevented by pretreating the patient with antihistamine (H_1 blockers), but the vascular headache continued to occur unless the patient was pretreated with ergotamine, which blocked the headache but had no effect on the respiratory tract reactions. These very interesting observations suggest that mediators released during IgE-mediated anaphylaxis can produce vascular headaches, possibly by stimulating the second (or vasodilator) phase of a vascular-type headache. If this mediator is histamine, it would need H_2 cerebral arterial receptors, since H_1 antihistamines do not block vascular headache.

The role of histamine in vascular headaches was first reported by Pickering (1933), who injected 0.1 mg of histamine intravenously, producing vascular headaches in all subjects. Keeney (1946) systematically reviewed this subject and studied 37 patients with periodic vascular headache. Twenty-four developed typical vascular headaches after subcutaneous injections of 0.1 mg histamine. In 7 of 10 patients, 0.6 mg of nitroglycerine sublingually also produced vascular headache, suggesting that vasodilatation, rather than a specific susceptibility to histamine, represented the pathogenic event in vascular head pain.

Although it is clear that subcutaneous or intravenous injections of large dosages of histamine or other vasodilators will produce cerebral vascular dilatation and headaches in susceptible individuals, it is not clear if these observations have any relevance to spontaneous migraine occurring as a consequence of IgE-mediated rhinitis, asthma, or urticaria.

In an important study by Kaliner et al. (1982), plasma and histamine levels were measured during continuous infusions of histamine into 8 normal volunteers and 4 asthmatics not taking any medications. Resting or baseline plasma histamine levels were $.62 \pm 0.12$ ng/ml and rose progressively in direct proportion to the concentration of infused histamine. Plasma levels of histamine required to elicit symptoms were as follows: 1.61 ± 0.30 ng/ml eg 30% increase in heart rate, 2.39 ± 0.52 ng/ml = significant flush and headache. Pretreatment with hydroxyzine (H_1 blocker) or cimetidine (H_2 blocker) failed to influence the amount (level) of histamine associated with flush and headache. However, pretreatment with both an H_1 and H_2 blocker raised the threshold whereby histamine produced the same symptoms (5.76 ± 0.78 ng/ml) when compared with the lower levels of histamine previously associated with headache and flush (2.39 ng/ml) when pretreatment was not carried out.

Another interesting study of intravenous histamine infusion (Krabbe & Olesen, 1980) was conducted in three patient groups: 13 normal, nonheadache prone volunteers, 10 patients who suffered from muscle contraction headaches, and 25 patients with recurrent migraine headaches. Histamine infusions of 0.16, 0.33 and 0.66 μg/kg/minute were used. The results showed that no normal volunteers developed headache, although flushing and other systemic symptoms prevented maximum infusion of histamine in 4 out of 13 subjects. In the 10 muscle contraction patients, 5 had mild throbbing headache and 4 experienced a pressing type of head pain during the histamine infusion. One patient did not experience head pain despite maximum histamine infusion. In the 25 migraine patients, all but one developed severe pounding head pain during histamine infusions that were often less than 0.66 μ/kg. In 15 out of 18 migraine patients, simultaneous infusion of the H_1 blocker mepyramine diminished or blocked the headache. Cimetidine (H_2 blocker) also decreased headache significantly. Pretreatment with H_1 and H_2 blockers was not attempted.

The relevance of these artificial laboratory experiments to naturally occurring migraine headaches is not clear. For instance, Anthony et al. (1978) conducted a clinical trial using both chlorphenaramine (H_1 blocker) and cimetidine (H_2 blocker) in the chronic prophylaxis for prevention of migraine headaches. They found no benefit over the placebo treatment regimen.

In patients with allergic diseases such as asthma, neither spontaneous exacerbations of asthma with elevated plasma histamine, 1 to 5 ng/ml (Simon et al., 1977), nor antigen inhalation–induced asthma with plasma histamine of 1 to 6 ng/ml (Bhat et al., 1976) were associated with any headaches despite other systemic symptoms of histaminemia, including significant asthma and flushing.

In spontaneous rhinitis, asthma, or urticaria, it seems unlikely that enough histamine molecules spill into the vascular space, escape active degradation enzymes, and become available to vascular receptors in the cerebral arteries to effect significant vasodilatation in most normal people. However, in patients with vascular headaches and significant target organ susceptibility to any vasodilators, such mechanisms may play an occasional role in producing head pain.

There are several artificial systems with which a large intravascular discharge of mediators can occur. In systemic anaphylaxis, antigen is circulating in the vascular space and interacting with IgE fixed to circulating basophils. This leads to the release of mediators from storage cells that are within the vascular spaces. Under such circumstances, 100 ng/ml of histamine may be measured in the plasma and patients frequently develop generalized peripheral vasodilatation and hypotensive·shock. Selected patients also develop vascular headache. These have been recorded in the absence of treatment with epinephrine, another pharmacologic cause of head pain. Systemic anaphylaxis occurs in the following instances: after a bee sting, after injection of drugs (penicillin) or proteins (horse serum), with food anaphylaxis, and as a side effect of desensitization injections for the treatment of hay fever and asthma.

In 1950 Loveless studied the occurrence of headache, as well as other effects of overdosage of allergens, in 177 pollen-sensitive persons. Headache, when it occurred in these subjects after allergen injection overdosage, was generalized and not hemicranial. It occurred in both those with and those without histories of frequent headache attacks. Of the 177 subjects, there were 925 overdosage reactions. Twelve of the 177 subjects experienced headaches as part of such overdosage reactions on one or more occasions. Indeed, these 12 persons experienced 26 headaches during 121 overdosage reactions, or 21% of the time. For the entire group, the incidence of headache as an aspect of allergen overdosage effects was 2.8%, and then always as part of a widespread allergen overdosage syndrome, including urticaria, rhinitis, asthma, and/or hypotension. In the Loveless study, headache never occurred as an isolated phenomenon during antigen IgE reactions.

Since most allergy practices have an incidence of systemic reactions to injected allergy extracts on the order of 1 in 500 injections, this artificial or iatrogenic event cannot begin to account for spontaneous vascular or migraine headaches, even in the small portion of atopic population receiving immunotherapy.

Walker (1960) again emphasized the insignificance of the effects of food allergens in the migraine headache attack. She was not able to demonstrate a significant therapeutic effect from elimination diets but was convinced that for some patients the occurrence of allergic phenomena is so disturbing and exhausting it is sufficient to precipitate migrane attack by psychoneural pathways. Sleep deprivation is a major problem in chronic allergic diseases.

SUMMARY

- Allergic reactions can be categorized into four types, according to Gell and Coombe.
- Any type of rhinitis can be associated with paranasal head pain. The headache is dull, deep, aching, and nonpulsatile. It is associated with nasal congestion. One type of rhinitis is IgE mediated and a legitimate cause of head pain.
- The mucosa covering the approaches to the paranasal sinuses was found to be the most pain sensitive of the nasal and paranasal structures and cavities, whereas the mucosa lining of the sinuses was of relatively low sensitivity.
- Inflammation and engorgement of the turbinates, ostia, nasofrontal ducts, and superior nasal spaces are responsible for most of the pain emanating from the nasal and paranasal structures.
- Most of the pain arising from faradic, mechanical, and chemical stimulation of the mucosa of the nasal and paranasal cavities was referred pain, that is, it was felt at a site other than that stimulated. It was referred chiefly to those areas supplied by the first division of the fifth cranial nerve.
- The phenomena of migraine and certain allergic responses are similar in many respects. In both, attacks are paroxysmal, with associated edema and hyperemia, presumably mediated by protein breakdown products and terminated by vasoconstrictor drugs. However, there is only marginal evidence that histamine or ingested allergens are implicated in the etiology of migraine or that migraine results from ingested of such allergens as a part of an antigen–antibody reaction.
- The role of stress, induced by chronic, sleep-depriving allergic diseases and medications used to treeat allergy, seems to be a more important linkage between allergy and headaches.

REFERENCES

Anthony, M., G.D.A. Lord, and J.W. Lance (1978). Controlled trials of cimetidine in migraine and cluster headache. *Headache 18:* 261–264.

Austen, K.F. (1984). The heterogeneity of mast cell populations and products. *Hosp. Pract. 19:* 135–146.

Atkins, C.J., J.J. Kondon, and F.P. Quismorio (1972). The choroid plexis in systemic lupus erythematosus. *Ann. Intern. Med. 76:* 165–172.

Balyeat, R.M. and F.L. Brittain (1930). Allegic migraine—based on a study of 55 cases. *Am. J. Med. Sci. 180:* 212–220.

Bassoe, P. (1933). Migraine, *JAMA 101:* 599–605.

Beall, G.N. and P.P. Van Arsdel (1960). Histamine metabolism in human disease. *J. Clin. Invest. 39:* 676–684.

Benveniste, J. (1974). Platelet-activating factor, a new mediator of anaphylxis and immune complex desposition from rabbit and human basophils. *Nature 249:* 581–582.

Bergstrom, S.H., H. Duner, U.S. Von Euler et al. (1959). Observations on the effects of infusions of prostaglandin E in man. *Acta Physiol. Scand. 45:* 144–153.

Bhat, K.N., C.M. Arroyave, S.R. Marney et al. (1976). Plasma histamine changes during provoked bronchospasm in asthmatic patients. *J. Allergy Clin. Immunol. 58:* 647–656.

Broder, E., M.W. Higgins, K.P. Mathews, and J.B. Keller (1974). The epidemiology of Asthma and hay fever in a total community: Tecumseh, Michigan (32). *J. allergy Clin. Immunol. 54:* 100–112.

Cochrane, C.G. and J.H. Griffin (1982). The biochemistry and pathophysiology of the contact system of plasma *Adv. Immunol. 33:* 241–305.

Dalessio, D.J. (1972). Dietary migraine. *Am. Fam. Physician 6:* 60–65.

Dalsgaard-Nielsen, T. (1974). The nature of migraine. *Headache 14:* 13–18

David, J.R. and R.R. David (1972). Cellular hypersensitivity and immunity: Inhibition of macrophage migration and lymphocyte mediators. *Prog. Allergy 16:* 300–332.

DeGowin, E.L. (1932). Allergic migraine: Review of sixty cases. *J. Allergy 3:* 557–564.

Fink, J.N. (1972). Urticaria and physical allergy. In *Allergic Diseases* (R. Patterson, ed.), p. 341. J.B. Lippincott, Philadelphia.

Fowler, P.B.S. (1962). Epilepsy due to angioneurotic edema. *Proc. Roy. Soc. Med. 55:* 13–15.

Gell, P.G.H. and R.R.A. Coombs (1968). The allergic response and immunity. In *Clinical Aspects of Immunology,* pp. 423–456. F.A. Davis, Philadelphia.

Gonzales, S. (1953). Association of asthma and headache of allergic origin. *Med./ Ibera 2:* 747–753.

Goth, A. (1978). Antihistamines. In *Allergy: Principles and Practice* (E. Middleton, C. Reed, and E. Ellis, eds.), pp. 454–463. C.V. Mosby, St. Louis.

Grant, E.C.G. (1979). Food allergies and migraine. *The Lancet I;:* 966–968.

Hahn, L. (1930). Relation between migraine and allergy. *Med. Klin. 26:* 1219–1226.

Hamburger, J. (1935). Migraine: Role of food allergy. *Rev. Immunol. (Paris) I:* 102–109.

Hazelman, B.L., I.C.M. MacLennan, and R.G. Earler (1975). Lymphocyte proliferation to artery antigen as a positive diagnostic test in polymyalgia rheumatica. *Ann. Rheum. Dis. 34:* 122–128.

Healey, L.A. and K.R. Wilske (1977). Manifestations of giant cell arteritis. *Med. Clin. North Am. 61:* 261–270.

Hyslop, G.H. (1934). Migraine: Suggestions for its treatment. *Med. Clin. North Am 17:* 827–842.

Kaliner, M. and K.F. Austen (1973). A sequence of biochemical events in the antigen-induced release of chemical mediators from sensitized human lung tissue. *J. Exp. Med. 138:* 1094–1102.

Kaliner, M., J.H. Shelhamer, and E.A. Ottesen (1982). Effects of infused histamine: Correlation of plasma histamine levels and symptoms. *J. Allergy Clin. Immunol. 69:* 283–289.

Kallos, P., and L. Kallos-Deffner (1955). Allergy and migraine. *Intern. Arch. Allergy Appl. Immunol. 7:* 367–392.

Kaplan, A. (1978). Urticaria and angioedema. In *Allergy: Principles and Practice* (E. Middleton, C. Reed, and E. Ellis, eds.), pp. 1080–1099. C.V. Mosby, St. Louis.

Kaplan, A.P. and K.F. Austen (1975). Activation and control mechanisms of Hagemen factor—dependent pathways of coagulation, fibrinolysis and kinin generation and their contribution to the inflammatory process. *J. Allergy Clin. Immunol. 5b:* 491–503.

Kay, A.B. and K.F. Austen (1971). The IgE-mediated release of an eosinophil leukocyte chemotactic factor from human lung. *J. Immunol. 107:* 899–906.

Keeney, E.L (1946). Periodic vascular head pain. *Clinics 5:* 550–567.

Klein, R.G., R.J. Campbell, G.G. Hunder, and J.A. Carney (1976). Skip lesions in temporal arteritis. *Mayo Clin. Proc. 51:* 504–510.

Kohler, P.F. (1978). Immune complexes and allergic disease. In *Allergy: Principles and Practice* (E. Middleton, C. Reed, and E. Ellis, eds.), pp. 155–176. C.V. Mosby, St. Louis.

Krabbe, A.E. and J. Olesen (1980). Headache provoked by continuous intravenous infusion of histamine. *Pain 8:* 253–259.

Lance, J.W. and M. Anthony (1966). Some clinical aspects of migraine. *Arch. Neurol. 15:* 356–361.

Lever, W.F. (1961). Urticaria and angioedema. In *Histopathology of the Skin,* pp. 114–120. J.B. Lippincott, Philadelphia.

Lewis, G.P. (1961). Bradykinin. *Nature 192:* 596–600.

Loveless, M.H. (1950). Milk allergy. A survey of its incidence: Experiments with a masked ingestion test. *J. Allergy 21:* 489–501.

Mathews, K.P. (1974). A current view of urticaria. *Med. Clin. North Am. 58:* 185–196.

May, C.D. and S.A. Bock (1978). Adverse reactions to food due to hypersensitivity. In *Allergy: Principles and Practice* (Middleton, Reed, and Ellis, eds.), pp. 1159–1171. C.V. Mosby, St. Louis.

Medina, J.L. and S. Diamond (1976). Migraine and atopy. *Headache 15:* 271–274.

Millonig, A.G., H.E. Harris, and W.J. Gardner (1950). Effect of autonomic denervation on the nasal mucusa. *Arch. Otolaryngol. 52:* 359–365.

Monro, J., J. Brostoff, C. Carini, and K. Zilkha (1980). Food allergy in migraine. *The Lancet I:* 1–4.

Neusser, E. (1892). Klinisch-hamatologische Mittheilungen. *Wein. Klin. Wscher.5:* 41–45.

Newball, H.H., R.C. Talamo, and L.M. Lichtenstein (1975). Release of leukocyte kallikrein mediated by IgE. *Nature 254:* 635–637.

Nutman, D.D. N. Kurata, and E.M. Tan (1975). Profiles of antinuclear antibodies in systemic rheumatic diseases. *Ann. Intern. Med. 83:* 464–469.

Ogden, H.D. (1951). The treatment of allergic headache. *Ann. allergy 9:* 611–619.

O'Neil, W.N. Jr., S.P. Hammar, and H.A. Bloomer (1976). Giant cell arteritis with visceral angiitis. *Arch. Intern. Med. 136:* 1157–1160.

Pagniez, P., P. Vallery-Radot and A. Nast (1919). Therapeutique preventive de certaines migraines. *Presse Med. 27:* 172–176.

Pickering, G.W. (1933). Histamine headache. *Clin. Sci. I:* 77–101.

Plaut, M. and L.M. Lichtenstein (1983). Cellular and chemical basis of the allergic inflammatory response. In *Allergy: Principles and Practice* (Middleton, Reed, and Ellis, eds.), pp. 119–146. C.V. Mosby, St. Louis.

Ralston, H.J. and W.J. Kerr (1945). Vascular responses of the nasal mucosa to thermal stimuli with some observations on skin temperature. *Am. J. Physiol. 144:* 305–312.

Rinkel, H.J. (1933). Considerations of allergy as factor in familial recurrent headache. *J. Allergy 4:* 303–312.

Rowe, A.H. (1932). Allergic migraine. *JAMA 99:* 912–917.

Ruddy, S., I.Gigli, and K.F. Austen (1972). The complement system in man. *N. Engl. J. Med. 287:* 489–495.

Ryan, R.E. Sr., and R.E. Ryan, Jr. (1979). Headache of nasal origin. *Headache (April):* 173–177.

Schwartz, M. (1952). Is migraine an allergic disease? *Acta Allerg. 5 (Suppl. II):* 426–432.

Simon, R.A., D.D. Stevenson, D.M. Arroyave, and E.M. Tan (1977). The relationship of plasma histamine to the activity of bronchial asthma. *J. Allergy Clin. Immunol. 60:* 312–316.

Smith, J.M. (1978). Epidemiology and natural history of asthma, allergic rhinitis and atopic dermatitis (eczema). In *Allergy: Principles and Practice* (Middleton, Reed, and Ellis, eds.), p. 637. C.V. Mosby, St. Louis.

Solomon, W.R. (1967). Hay fever, allergic rhinitis and asthma. In *A Manual of Clinical Allergy* (J.M. Sheldon, ed.), pp. 78–88. W.B. Saunders, Philadelphia.

Speer, F. (1975). The many facets of migraine. *Anne. Allergy 34:* 273–285.

Stanson, A.W., R.G. Klein, and G.G. Hunder (1976). Extracranial angiographic findings in giant cell arteritis. *Am. J. Roentgen. 137:* 957–963.

Tennenbaum, J.I. (1972). Allergic rhinitis. In *Allergic Diseases* (R. Patterson, ed.), p. 172. J.B. Lippincott, Philadelphia.

Trousseau, A. (1873). Clinique medical de L'Hotel-Dieu de Paris. 4th ed., Vol. 2, p. 460. Baillieu, Paris.

Unger, L. and J.L. Cristol (1970). Allergic migraine. *Ann. Allergy 28:* 106–112.

Unger, L. and M.C. Harris (1974). Stepping-stones in allergy. *Ann. Allergy 33:* 353–363.

Unger, A.H., and L. Unger (1952). Migraine is an allergic disease. *J. Allergy 23:* 429–436.

Vahlquist, B. (1955). Migraine in children. *Int. Arch. Allergy 7:* 348–360.

Vane, J.R. (1976). The mode of action of aspirin and similar compounds. *J. Allergy Clin. Immunol. 58:* 691–712.

Van Leeuwen, W. and Z. Zeydner (1922). Occurrence of toxic substance in blood in cases of broncial asthma, urticaria, epilepsy and migraine. *Br. J. Exp. Pathol. 3:* 282–287.

Vaughan, W.T. (1934). Analysis of allergic factor in recurrent paroxysmal headache. *Trans. Assoc. Am. Physicians 49:* 348–358.

von Pirquet, C. (1906). Allergie. *Munchen. Med. Wsch. 53:* 1457–1465.

Waaler, E., O. Tonder, and E.J. Milde (1976). Immunological and histological studies of temporal arteries from patients with temporal arteritis and/or polymyalgia rheumatica. *Acta Pathol. Microbiol. Scan. 84:* 55–63.

Walker, V.B. (1960). *Report to the Ciba Foundation Conference on Migraine*. London, England.

Wasserman, S.I. (1983). Mediators of immediate hypersensitivity. *J. Allergy Clin. Immunol. 72:* 101–115.

Wasserman, S.I., N.A. Soter, D.M. Center, and K.F. Austen (1977). Cold urticaria: Recognition and characteristics of a neutrophil chemotactic factor which appears in serum during experimental and cold challenge. *J. Clin. Invest. 60:* 189–196.

Wolf, A.A. and L. Unger (1944). Migraine due to milk; Feeding tests. *Ann. Intern. Med. 20:* 831–843.

Wolff, H.G. (1955). Headache mechanisms. *Int. Arch. Allergy 7:* 210–225.

Ziegler, D.K., R. Hassanein, and K. Hassanein (1972). Headache syndromes suggested by factor analysis of symptom variables in a headache prone population. *J. Chron. Dis. 25:* 353–362.

14

The Teeth and Jaws as Sources of Headache and Facial Pain

FRANCIS V. HOWELL

Both odontalgia and the broad area of motion-related disturbances (referred to as TMJ syndrome) are of considerable interest to the physician and the dentist. The fifth cranial nerve or trigeminal nerve has wide distribution in the anterior portion of the head, and disturbances over this distribution may produce variable responses that are often difficult to evaluate. All too often, trigeminal neuralgia will mimic toothache, and many teeth have been removed or pulps extirpated for root canal therapy by the uninitiated clinician. On the other hand, odontalgia can, in certain instances, produce many of the symptoms of trigeminal neuralgia. Conversely, before anticonvulsant or antidepressant drugs are prescribed and before surgical disruption of a peripheral nerve is considered, the possibility of local and reversible sources of nerve excitation must be ruled out.

Ruling out dental disease and temporomandibular joint dysfunction is mandatory in evaluating headache and other facial pain, particularly when it is unilateral. Bilateral pain is frequently associated with emotional disturbances.

Pain due to inflammatory and retrograde pulpal disease and to independent or concomitant periodontal disease is relatively common. It is not difficult to eliminate, particularly if the specific lesion can be demonstrated clinically or radiologically. However, in some typical manifestations of pulpal disease and the TMJ syndrome direct etiology is not evident.

The dental profession is well aware of the important role that apprehension of impending dental procedures constitutes as a real barrier to adequate diagnosis and the ways pain may be altered by affecting the threshold of response when a patient is to undergo nerve testing, digital palpation, percussion, or some other painful procedure. In the TMJ syndrome, emotional factors are often of extreme importance and are an integral part of the painful condition because of nervous habits or bruxism, for example.

Anatomic and Physiologic Considerations

Impulses from the teeth and temporomandibular joint area are carried by branches of the second and third divisions of the fifth cranial nerve. Nerves enter the pulp through the apex and accompany the larger vessels to form an almost complete mantle around the arteries (Berkelbach, 1935–36). These nerve fibers form a complicated network between the odontoblasts and extend partially into the calcified portion of the dentinal tubule, permitting the surface of dentin, wherever exposed, to transmit pain as in caries or dentin fractures (Lewinsky & Stewart, 1935–36). Brashear (1936) found that more than half of the unmyelinated and small myelinated nerve fibers were less than 6 μ, with the remainder varying in size up to 10 μ. Thermal, mechanical, and chemical stimulation of dentin in a normal tooth results only in pain with the patient unable to differentiate its exact cause. Therefore, a tooth that is "alive" can be stimulated by numerous irritants, and the resultant pain can be described by the patient only as "pain." On the other hand, sensations such as touch and pressure appear to be transmitted primarily to the nerve endings in the periodontal ligament and the alveolar bone. These senations are often easily described by the patient.

A classic study by Robertson et al. (1947) demonstrated the distribution and pathophysiology of headache and other pain in the face and head resulting from afferent impulses originating in the teeth. Comparisons were made between experimental stimulation of the teeth and clinical situations in which morbid processes were present. In the study, two different electrical methods were employed: one, for inducing toothache well above the pain threshold, and the other, for inducing pain only at the threshold. For highintensity toothache, a 60-cycle, 110-V stimulator was used with a step-down transformer giving a voltage from 0 to 25 V. A bipolar electrode was insulated to the tips. The handle of the electrode was held by the subject and the tips were place securely against the tooth, utilizing small traumatic chips in the enamel and areas in which pit cavities were present. With the subject sitting in a chair, a rheostat was gradually advanced from zero to a voltage sufficient to induce toothache of 4 to 8 plus intensity. Pain was estimated on an arbitrary basis of 1 to 10, with 10 plus being extremely high intensity or the point at which patient experienced the "worst" pain. Toothache was held at the 4 to 8 intensity for a period of 10 minutes. In the lower ranges of intensity, initial current inducing toothaches had to be increased to continue to induce pain. Thus, the volatage was gradually increased and current was momentarily interrupted every 5 to 10 seconds to keep the toothache in the 4 to 8 plus range.

The second method used to induce pain at its threshold employed a "vitalometer," as described by Ziskin and Wald (1938). This is a method similar to the pulp testing procedures performed clinically by most dentists. A single electrode is applied to the tooth and the circuit is complete through a coupling held in the hand of the subject. The pain threshold in this phase of the experiment was expressed as the smallest voltage that would elicit a painful sensation.

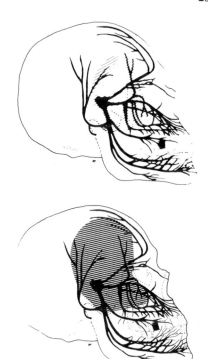

Figure 14-1A. The distribution of sensations of fullness, numbness, and stiffness 5 minutes after noxious stimulation of the upper right second bicuspid *(4)*.

Figure 14-1B. The distribution of headache 20 minutes after noxious stimulation of the upper right second bicuspid *(4)*.

DESCRIPTION OF HEADACHE RESULTING FROM NOXIOUS STIMULATION OF THE TEETH

In a study conducted at the New York Hospital, headache that occurred after experimental induction of toothache in the manner described above was divided into *Series 1, Noxious Stimulation of Teeth in the Upper Jaw,* and *Series 2, Noxious Stimulation of Teeth in the Lower Jaw.* In Series 1, the stimulation to a premolar or first molar tooth in the maxilla, pain of 4 to 8 plus intensity and was manifested by pain in the tooth. However, following a break in the stimulating current, a jab of more intense pain was experienced as a "narrow column of pain which spread vertically into the eye, the orbital ridge, and the temple." With extremely intense toothache (10+), pain spread into adjacent teeth and along the maxilla. During the period of toothache, intense apprehension, profuse salivation, lacrimation, and flushing of the face on the side of stimulation were noted with generalized sweating. On termination of stimulation, pain decreased quickly to 1 plus intensity with only a sensation of pressure between the teeth. After toothache completely diminished, there was a continuing sensation of tightness, slight numbness, and fullness over the cheek, and a tight, stiff sensation in the skin and deep tissues in the temporal region, the forehead, and scalp on the same side. Some stiffness in the temporomandibular joint and fullness in the ear was described. Within 5 to 10 minutes after all pain in the tooth was terminated, a steady aching and diffuse pain of 1 plus intensity was experienced in the temporal region, along the zygomatic ridge, and for a short distance over the eye. Graphic demonstration of the pattern of head pain was expressed (Fig. 14–1) 5 minutes and

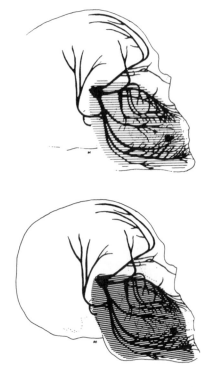

Figure 14-2A. The distribution of fullness, numbness, and stiffness 5 minutes after noxious stimulation of the lower right second bicuspid *(29).*

Figure 14-2B. The distribution of headache 20 minutes after noxious stimulation of the lower right second bicuspid *(29).*

20 minutes after stimulation. Most headache persisted from 1 to 8 hours and in one instance for up to 24 hours with gradually diminishing intensity. Although the sensation of tightness, fullness, and numbness was rather short lived, during the period of diminishing intensity there was photophobia and injection of the conjunctiva, with tenderness to the temporal muscle and overlying tissues on palpation. Sensation to a pinprick was sharper.

In Series 2, a lower premolar or first molar tooth was stimulated in the same manner as in Series 1, maintaining the 4 to 8 plus toothache for a period of 10 minutes. During the stimulation, there was intense aching pain in the tooth with a less intense pain throughout the lower jaw extending into the anterior wall of the ear canal. At the end of the stimulation, the high-intensity pain was quickly terminated, but a persistent sensation of pressure in the tooth was noted, often accompanied by a dull, diffuse, aching pain of low intensity throughout the lower jaw on the same side. Subsequently, a sensation of fullness and heaviness developed, and a 2 to 3 plus intensity of pain that extended throughout the upper and lower jaws into the zygoma and temporal area and extending over the top of the ear. There was also fullness and aching in the ear. This "lower-half" headache was increased in intensity by biting and bending over. The pattern is well demonstrated in Fig. 14-2. Many of the same effects were noted as in Series 1—apprehension, lacrimation, salivation, flushing of the face, photophobia, and generalized sweating as well as stiffness of the masseter muscle. The quality of pain in response to aspirin was the same in Series 1 and in Series 2. In each series, the effects of noxious stimulation were completely reversible and no sequelae were noted. Results of this classic and extensive study are well documented by the clinical pattern of odontology resulting from retrograde and inflammatory odontalgia. In the same experiment, the effect of local anesthetic to the source of noxious stimulation adjacent to the tooth was applied in two phases. In the first, procaine injections, there was direct injection into the area of headache, and pain persisted in scattered fashion with greatest area of pain diminished. However, there was complete absence of pain following the local anesthetic injection by an infiltrative procedure (tuberosity injection). Some pain returned following the cessation of anesthesia to the area; in some cases, the area remained free when normal sensation returned to the tooth.

In conclusion, it is obvious that the elimination of the headache after blocking the path of afferent impulses from the tooth and adjacent tissues allows one to assume that the experience was caused by afferent impulses arising from the stimulted tooth. These afferent impulses thus gave rise to excitatory processes in the brain stem, which spread to exert effects on many trigeminal structures.

Practical Clinical Considerations

Although it can be demonstrated by the described experiments of toothache-induced headache and by clinical manifestation of odontalgia that the headache follows certain prescribed patterns, there is an obvious and practical clinical consideration. Only under unusual circumstances can this type of headache be seen without accompanying odontalgia from a disease pulp or an inflamed periodontal condition. A relatively easy elimination of this pain by nerve blockage or infiltrative local anesthesia produces a fairly clear-cut *cause and effect* relationship. Unfortunately, the observation made experimentally that the headache can return when the local anesthetic effect dissipates often leads, in a clinical situation, to discomfort for the patient. The present practice of using short-acting, local anesthetics for all dental operative procedures should possibly be modified by the clinician. Certainly, the patient who is undergoing routine filling procedures on the teeth does not want local anesthetic effects for a long period of time. However, when the clinician is aware that nerve tissue has been subjected to considerable agitation, the use of long-acting, local anesthetics such as bupivacaine hydrochloride should be considered.

CRACKED TOOTH SYNDROME

Odontalgia from the usual degenerative and inflammatory etiologies produces fairly predictable patterns of pain, which become obvious when local anesthesia is used and the pain dissipates. Occasionally, the localization of the tooth involved in the odontalgia may be difficult because in the early degenerative stages the tooth is often not sensitive to percussion or other evidence of pressure building up within. All dentists are aware that analgesics may be required for the patient until the exact culprit can be determined in a few hours or even a few days.

Another type of pain termed the cracked-tooth syndrome (incomplete tooth frac-

Table 14-1 Locations of cracked teeth

Tooth	No.	Percentage
Mandibular		
Second molars	17	34
First molars	9	18
Third molars	1	2
Bicuspids	1	2
Maxillary		
First molars	12	24
Second molars	2	4
First bicuspids	6	12
Second bicuspids	2	4
Totals	50	100

ture, greenstick fracture, etc.) is of considerable clinical significance to the physician as well as to the dentist in evaluating pain because the pain does not follow the "usual" patterns of directly induced and referred pain. Frequently, the patient is seen by the dentist who can find no organic evidence of dental disease and then seeks referral from a physician, often from a neurologist. At Scripps Clinic's Department of Oral Medicine, almost half of the patients who are seen with this syndrome are referred by physicians.

The condition has been recognized in the dental literature for a number of years, and Gibbs, in 1954, termed the condition cuspal fracture odontalgia. Sutton, in 1962, described the condition as greenstick fracture, and Cameron, in 1964, coined the term *cracked tooth syndrome,* which appears to predominate in the dental literature. The term *incomplete tooth fracture,* suggested by Maxwell and Braly in 1977, indicated that the syndrome itself resulted because the tooth did not fracture completely but only dentinal tubules were involved. The most comprehensive study to date, Cameron (1964) presented a series of significant cases (Table 14-1). This makes it obvious that more than half of all cracked teeth are mandibular molars, with the second molar being the most commonly involved. There has been considerable speculation as to the preponderance of involvement of the lower molar teeth—possibly the motion of the mandible and the position of the lingual cusps of the maxillary molars produce a cleavage action. Unlike ordinary odontalgia due to retrograde pulpal disease, most of the teeth involved in this syndrome have few, if any, restorations. The cusps are usually normal in appearance. Examination of prehistoric skulls does not reveal significant incidence of cracked teeth, and it has been speculated that the popularity of hot liquids, such as coffee and soup and the ready availability of cold and frozen foods, such as ice cream, combine to produce extensive expansion and contraction of the enamel and dentin, thus making the coronal structure susceptible to fracture. In the Department of Oral Medicine at Scripps Clinic, it has been observed that many of these patients are ice chewers, and it is felt that the melting of the ice cube into the fossae between the cusps can produce considerable lateral pressure against the cusps as the ice crystal fractures under pressure. Ice chewing appears to be a definite hazard to all patients who have small fillings within the central grooves between the cusps or to those who have no restorations whatever.

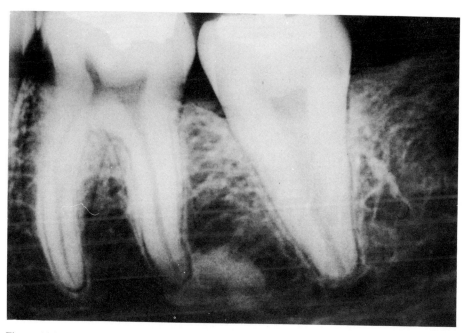

Figure 14-3. Second molar (single rooted tooth) exhibits thickening of periodontal ligament on sides near apex. This is an indication of a split tooth.

Again, ready availability appears to be a factor in ice chewing, since beverages, until recently, seldom contained ice.

In Figure 14-3 (a dental radiogram from a patient who is an ice chewer), the second molar tooth (to the right) contains an anterio-posterior (mesiodistal) crack beneath the small occlusal restoration. The pulp tests were "normal." In this particular case, the patient presented with pain to cold and pressure, particularly compression of tough foods. Pain was present only at certain times, and the patient could be free of pain for weeks at a time. As the crack was subjected to more occlusal pressure, particularly from ice chewing, the pain became more intense until finally the crack was discovered and a crown was placed on the tooth. This completely eliminated the symptoms, and, after 5 years, the tooth is completely normal.

The symptomatology of a cracked tooth is summarized in Table 14-2, taken from Cameron (1964). Typically, a patient will complain of pain radiating to the side of the head after biting on compressible food, such as nuts, meat, or bread crusts. The pain is often sudden, and after the initial impulse cannot be localized to a specific tooth by the patient. Following such an incident, there is extreme sensitivity to cold. This sensation will continue to be an important diagnostic consideration because the electric pulp tester often does not differentiate between the normal tooth and the cracked tooth. Cold applied to a tooth can be a distinguishing feature.

As the cracked tooth syndrome proceeds, if not discovered, the traumatization to the dental tubules will allow direct penetration of the dental pulp and actual pulpal death with the usual sequelae. It is extremely important for the dentist as well as the physician to realize that when the condition is first discovered coronal protection is

Table 14-2 Symptoms
of cracked teeth

Pain	No. of patients
Pressure	27
Cold	16
Heat	14
Ache	9
Cellulitis	5
Sweet	1
None reported	6

indicated to preserve the vitality of the pulp tissue. Without preserving the pulp, no repair can take place. Many dentists, on finding such a tooth, resort to root canal therapy, which essentially condemns the tooth to eventual extraction. This is because oral fluid will continue to seep into the cracked areas, making the endodontic treatment unsuccessful.

TEMPOROMANDIBULAR JOINT SYNDROME (MYOFASCIAL PAIN DYSFUNCTION SYNDROME)

Costen's concept (1934) of occlusal disharmony with resultant damage to the temporomandibular joint was attributed to a wide variety of signs and symptoms; this has now been totally discarded and replaced by concepts probably first delineated by Schwartz in 1955. The term *temporomandibular joint pain dysfunction syndrome*, along with a plausible explanation of pain patterns, correlates well with muscular and articular disturbances. The more popular term is myofascial pain dysfunction syndrome (MPD), used by Laskin (1969). Certainly, the clinical features ascribed to this syndrome have fairly definite signs and symptoms as delineated from organic diseases of the temporomandibular joint itself.

Bell (1982), responding to the rather confusing numbers of TMJ disturbances and disorders, developed a useful classification (Table 14-3). It is interesting to note that not all the conditions have pain that involves large areas of the distribution of the fifth nerve; only in the area of acute muscle disorders is the pain not readily apparent

Table 14-3 Classification of
temporomandibular disorders

Class	Disorder
A	Acute muscle disorders
B	Disk—interference disorders of the joint
C	Inflammatory disorders of the joint
D	Chronic mandibular hypomobilities
E	Growth disorders of the joint

as to etiology. In addition, the disorder has a definite symptom complex. A review of all temporomandibular joint disorders is therefore not necessary. Only the masticatory muscle spasm disorder (MPD) need be discussed here because of its complexity and wide spectrum of symptoms. Again, the rather narrow criteria make this disorder unique. MPD is unique because it is frequently associated with the type of pain seen in headache or confused with disturbances of the fifth nerve. Pain in this syndrome is due to spasm of the masticatory muscles and not to disease of the joint itself. This is often precipitated by an overextension of the jaw, which stretches the muscle and then produces spasm upon contraction. Although muscle overextension can be produced by encroachment by prosthetic appliances or dental restorations or may result from space between the mandible and the maxilla resulting from overclosure, these features are not as important as oral habits coupled with psychophysiological characteristics of the patients. The median age of patients with this syndrome is 32, and nearly 85% are female in most studies. Patients often exhibit features of emotional stress.

There are varying clinical features, but four signs and symptoms must be present for the diagnosis: (1) muscle tenderness, (2) clicking or popping noise in the joint, (3) limitation of jaw motion, (4) pain. Two negative findings must be present to differentiate this syndrome from organic disease of the joint: (1) no clinical, radiographic, nor laboratory evidence of joint disease; (2) lack of tenderness in the joint itself on palpation through the external auditory meatus, thus demonstrating the muscular nature of the condition.

Specific muscles are involved. In Greene et al.'s study (1969), the following were involved:

Lateral pterygoid	84%
Masseter	70%
Temporalis	49%
Medial pterygoid	35%
Cervical, scalp, and facial	43%

Tenderness in these muscles usually produces a high percentage of limitation of movement. Vertigo and subluxation occur infrequently.

Sudden onset is often described by patients, but this may be due to threshold effects. Intensification of pain often occurs as a distinctive feature because of the contralateral nature of the masticatory apparatus. For this reason, a patient who has pain on the right side of the face favors that side by chewing on the left, thereby increasing the luxation of the apparatus on that side and, naturally, increasing the muscle spasm. Because of the distribution of the fifth nerve, patients often describe the resulting pain as toothache, earache, sore neck, headache, sinus, and neuralgia. The clinician, utilizing the pressure points of muscle attachment, should have little difficulty in diagnosing the condition.

Treatment is controversial, as many dental clinicians feel that the cause of the muscle tenderness is malocclusion, lack of proper vertical dimension of the jaws, or some other factor. Most clinicians today feel that, in the absence of organic disease of the joint itself, conditions that fit this category should be treated conservatively and the patient is instructed concerning contralateral aspects of muscle function and the pattern of pain in these muscles. Pain can often be brought under control rapidly.

Establishing a hinge relationship, banning forward movement of the jaw, will often eliminate muscle spasm, pointing out that favoring the more painful side can intensify the problem by leading to more extensive muscle spasm and aggravating already overextended muscles helps the patient understand the difficulty. The judicious use of muscle relaxants for patients who have severe spasm and anxieties has proven effective as well. Utilization of the physical therapist to provide instruction on balanced muscular motion has proved to be helpful. Biofeedback techniques have also been of value. Of considerable importance to the physician is the recognition that these patients are often under stress or have emotional disturbances that must be given appropriate therapeutic consideration.

SUMMARY

- With noxious stimulation of healthy and diseased teeth, it is possible to analyze a variety of face and head pains that stem from the teeth.
- Use of locally acting anesthetics to interfere with toothache-induced headache allows one to assume that the painful experience was caused by afferent impulses arising from the stimulated tooth.
- The cracked-tooth syndrome (incomplete tooth fracture) may produce pain radiating to the head following mastication. Appropriate therapy will resolve the matter.
- The temporomandibular joint syndrome represents a dysfunction of the entire masticatory apparatus. It is associated with muscle tenderness, clicking or popping noises in the joint, limitation of joint movement, and pain. Much of the pain is related to muscle spasm. Treatment should invariably be conservative.

REFERENCES

Bell, W.E. (1982). *Clinical management of temporomandibular disorders.* Year Book Medical Publishers, Chicago, London.

Berkelbach van der Sprenkle, S. (1935–36). Microscopical investigation of the tooth and its surroundings. *J. Anat.70:* 233.

Brashear, A.D. (1936). Innervation of the teeth. *J. Am. Dent. Assoc.23:* 662.

Cameron, C.E. (1964). Cracked tooth syndrome. *J. Am. Dent. Assoc.68:* 405.

Costen, J.B. (1934). A syndrome of ear and sinus symptoms dependent upon disturbed function of the temporomandibular joint. *Ann. Otol. Rhinol. Laryngol. 43:*1.

Gibbs, J.W. (1954). Cuspal fracture odontalgia. *Dental Digest 60:* 158.

Greene, C.S., M.D. Lerman, H.D. Sutcher, and D.M. Laskin (1969). The TMJ pain-dysfunction syndrome: Heterogeneity of the patient population. *J. Am. Dent. Assoc 79:* 1168.

Laskin, D.M. (1969). Etiology of the pain-dysfunction syndrome. *J. Am. Dent. Assoc. 79:* 147.

Lewinsky, W., and D. Stewart (1935–36). The innervation of the dentine. *J. Anat. 70:*349.

Maxwell, E.H. and B.V. Braly (1977). Incomplete tooth fracture. *J. Calif. Dental Assoc., October:*pp. 51–55.

Robertson, H.S., H. Goodell, and H.G. Wolff (1947). Studies on headache: The teeth as a source of headache and other pain. *Arch. Neurol. Psychiat. 57:*277.

Schwartz, L. (1955). Pain associated with the temporomandibular joint. *J. Am. Dent. Assoc. 51:*394.

Silvestri, A.R. (1976). The undiagnosed split-root syndrome. *J. Am. Dent. Assoc. 92:*930.

Sutton, P.R.N. (1962). Greenstick fracture of the tooth crown. *Br. Dent. J. 112:*362.

Ziskin, D.E. and A. Wald (1938). Observations on electrical pulp testing. *J. Dent. Res. 17:*79.

15

The Major Neuralgias, Postinfectious Neuritis, And Atypical Facial Pain

DONALD J. DALESSIO

Perhaps no subject in medicine is as confusing to patient and physician alike as that of recurrent chronic facial pain. Often unilateral, frequently unresponsive to therapy, long-lasting, and discomforting, some chronic facial pains have resisted even simple nosologic classification. Some patients with severe protracted facial pain will develop complications related to attempts at pain relief as significant as the original problem. Drug addiction or dependence, serious (even suicidal) depression, disability, and invalidism are among the most frequently encountered complications of long-term intense facial pain. Nonetheless, a physician who understands how to deal with patients with chronic facial pain, and who understands the mechanisms behind their pain-centered behavior, may be able to help make a significant improvement in the lives of many of these patients by using a judicious combination of drug therapy, surgery, and other modalities.

CLINICAL FEATURES OF TRIGEMINAL NEURALGIA PAIN

Trigeminal neuralgia almost always begins after the age of 30 years, unless the patient has concomitant multiple sclerosis. The pain is of high intensity and occurs particularly in association with trigger zones (i.e., areas of increased sensitivity on the face), especially about the nares and mouth, which set off the attack when they are stimulated—often by trivial sensations (Figure 15-1). Thus, the behavioral characteristics of patients with trigeminal neuralgia are avoidance of touching the face, or washing, shaving, biting, or chewing, or any other maneuvers that stimulate the trigger zones and produce the pain. This avoidance technique is an invaluable clue to the diagnosis. With almost every other facial pain syndrome, patients will be found massaging the painful area, abrading it, or applying heat or cold, but in trige-

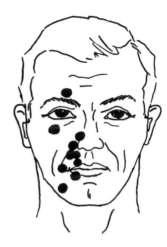

Figure 15-1.   Trigger zones in tic douloureux.

minal neuralgia exactly the opposite occurs; the patient goes to great lengths to avoid any stimulation of the face or mouth whatsoever.

The pain paroxysm is usually a high-intensity jab lasting less than 20 to 30 seconds, followed at times by a period of relief lasting a few seconds to a minute, again followed by another jab of pain. Repeated episodes of pain may occur, but the pain is not long-lived as is usual in other chronic facial pains.

Medical Treatment

The medical treatment of trigeminal and other cranial neuralgias is based on the capacity of the drugs employed to interrupt the temporal summation of afferent impulses that set off the painful attack. If the trigger zones are touched, and repeatedly, a curve can be developed demonstrating a spatial and temporal relationship of repetitive stimuli to pain (Figure 15-2). If carbamazepine is then given for 24 hours, the shape of this curve will be altered, and as the responsiveness of the trigger zones becomes less evident, the condition is gradually relieved.

Most authorities agree that medical treatment is indicated first, if for no other reason than that its use constitutes a therapeutic challenge to the diagnosis. If, for example, a patient presumed to have trigeminal neuralgia does not rapidly respond to carbamazepine, in 24 to 48 hours, the diagnosis is seriously in doubt. The diagnosis is, after all, made on the basis of history alone, and patients are generally not good observers of their own pains or sensations.

If the patient does respond to carbamazepine, then clearly this is the treatment of choice. Those clinicians who have followed patients with trigeminal neuralgia for more than a decade realize that the disease is often remitting, and it may be possible, using drugs, to nudge the patient into another remission, following which, medication can sometimes be stopped. If this is not the case, and the response to carbamazepine is only partial, other drugs may also be useful in treating this condition, including phenytoin, baclofen, and chlorphenesin. Some neurosurgeons suggest that unpleasant side effects occur frequently with carbamazepine and that up to 20 to 30%

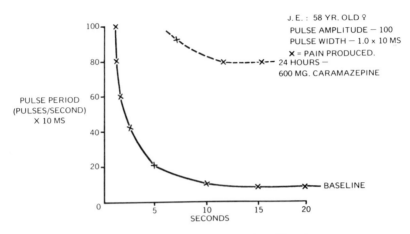

Figure 15-2. Temporal summation of impulses.

of patients taking this drug need to stop it; this is surprising, because the drug seems to be better tolerated when used in epilepsy.

Nonetheless, one cannot deny that carbamazepine may produce undesirable sedation or idiosyncratic reactions, including blood dyscrasias (rarely). Thus, caution needs to be employed when using it.

Tomson and Bertilsson (1984) have assessed the therapeutic effect of carbamazepine-10,11-epoxide in trigeminal neuralgia, and find it comparable to the parent compound. A major metabolic pathway for carbamazepine is the formation of the aforementioned epoxide, which is thereafter further metabolized to 10,11-dehydroxy-10,11-dihydro-carbamazepine before it is excreted in the urine (Faigle & Feldmann, 1982). The authors suggest that the epoxide metabolite has a higher pain-relieving potency than the parent compound, but clinically, the effect is the same. It should be noted that the number of patients treated in this study (six) was very small, they were not treated identically, and the observation periods were short. The epoxide compound is an experimental drug and is not generally available.

Specifics of Medical Treatment

To inhibit or reduce synaptic transmission and relieve pain, one naturally turns to the anticonvulsants. These drugs reduce the sensitivity of the trigger zones and relieve the pain within 4 to 24 hours, often dramatically. Generally, treatment is begun with carbamazepine, 100 to 200 mg two or three times daily. If this dosage is well tolerated and if the pain is rapidly relieved, it may be continued for several weeks or months, depending on the course of the disease. One should attempt to titrate the medication to the severity of the patient's pain. To keep the patient pain-free, it may be necessary to continue the carbamazepine at a maintenance level such as 200 mg per day.

If symptoms persist with the patient on carbamazepine, phenytoin may be added to the regimen, up to 400 mg per day, and if there is no response to both drugs, we

Table 15-1 Drugs commonly used in medical therapy of trigeminal neuralgia

Drug	Route of administration	Dosage (mg/day)	Side effects/precautions
Carbamazepine	Oral	200–600	Drowsiness, ataxia, confusion. Monitor for blood disorders weekly at first, then monthly
Phenytoin	Oral	200–400	CNS, haemopoietic, oral
Chlorphenesin	Oral	800–2400	Drowsiness
Baclofen	Oral	30–80	Drowsiness, weakness, nausea, vomiting

commonly employ a third agent, usually chlorphenesin, 400 mg three to four times daily (Table 15-1).

By the time the three-drug treatment level is reached, one should be considering referring the patient for appropriate surgery. Generally, parenteral doses are not used.

Other drugs, including sodium valproate, chlorazepate and baclofen, have also been employed. Of these, baclofen is the best studied (see below).

Monitoring Serum Levels

Serum levels of anticonvulsants are a useful means of monitoring treatment. For carbamazepine, at least initially, levels of 6 to 12 μg/ml are usually required to relieve the pain. For phenytoin, therapeutic levels are 10 to 20 μg/ml.

Use of Baclofen

Fromm et al. (1984) have reported on the use of baclofen in refractory trigeminal neuralgia. These authors treated 14 patients who were refractory to or unable to take carbamazepine, starting with 10 mg tid, and they achieved pain relief in 10 patients. At two subsequent visits a week apart, baclofen was increased to 60 to 80 mg per day, or a mean dose of 1.03 mg/kg. Concomitant drugs were carbamazepine in five patients, phenytoin in one, and carbamazepine and phenytoin in two. Although side effects occurred (especially drowsiness), some patients did achieve satisfactory control.

A combination of carbamazepine and baclofen seems a sensible alternative in refractory cases unresponsive to the other combinations mentioned above.

Mechanisms of Action of Drugs Used in Medical Treatment

The pharmacologic effects of the four most commonly employed drugs in the medical treatment of trigeminal neuralgia are similar (see Table 15-2).

Table 15-2 Pharmacologic activity of baclofen, chlorphenesin, phenytoin, and carbamazepine

Effect	Baclofen	Chlorphenesin	Phenytoin	Carbamazepine
Anticonvulsant activity	+	+	+ + +	+ +
Muscle relaxant effect	+ + +	+ + +	+	+ +
Sedative effect	+ +	+ +	+	+ +
Anaesthetic activity	0	0	0	0
Analgesic effect	0	±	0	±

Carbamazepine and Phenytoin

Phenytoin reduces post-tetanic potentiation of synaptic transmission within the spinal cord as well as the stellate ganglion of animals. Post-tetanic potentiation can be considered as an enhancement of synaptic transmission following rapid, repetitive, presynaptic stimulation. Carbamazepine also depresses post-tetanic potentiation at the spinal cord level in animals, and significantly inhibits polysynaptic reflex activity in the spinal cord (Fromm, 1969). Both drugs depress synaptic transmission in the spinal trigeminal nucleus. Laboratory studies have shown that these anticonvulsants depress synaptic transmission in the trigeminal system, as evidenced by decreasing amplitude and increasing latency of evoked potentials (Fromm & Landgren, 1963).

Chlorphenesin

Chlorphenesin depresses transmission to a number of spinal and supraspinal polysynaptic pathways. It also depresses polysynaptic potentials in the spinal cords of animals and inhibits convulsions induced by strychnine (Matthews et al., 1963). Our laboratory studies have demonstrated depression of synaptic transmissions by chlorphenesin in the trigeminal system of the cat.

Baclofen

Baclofen depresses exitatory synaptic transmission in the spinal trigeminal nucleus and resembles the actions of the other drugs in this respect. It increases the latency of response and decreases the number of spikes in trigeminal nucleus neurons elicited by maxillary nerve stimulation (Fromm et al., 1984).

Note that all four drugs have anticonvulsant, muscle-relaxant, and sedative properties, which could be predicted from the preceding evidence. None is anesthetic or analgesic. Despite this paradox, pain relief is achieved by interrupting the neurophysiologic state that produces the pain.

Side Effects of Medical Treatment

Carbamazepine

The side effects of carbamazepine that most frequently limit therapy include ataxia, drowsiness, and fatigue. Older patients may note confusion while taking the drug.

Idiosyncratic side effects include leukopenia, agranulocytosis and, rarely, aplastic anemia. It is therefore advisable to obtain pretreatment baseline values of blood and platelets and to repeat these tests at regular intervals (e.g., monthly) during treatment.

Phenytoin

The most common side effects of this drug are drowsiness, dizziness, and diplopia, which can be reduced by appropriate dosage modification. More severe CNS effects such as ataxia, nystagmus, and slurred speech are an indication for immediate reduction of the dosage. Idiosyncratic side effects of phenytoin include gum hypertrophy and occasionally megaloblastic anemia.

Chlorphenesin and Baclofen

The most common side effect noted with chlorphenesin is drowsiness. Similarly, drowsiness, weakness, nausia, and vomiting may occur with baclofen.

Pathophysiology

Kugelberg and Lindblom (1959) have studied the neuropathophysiology of trigeminal neuralgia. Their results indicate that the excitatory state necessary to fire an attack may be built up over a considerable time by temporal summation of afferent impulses. Antiepileptic drugs, when effective, raise an attack threshold and shorten the duration of attacks by diminishing the self-maintenance of the excitation. They postulate that periodic discharges in the brainstem, in structures related to the spinal nucleus of the fifth cranial nerve, may explain the suddenness, intensity, and brevity of the attack.

Fromm, Terrance, and Maroon (1984) suggest that trigeminal neuralgia has a peripheral cause and a central pathogenesis. In other words, both peripheral and central factors are operative in this disease. For example, chronic "irritation" of the peripheral trigeminal nerve, from whatever cause, leads to failure of segmental inhibition in the trigeminal nucleus and to the production of ectopic action potentials in the trigeminal nerve. This consideration, of increased neuronal discharges and reduced inhibitory mechanisms, produces a hyperactive sensory circuit, leading eventually to paroxymal discharges in the trigeminal nucleus. These antidromic jolts, if you will, are perceived by the patient as painful attacks of trigeminal neuralgia.

TRIGEMINAL NEURALGIA AND MULTIPLE SCLEROSIS

Sensory disturbances in the distribution of the trigeminal nerve are relatively common in multiple sclerosis and may even involve the inside of the mouth. The usual descriptions of facial hypesthesia are nonspecific. Often patients speak of numbness or deadness of the face, or of a feeling that part of the face has been anesthetized by novocaine. Pain may or may not be associated with these sensations, which may be quite transient, last for a day or two or more, or sometimes become permanent. Objective signs of sensory loss are difficult to elicit but there may be associated impairment of pain and temperature sensitivity, and loss of touch in the region involved. The corneal reflex may be diminished or absent when the loss of sensation affects the first division of the trigeminal nerve.

Intermittent trigeminal neuralgia, as opposed to the condition described above (which might be termed trigeminal neuritis), is uncommon in multiple sclerosis; incidence varies between a 1 and 2% (Harris, 1950; Garcin et al., 1960). Conversely, the incidence of the multiple sclerosis among patients with trigeminal neuralgia is approximately 3%. Typically, the classic history of trigeminal neuralgia (Parker, 1978) will be obtained in patients with multiple sclerosis except that it may appear at a younger age than is usual when the disease occurs in its idiopathic form. Some patients with multiple sclerosis manifest recurrent episodes of face pain, generally long-lasting and not stabbing or lancinating, without associated trigger zones. These patients are assumed to have a form of atypical facial pain and not true trigeminal neuralgia.

In our experience, trigeminal neuralgia almost never occurs as the first manifestation of the disease, and all of the patients seen with trigeminal neuralgia in association with multiple sclerosis have had very significant physical signs of multiple sclerosis before the facial pain began. Most, for example, have paraparesis or paraplegia, disorders of sensory function including posterior column signs, and the like. Cases of trigeminal neuralgia appearing as the first manifestation of multiple sclerosis are rare.

The treatment of trigeminal neuralgia occurring in association with multiple sclerosis is the same as that given for the idiopathic variety.

Regarding the pathogenesis of trigeminal pain in multiple sclerosis, demyelinating plaques may be found at the point of entry of the fifth root, or involving the main sensory nucleus or the descending root of the trigeminal nerve.

Demyelinating plaques may also be found in the gasserian ganglion. If this is the case, plaques are often found in adjacent structures also involving the facial nucleus, sometimes producing facial weakness and continuous rhythmic fascicular contractions, termed facial myokymia. Presumably, the plaques occurring either in the ganglion or in the main sensory nucleus alter the electrophysiology of facial sensation, allowing hyperactive sensory circuits to appear, producing trigger zones and the characteristic manifestations of trigeminal neuralgia, as we have come to know them.

GLOSSOPHARYNGEAL NEURALGIA

Glossopharyngeal neuralgia (tic) is characterized by severe pain in the region of the tonsil and ear. Its timing features are like those of trigeminal neuralgia, and it may be initiated by yawning and swallowing or contact of food with the tonsillar region. Rarely, the patient may become unconscious during a paroxysm of pain (probably due to asystole). Examination reveals no evidence of reduction in perception of pin-prick or touch or of motility function in the nasopharynx.

The pain of glossopharyngeal neuralgia is often relieved by temporary cocainization of the involved side of the throat. Extracranial block of the glossopharyngeal nerve with alcohol is not recommended because the injection of alcohol in the region of the jugular foramen might well cause paralysis of the 10th , 11th, and 12th cranial nerves and could conceivably also involve the sympathetic trunk.

If the patient does not respond to carbamazepine, the treatment of choice for glossopharyngeal neuralgia is intracranial section of the nerve. Usually the exposure is through a unilateral suboccipital craniectomy. The nerve can be identified as it passes along the floor of the posterior fossa to emerge through the jugular foramen.

Some authors use the terms glossopharyngeal and vagal neuralgia or vagoglossopharyngeal neuralgia instead of glossopharyngeal neuralgia, implying that the pain can radiate into the distribution of the vagus nerve as well as that of the glossopharyngeal nerve. The original term, glossopharyngeal neuralgia, is recognized by most neurologists and is more commonly used.

Because the ear and its adjacent structures are supplied by pain fibers from the 5th, 7th, 9th, and 10th cranial nerves, neuralgias of these structures often closely resemble each other and sometimes become inseparable. It is therefore not surprising that there has been controversy concerning the existence of separate neuralgias of these nerves and conflict as to the best surgical procedures. It is likely that the mechanism of the pain in all is the same.

SURGICAL PROCEDURES FOR THE ELIMINATION OF MAJOR TRIGEMINAL NEURALGIA

A number of patients with trigeminal neuralgia, between 25 and 50%, will eventually fail on medical therapy and will need some form of neurosurgical treatment (see also Chapter 21). The type of operation performed varies widely from place to place. Patients need to be completely and clearly appraised of the nature of the operations proposed, the procedures to be undertaken, possible side effects, costs, and morbidity and mortality. Informed consent regarding these neurosurgical procedures, given their many differences, is mandatory (Table 15-3).

Two operations, including local ablation of peripheral nerves, and wide section of the sensory roots of the trigeminal nerve, are rarely done any longer, since better methods are usually available for surgical pain relief.

Selective lesion or lesions of the trigeminal root using a radio frequency electrode placed in the root under radiographic control (radio frequency rhizotomy) is an operative procedure that has gained wide acceptance (Sweet & Wepsic, 1974) (Tew & Keller, 1977). It has the advantages of safety and simplicity. The anesthesia used is light, the patient is awake during some of the procedure, recovers rapidly,and is often found eating supper a few hours after the operation. Almost always, the patient can be discharged the next day.

However, there is a recurrence rate of about 25%, corneal anesthesia occurs occasionally, and rarely, uncomfortable dysesthesias or jaw weakness results. Altered sensation in the face is reported by many patients, but only a few are bothered by it. To the present, no mortality has been associated with this operation.

A variation on this procedure has been proposed by Hakanson (1981). He injects

Table 15-3 Comparison of operative techniques for trigeminal neuralgia[a]

Technique	Description	Complications
Radio-frequency rhizotomy	90% effective minor percutaneous needle procedure, brief hospital stay	Facial sensory loss is frequently quite severe, corneal hypesthesia (10–15%), occasional masseter weakness)
Glycerol injection	85% effective minor percutaneous needle procedure, brief hospital stay	Facial sensitivity loss is slight; persistent corneal hypesthesia and masseter weakness is rare
Microvascular decompression	90% effective major craniotomy, 4–10 day hospital stay	+4% serious postoperative complications, 1% mortality

[a]Each of the procedures is associated with a modest recurrence rate. The recurrence rate is least with microvascular decompression and modestly greater with radiofrequency rhizotomy and glycerol injection.

0.3 to 0.4 ml of glycerol by the anterior percutaneous route in the trigeminal cistern (Meckel's cave), which is visualized by aid of contrast medium (metrizamide). Hakanson reports excellent response to this procedure, with only minimal disturbance of facial sensitivity. Sweet and his colleagues (1981) have also reported their experience with this procedure. They describe greater pain on injection, and more sensory loss than Hakanson reported. The presumption is made that glycerol is neurotoxic, acts on partially demyelinated nerve fibers, and eliminates the compound action potential in the trigeminal rootlets that are associated with pain.

An alternative procedure is microvascular decompression of the trigeminal root (Jannetta, 1977); (Voorhees & Patterson, 1981). Here, the neurosurgeon assumes that he or she will find a lesion (usually an arterial loop) compressing the trigeminal root close by the brain stem. Thus, in effect, the operation is exploratory, for *none* of our current sophisticated neurodiagnostic studies, including arteriography, computerized tomography of the head, or other special views, actually allows the surgeon to predict with certainty before the operation that such a lesion will be found. If and when it is found, the offending, compressing lesion is lifted from the trigeminal root, often by interposing a sponge. This approach, thus, assumes that, in most cases, trigeminal neuralgia is a compressive cranial mononeuropathy.

These various operations, of course, have significant differences in costs. Radio frequency lesions and glycerol injections are done rapidly and the patient is almost always quickly discharged. With microsurgical decompression of the trigeminal root, a formal craniotomy is required, and the patient frequently spends 4 to 10 days in the hospital and a similar period of time in convalescence.

PATHOLOGIC ANATOMY OF THE TRIGEMINAL (GASSERIAN) GANGLION IN TIC DOULOUREUX

Alterations in the anatomy of the gasserian ganglion and sensory root have been reported for years. In 1934 Dandy found aberrant arteries and other vascular anomalies in 40% of patients with tic douloureux as he exposed the fifth nerve root through the posterior fossa. More recently, Jannetta (1967) has demonstrated small arterial loops impinging on nerve fibers during subtentorial microdissection of the trigeminal root in patients with tic douloureux. Separation of these vessels from the root, combined with partial rhizotomy, relieved the neuralgia without producing a major sensory abnormality. Following an anatomic study, Kerr (1963) has proposed that contact between the internal carotid artery and the undersurface of the gasserian ganglion may be a significant factor in the development of tic douloureux. He based this proposal on sections of the petrous tip, which demonstrated that a lacuna in the bony root of the carotid canal is frequently present in normal patients. He found considerable variability in the fascial reinforcements of this lacuna, with a tendency for it to become reduced in thickness with age. Kerr felt that this structural variant was compatible with features peculiar to tic douloureux. In addition, electron-microscopic abnormalities in the gasserian ganglion itself have been described.

TICLIKE NEURITIDES OF THE FIFTH CRANIAL NERVE ASSOCIATED WITH BRAIN TUMORS AND OTHER PATHOLOGIC PROCESSES

Ticlike neuritides, relatively uncommon painful states resembling tic douloureux, can usually be differentiated, because each painful paroxysm is commonly a sustained high-intensity ache of several minutes' duration, whereas the true tic is characterized by recurrent, brief, painful jabs lasting approximately 30 seconds. Cushing (1920), in describing these neuralgias resulting from tumor involvement of the sensory root, the trigeminal ganglion, or the fifth nerve, has divided them into four groups on the basis of the site of the precipitating cause:

1. Tumors of the cerebellopontile recess upon the trigeminal root may rarely be accompanied by paroxysms of pain that resemble tic douloureux. The pain is not eliminated by trigeminal ganglion operation. Sometimes there is a low-intensity, steady, dull ache, but usually little or no pain is produced by such tumors, and a gradual hypesthesia in the distribution of the fifth cranial nerve occurs.
2. Tumors of the middle fossa that involve the trigeminal ganglion by direct pressure from above, mainly on the dura overlying the ganglion, are growths with a meningeal attachment, such as endothelial tumors, granulomas, and occasional gliomas. The pain, again, rarely resembles tic douloureux in its temporal features. Furthermore, it is an inconspicuous symptom of the underlying disorder. Usually when pain occurs it is of a sustained aching and burning character, and is associated with hypesthesia of an appropriate area of the skin. Paroxysms of high-intensity pain lasting 10 to 15 minutes may occur.
3. Tumors that arise in the cranium or in the extracranial tissues beneath the ganglion, often metastatic, are almost certain to involve the ganglion in the course of time. Occasionally, the nerve is completely destroyed, resulting in total anesthesia in its territory, without production of pain; but more often the process is accompanied by aching and burning pain of high intensity occurring in paroxysms lasting 10 to 15 minutes.

4. Endothelial tumors originating from the envelopes of the trigeminal ganglion give rise to pain in the region supplied by one or more branches of the fifth nerve. The character of the pain, a more or less sustained, steady ache, readily distinguishes it from true trigeminal neuralgia. It is also inevitably accompanied by a hypesthesia, if not anesthesia, and motor paralysis. Also, the third, sixth, and eighth nerves may be involved by the tumor. Avulsion of the sensory root on the side affected, resulting in total anesthesia, eliminates the pain.

When true tic douloureux is found to occur in a young person, particularly a young woman, the patient should be carefully examined for evidence of a demyelinating disease or multiple sclerosis. Pain usually persists between paroxysms, but the symptoms may be indistinguishable from those of true tic. Every opportunity for remission should be exploited, but if the pain becomes intractable, the patient should be treated in much the same way as patients with true tic douloureux. The symptom is sometimes associated with a plaque in the pontine and adjacent regions of the brain stem.

Thus, a specific gross pathologic lesion is only rarely associated with true trigeminal neuralgia. Some patients with persistent burning sensations involving one of the three divisions of the trigeminal nerve may be said to have a form of trigeminal neuritis related to such a lesion. For example, advanced multiple sclerosis can produce a syndrome indistinguishable from idiopathic tic douloureux. Occasionally, posterior fossa lesions, extracerebral in type such as arteriovenous malformations, epidermoids, acoustic neuromas, meningiomas, arachnoiditis, and basilar artery aneurysm will produce similar complaints, but almost always in the context of other neurologic findings. Even more rarely, osteomas of the foramen ovale may evoke facial pain. In general, it may be said that such lesions are rare and usually, if the history is carefully obtained, the character of the pain will be seen to be somewhat different from that of idiopathic tic douloureux.

GENICULATE NEURALGIA OF HERPETIC ORIGIN

Generally, geniculate neuralgia is related to herpes zoster infection of the geniculate ganglion and is characterized by severe pain in the tympanic membrane, the walls of the auditory canal, the external auditory meatus, and the external structures of the ear. The pain is typically deep, and may be associated with a herpetic rash in the auricle, or the rash may be present in the external auditory canal. The disease may be associated with facial palsy, difficulty with hearing, vertigo, and tinnitus. Treatment is symptomatic.

HEMIFACIAL SPASM

Maroon (1978) has reviewed the literature on hemifacial spasm and described his therapy of this syndrome. Recent surgical observations indicate that hemifacial spasm is most likely caused by normal or pathologic vascular structures that cross-compress the facial nerve. The critical area of compression is found at the brain stem exit zone of the seventh nerve. In this area the central glial investment of the facial nerve changes to peripheral or Schwannian myelin. It is suspected that this anatomic junction zone may be of pathophysiologic significance when directly compressed or irritated. Maroon recommends a retromastoid craniectomy and vascular decompression operation to relieve hemifacial spasm, while at the same time preserving facial nerve function. This is in contrast with commonly used destructive operations for hemifacial spasm. He emphasizes, however, that microsurgical techniques must be employed, using the retromastoid approach, or high morbidity and mortality may occur. Interestingly, in Maroon's series of cases, facial pain or headache associated with clonic facial spasm was extremely rare. He emphasizes that the problem is primarily a muscular one related to predominant contraction of the orbicularis and zygomatic muscles.

Hemifacial spasm should be differentiated from blepharospasm and the synkinesis that may occur following Bell's palsy. In our experience, blepharospasm is almost always bilateral, affects primarily the periorbital muscles, but may spread to the upper facial muscles as well. In a small number of patients with Bell's palsy, hemifacial synkinetic movements may develop as the patient recovers from the episode but is left with persisting weakness. This history is clearly different from that of hemifacial spasm. Also, facial myokymia may appear as a form of fascicular twitching of the facial muscles, especially the orbicularis oculi.

In none of these conditions is facial pain common.

HEADACHE AND DIABETIC NEUROPATHY

Isolated cranial nerve palsies, especially of the third and sixth nerves, are known to occur in diabetics. Neuralgia of the fifth nerve with diabetic ocular paresis may occur.

No suitable explanation for the pain is available. It appears likely that the third, fourth, and sixth cranial nerve defects stem from vascular occlusive disease of the vasa nervorum and that, rarely, the fifth cranial nerve becomes similarly involved.

HERPETIC AND POSTHERPETIC NEURITIS

Herpes Zoster Involvement of the Gasserian Ganglion and Trigeminal Nucleus

The pain of herpes zoster, in contrast with that of tic, is steady and sustained. Although the pain often spontaneously regresses within 2 or 3 weeks, it may persist for several months, and when it occurs in persons past the age of 70, as it frequently does, its duration may be a year or more. Rarely, it persists indefinitely. The pain is unilateral and the quality of the pain is both burning and aching. It may be experienced in any part of the distribution of the fifth cranial nerve, although involvement of the forehead is most common. The pain is nonthrobbing, relatively uniform, and usually diminished gradually in intensity. Examination soon after onset reveals erythema and the typical herpetiform lesion of the skin associated with hyperalgesia and parasthesia. Examination later reveals hypesthesia and paresthesia of the involved areas, and sometimes scarring and pigmentation of the skin. There may be weakness of the masseter muscle and pterygoid muscle on the homolateral side. The judicious use of codeine and salicylates, with reassurance of better days to come, makes the period of spontaneous regression tolerable. Sensory root section does not usually give complete relief. Often it has no effect.

Herpes Zoster and Involvement of Other Dorsal Root Ganglions and Nerve Tissues

Steady pain in the face and ear, the back of the head, and the neck, associated with vertigo and palsy of the homolateral side of the face, results from widespread inflammation involving the gasserian and glossopharyngeal and the first two or three dorsal root ganglions and the dorsal horns of the cervical portion of the cord. The pain has the qualities and duration previously described. As with all herpes, there may be a slight or moderate palsy. Herpetiform lesions may or may not be present.

Occipital Neuritis Due to Herpes, Other Infections, and Cervical Cord Tumors

Occipital headache due to inflammation, injury, or pressure on the occipital nerves, upper cervical spinal roots, dorsal horn, or root ganglions, is a long-lasting, sustained, nonthrobbing ache of moderate intensity. It is difficult to separate from muscle contraction headache, because it also is always associated with muscle contraction and tenderness. The characteristic feature is paresthesia or algesia of the tissues of the scalp and the skin of the neck. Discoloration or scarring of the skin, such as follows herpes, may also occur. When the headache is postherpetic, section of nerves or roots will probably not eliminate the pain, although it may be somewhat reduced. Procaine injections about the sensory roots have a similar slight effect in reducing the intensity of pain.

Occipital headache due to tumors of the upper cervical cord, especially to those masses attached or adjacent to the first two or three roots, closely resembles that already described. In most such instances, in addition to the pain there is disturbance in sensory perception within the dermatomes involved. Enhanced computerized tomography (CT) is the diagnostic procedure of choice, after plain cervical spine films are done. Removal of the tumor or rhizotomy, when removal is possible, eliminates or reduces the intensity of headache.

Sustained contraction of the neck with the x-ray picture of a straight cervical spine may also be associated with a variety of cervical defects, including displaced cervical intervertebral disk nuclei. Unilateral neck ache extending to the occiput, and sometimes also including the temple and forehead, may appear in patients with mid- and upper-cervical joint disorders.

Cautious extension of the neck by manual or other traction may have a therapeutic effect.

Patients who survive after rupture of the odontoid ligament have severe headache in the neck and the suboccipital region.

HEADACHE AND DISEASES OF THE CERVICAL SPINE

Brain et al., in 1952, called attention to the headache and other clinical manifestations of cervical spondylosis (see also chapter 24). Pain is commonly referred to the deep structures about the neck and back of the head, as well as into the arms and digits, which is likely to be worsened by moving the neck and pulling on the arms. Hyperalgesia, wasting, and fasciculations may be present. In addition, symptoms may arise from the impairment of function of the cervical spinal cord. Brain and his colleagues defined cervical spondylosis as a degenerative disorder of the cervical spine, leading to narrowing of the intravertebral spaces and protrusion of the intravertebral disks. These changes can cause pressure on the spinal nerves in their foramina as well as pressure on the spinal cord. Because the disorder is degenerative rather than inflammatory, he selected the term spondylosis rather then spondylitis. He considers trauma and the degeneration of the intravertebral disks with age to be the main precipitating factors. It is more common in men than in women and produces symptoms chiefly in the fifth and sixth decades. As a result of the morbid process, the nerve roots are compressed in the foramina, now the site of a secondary formation of fibrous tissue. Thus, nerve fibers undergo degeneration. The cord is directly compressed and tethered by the adhesions around the nerve roots, and normal neck movement causes continual mild injury. Blood supply may be affected by compression of the spinal veins and the anterior spinal artery. Spinal fluid may show a slight rise in protein, and when the neck is extended there may be a demonstrable obstruction on manometric tests. Brain finds that rest by immobilization with a plastic collar for 3 months usually eliminates the pain, rendering operative intervention unnecessary. When the spinal cord in compressed, however, surgical procedures are sometimes helpful if the operation takes place early in the course of the disorder.

A number of other workes have called attention to the occurrence of headache with pathologic changes of the cervical spine, and especially to the possibility of painful implication of the frontal part of the head.

Headache is said to be a common accompaniment of cervical disk lesions. High cervical bony defects or root damage do indeed become linked with headache, which may become frontal. Conspicuous in this category is the headache that accompanies the development of Paget's disease, involving the bones of the base of the skull and the upper cervical spine. The distortions and the displacements that occur under these circumstances may also be linked with occipital headache.

PAINFUL TIC CONVULSIF

Painful tic convulsif is characterized by periodic contractions of one side of the face, accompanied by great pain. It may be confused with the facial contortions and masticatory movements on the involved side that rarely accompany the paroxysms of true trigeminal neuralgia. Cushing (1920) has reported five cases of the disorder, which is extremely rare.

Painful tic convulsif is reported to be more severe in women than in men. It may begin in or about the orbicularis oculi as a fine intermittent myokymia, with some spread thereafter into the muscles of the lower part of the face. Occasionally, strong spasms may involve all of the facial muscles on one side almost continuously. Rarely, the face may become weak and some of the facial muscles may atrophy.

ATYPICAL FACIAL PAINS

The head and face pains included for consideration in this section differ from the typical or major facial neuralgias chiefly as follows:

1. In the atypical neuralgias, the pain is seldom limited to the distribution of the fifth or ninth cranial nerves but usually spreads over the area supplied by the cervical roots.
2. The pain is not significantly reduced or elminated by division of the fifth or ninth cranial nerves.
3. The pain is of a steady, diffuse, aching quality lasting for hours or days; it does not occur in paroxysms of short duration (1 to 30 seconds) followed by freedom from pain, as in tic douloureux.
4. The atypical facial neuralgia syndromes do not present trigger zones.
5. These disorders occur in a younger age group than the major neuralgias, and far more commonly in women.
6. Attacks are not precipitated by cold, drafts, cold water in the mouth, swallowing, talking, chewing, shaving, or washing the face, as in typical neuralgias considered in the previous sections.

Atypical Facial Neuralgia (Episodic)

A group of patients with so-called atypical facial neuralgia has been carefully studied. There is unilateral spread of pain from the nose, eye, cheek, and ear, ultimately involving the neck and shoulder. Such patients have recurrent attacks of variable duration. There may be associated redness of the nasal mucous membranes, swelling of the turbinates, and increased secretion and obstruction in the nose. Serious disturbances in mood, attitude, and behavior were conspicuous.

The pain had an aching quality and seemed to arise deep within the bones or the eyeball, in contrast with that of trigeminal neuralgia, which has both an aching and a burning component. The pain emanated from the region of the nose, the upper and lower jaws, the eyeball and above it, the ear and behind it, and the occipital region, the suboccipital region, and the neck and shoulder. The distribution varied considerably. The pain was not eliminated by any of the following procedures: section or alcohol injection of any branch of the trigeminal nerve; operations on structures in the painful areas, such as teeth, nasal structures, and sinuses; cocainization of the sphenopalatine ganglion; resection of the superior cervical sympathetic ganglion; supraorbital and infraorbital nerve evulsion; stripping of the periarterial (carotid) plexus; subtotal section of the sensory root of the trigeminal nerve; mastoid operations; or pelvic operations.

A series of patients with painful disorders in this distribution and of the nature described in the preceding paragraphs were studied at the Scripps Clinic and Research Foundation. The investigators determined that it is not possible to further define this bewildering group of facial pains and syndromes on the basis of any consistent history, and since the diagnosis rests entirely on the history, we choose to consider all unfortunate patients with these syndromes as having, simply, atypical facial neuralgia. We recognize that multiple factors may be responsible for the production of this syndrome, and when this diagnosis is made, we suggest a careful search be made for local pathology of the nose, eyes, teeth, sinuses, and pharynx. Cryptic tumors of the parotid gland should be sought. Atypical facial neuralgia may be associated with autonomic symptoms including cutaneous pallor, sweating, flushing, lacrimation, pupillary changes, rhinitis, and the like.If vasodilator phenomena are obvious, a trial on a vasoconstrictor agent of the ergot type may be worthwhile. But the physician should not be surprised if the patient does not respond to this or other forms of therapy.

Carotidynia

Fay (1932) introduced the word *carotidynia* to describe a variety of pain that arises in the neck. He suggested that the pain originated in the common carotid and external carotid arteries and its maxillary branches, and that the course of afferent impulses to the central nervous system was indirect, involving in part the vagus nerve. Carotidynia is a syndrome that features tenderness, swelling, and sometimes conspicuous pulsation of the common carotid artery on the affected side. Placing the thumbs on the common carotid arteries just below the bifurcation, and pressing the structures back against the transverse cervical processes with a rolling movement produces a severe pain. In patients who already have a dull aching pain referred to the eye, deep in the malar region, spreading back to the ear, behind the ear, and down the neck, the pain is accentuated. The attacks are usually periodic, are more likely to occur on the same side, and are not associated with visual disturbances.

Roseman (1967) has reviewed the literature on carotidynia and reported his observations in young and middle-aged adults. He describes a unilateral or bilateral neck pain of high intensity but of relatively short duration, lasting 11 days on the average. In 90% of the cases the disease was self-limited. Systemic signs of illness were absent. Treatment of carotidynia is usually supportive. Simple analgesics such as aspirin may be helpful. Corticosteroids are rarely necessary.

Lovshin (1977) has reported on a series of 100 cases of carotidynia from the Cleveland Clinic. All of the patients were examined, treated, and followed by the author. There were 82 females and 18 males, and 67 patients had a history of vascular headache. Forty-five patients volunteered the information that the glands in the neck had been swollen. Lovshin finds that the most common form of carotidynia is related to overdistention, relaxation, and increased pulsation in the carotid artery.

This syndrome of vascular neck pain is closely associated with various forms of extracranial vascular headache. It is more common in women than in men, the ratio being about 4 to 1. The syndrome occurs at almost any age but is most prevalent during the fourth and fifth decades, and there is often a history of vascular headache. The only significant abnormality found on physical examination is the presence of a tender, throbbing, often dilated carotid artery. The condition is frequently misdiagnosed and therefore not properly treated. Lovshin states that the preferred treatment is similar to that of migraine and other painful vasodilating conditions of the head. In particular, he suggests various oral preparations of ergotamine tartrate, or methysergide, 2 mg three or four times daily, in a short course. Apparently carotidynia is not characterized by an inflammatory arteritis. The condition is not related to cranial arteritis.

Raeder's Syndrome and the Pericarotid Syndrome

Raeder's paratrigeminal syndrome (1924) is a rare illness characterized by oculosympathetic paralysis, the sudden onset of severe frontotemporal burning, aching pain of rapid onset, with associated ptosis and meiosis, often in a periorbital distribution, no previous history of headache, and normal sweating in the supraorbital area of the ipsilateral forehead. Raeder based his conclusions on five cases in which there were cranial nerve dysfunctions, usually involving the optic, oculomotor, trochlear, trigeminal, and abducens nerves. Raeder's first patient had a tumor arising from the region of the trigeminal ganglion infiltrating all of these cranial nerves. Two of his cases had multiple cranial nerve lesions and sympathetic paralysis related to head injury. In two cases, no particular cause could be identified. In essence, then, Raeder's patients had multiple cranial nerve involvements, primarily parasellar, associated with oculosympathetic paralysis and intact facial sweating. Others have since described almost any lesion in which there is oculosympathetic paralysis associated with head pain as a Raeder's syndrome. Given this confusion, it would probably be best to abandon the eponym and more precisely classify patients with oculosympathetic paralysis and headache, who may or may not have disturbances of sweating as well.

Many patients with cluster headaches have an associated oculosympathetic paralysis, but in this situation the tempo of the cluster headache establishes the diagnosis, rather than the automatic dysfunction.

Vijayan and Watson (1978) have described a pericarotid syndrome characterized by oculosympathetic paralysis, ipsilateral head pain, and anhidrosis over the forehead with otherwise intact facial sweating. They suggest that the site of the lesion involving the oculosympathetic fibers in their patients is pericarotid. Their patients had no previous history of headache. They were able to establish a pathogenesis in only one of their six patients in whom a left internal carotid artery occlusion had occurred. In the other five patients, the etiology was unknown.

Long-Sustained or Chronic Atypical Facial Neuralgia (Psychogenic)

In contrast with the probable vascular origin of pain in the episodic variety of atypical facial neuralgia, the pathophysiology of long-sustained or continuous atypical facial neuralgia is ill defined. The failure of ergotamine tartrate to eliminate or reduce the pain, the inconstancy of the edema, and the persistence of the pain for months or years invalidate the vascular hypothesis regarding patients with this chronic syndrome. Long-lasting alterations in mood, attitude, and behavior in this latter group of patients are conspicuous. The depressive, hypochondriacal, or hysterical features support the view that the pain is of a delusional nature, or at least that the delusion of pain is the outstanding feature of the patient's illness and is far more significant than any peripheral changes that might give rise to pain. The prognosis in this latter group of patients is grave regardless of therapy.

In a psychiatric study of atypical facial pain, Smith et al. (1969) from the Mayo Clinic found evidence of significant psychopathology. They studied 32 patients with atypical facial pain seen in the Neurology and Dentistry sections of the Mayo Clinic during an 8-month period. Psychiatric diagnoses grouped the majority of the patients into three categories: depressive reaction, conversion reaction, and hysterical personality with a conversion reaction or a depressive equivalent. In general, the patients were found to be perfectionistic, striving, success-oriented, hypochondriacal, and depressed. Smith and his associates postulate that the patients demonstrate a considerable resentment and anger that is repressed and internalized, resulting in depression as well as in the painful condition of atypical facial pain. The writers concur with the literature indicating that the condition is psychiatric and conclude that patients with this syndrome seem to be in need of an understanding, reassuring medical regimen with psychotherapy made available for those who would benefit from this approach.

CENTRAL PAIN, POSTHERPETIC NEURITIS, AND TRANSCUTANEOUS NEUROSTIMULATION

Recent reports of the analgesic effects of transcutaneous electrical neurostimulation (TNS) have emphasized peripheral mechanisms (Ignelzi & Nyquist, 1976; Loeser et al., 1975). Although the possibility of a central effect remains open, these reports noted an apparent "fatigue" of peripheral nerve fibers, which could account for the analgesia obtained.

We have recently had some success with TNS in reducing the severity of central pain states in a small series of patients. It would be of interest to review these cases because they demonstrate a central inhibitory effect of TNS.

Method and Results

The eight patients whose experience is charted in Table 15-4 have had either thalamic pain following a cerebrovascular accident (CVA) or postherpetic neuralgia. Three of

Table 15-4 Patients with central pain partially relieved by TNS

Case No.	Age	Sex	Diagnosis	Pain distribution	Pain duration pre-TNS	Pain severity pre-TNS (0–100)
1.	73	Male	Post-CVA	Right foot	1½ yrs	75
2.	40	Female	Post-CVA	Left arm, left leg, left side of head	6 mo	95
3.	61	Male	Post-CVA	Entire left side except abdomen	4 yrs	60 (if inactive) 90 (if active)
4.	79	Female	Postherpetic	T4–5, left	3½ yrs	?
5.	65	Male	Postherpetic	T8–10, left	5 yrs	50
6.	76	Male	Postherpetic	C1–2, right	5 yrs	50
7.	16	Male	Postherpetic	C2–3, right	1 yr	60
8.	68	Male	Postherpetic	L4–5, left	14 mo	80

four patients who had thalamic pain have obtained some relief with TNS (cases 1–3), and 5 of 14 patients with postherpetic neuralgia have likewise obtained significant relief (cases 4–8). We have no clear explanation for the failures except that several of these patients reported that TNS made them "nervous," or expressed displeasure at wearing the device.

The thalamic pain patients required electrode placement in the distribution of their pain, and one (case 3) obtained additional benefit from adding electrodes to the contralateral side as well. However, none of the patients with postherpetic neuralgia could tolerate such a "peripheral" placement, as it exacerbated their pain; electrodes at either side of the spinal vertebras at the dermatomal level of their pain were better tolerated.

All the patients wore the stimulating device throughout the day, except for case 7, who did not wear it to school but applied it at home each day. Case 3 has tried, on several occasions, to determine how long he could do without TNS, and has found that after 3 or 4 days his pain is unbearable.

Discussion

In herpes zoster, a varicella virus causes an inflammatory reaction in peripheral nerve and dorsal root ganglion (Adams, 1976). Most cases appear to recover uneventfully, but a variety of complications may arise, including myelitis and encephalitis (Gard-

Analgesics pre-TNS	TNS electrode placements (pair)	Duration TNS follow-up	Pain severity post-TNS (0–100)	Analgesics post-TNS
Meperidine 100 mg prn	Right ankle	7 months (decreased)	0–10	None
Oxycodone q4h	1. Left wrist 2. High cervical	6 weeks (lost to follow-up)	0–45	None
Valium	1. Both legs 2. Both shoulders	1 yr, 9 mo	0 (if inactive), 60 (if active)	None
Acetaminophen 650 mg q4h	Thoracic paraspinals	5 mo	?	None
None	Thoracic paraspinals	1 yr	0–50 (intermittent use)	None
None	High cervical	8 mo	20	None
ASA 650 mg q4h	High cervical	18 mo	25	ASA occasionally
Fiorinal 2/day	Lumbar spine	2 mo	50	Occasional propoxyphene

ner-Thorpe et al., 1976). Lesions include inflammatory necrosis in the dorsal root ganglion and associated destruction of the nerve cells and fibers in the cord, particularly in the anterior horns, substantia gelatinosa, and Clarke's column (Denny-Brown et al., 1944). If there has been such severe inflammation and necrosis in the acute stage then the subsequent loss of neurons and fibrosis may be associated with postherpetic neuralgia (Gordon & Tucker, 1945). The vascular dilatation and hemorrhage, which are common findings at the spinal level of the neuraxis in herpes zoster, suggest that the pathologic lesions may be comparable to the thrombotic CVAs associated with thalamic pain (Mumenthaler, 1976).

The fact that lesions at various levels of the neuraxis may give rise to pain has stimulated a number of theories to account for the phenomenon: iritable foci, disinhibition of thalamic function, and/or alteration of functional balance in sensory systems. Irritability, resulting in epileptiform activity in partially damaged cells surrounding the area of destruction (sensory epilepsy), may occur in some cases; the condition sometimes responds to anticonvulsants, such as carbamazepine. However, the quality of pain and failure of the drug in many cases suggest this is not an adequate explanation. In recent years, a model emphasizing the loss of normal inhibitory input from the periphery has gained favor (Melzack & Wall, 1965).

Previous reports on the effectiveness of TNS in a variety of pain states have incidentally noted some success with central pain (Davis & Lentini, 1975; Ebersold et al., 1975), but the implications of this finding appear to have been overlooked. What the earlier reports and the present series demonstrate is precisely what the gate-control theory would predict, namely, that peripheral stimulation can produce a central pain-inhibiting effect (see Chapter 2). Although peripheral nerve fiber "fatigue" may also occur with TNS, the partial analgesia produced in these cases of central pain is consistent with an inhibition at the spinal or higher levels. Furthermore, it is unlikely that the results reported here are due to a placebo effect, inasmuch as our experience suggests that pain relief that is maintained for 2 to 4 weeks is likely to persist indefinitely (Sternbach et al., 1976).

SUMMARY

- Both medical and surgical therapies may be used in the individual patient with trigeminal neuralgia. Ordinarily, the treatment is medical. However, if a response to drugs is not forthcoming, or if the patient becomes toxic while taking medications or refuses to abide by an appropriate medical program, then surgical consultation should be obtained and the appropriate operation performed. The form and type of the neurosurgical procedure will probably depend to a considerable extent on the expertise of the neurosurgeon and his training. Generally, in the elderly the simplest procedures should be attempted first. It may be necessary to employ both medical and surgical procedures in the individual patient.
- The medical drug of first choice is carbamazepine.
- Anticonvulsants are not helpful in postherpetic pain syndromes.
- Atypical facial neuralgia is a general term used to cover a variety of head and face pains that are poorly defined and may not deserve separate clinical status.
- The pathogenesis of the atypical facial neuralgias is uncertain and multiple causation seems likely. Search for local inflammatory pathology, vasomotor phenomena, and depressive symptoms is indicated, with treatment being guided by the findings.
- Three cases of the thalamic pain and five cases of postherpetic neuralgia have shown a significant decrease in pain levels with transcutaneous electrical neurostimulation (TNS). Such a favorable response in central pain states suggests that, in addition to any peripheral nerve fiber "fatigue" that TNS may cause, it has central inhibitory effects as well.

REFERENCES

Adams, J.H. (1976). Virus diseases of the nervous system. In *Greenfield's Neuropathology* (W. Blackwood and J.A.N. Corsellis, eds.), pp. 301–302. Arnold, London.

Brain, W.R., D.W.C. Northfield, and M. Wilkinson (1952). The neurological manifestations of cervical spondylosis. *Brain 75:* 187.

Cassinari, V. and C.A. Pagni (1969). *Central Pain: A Neurosurgical Survey,* pp. 93–108, 139–158. Harvard University Press, Cambridge.

Cushing, H. (1920). The major trigeminal neuralgias and their surgical treatment, based on experiences with 332 Gasserian operations. The varieties of facial neuralgia. *Am. J. Med. Sci. 160:* 157.

Dalessio, D.J. (1982). Trigeminal neuralgia. A practical approach to treatment. *Drugs 24:* 248–255.

Dalessio, D.J. (1977). Medical treatment of trigeminal neuralgia. *Clin Neurosurg. 24:* 579–583.

Dandy, W.E. (1925). Section of the sensory root of the trigeminal nerve at the pons. *Bull. Johns Hopkins Hosp. 36:* 105.

Dandy, W.E. (1934). Concerning the cause of trigeminal neuralgia. *Am. J. Surg. 24:* 447.

Dandy, W.E. (1945). *Surgery of the Brain.* W.F. Prior, Hagerstown, MD

Davis, R. and R. Lentini (1975). Transcutaneous nerve stimulation for treatment of pain in patients with spinal cord injury. *Surg. Neurol. 4 (Suppl.):* 100–101.

Denny-Brown, D., R.D. Adams, and P.J. Fitzgerald (1944). Pathologic features of herpes zoster. *Arch. Neurol. Psychiatry 51:* 216–231.

Ebersold, M.J., E.R. Laws, Jr., H.H. Stonnington, and G.K. Stillwell (1975). Transcutaneous electrical stimulation for treatment of chronic pain: A preliminary report. *Surg. Neurol. 4 (Suppl.):* 96–99.

Faigle, J.W. and K.F. Feldmann (1982). Carbamazepine biotransformation. In *Antiepileptic Drugs,* 2nd ed. (D.M. Woodbury, J.K. Penry, and C.E. Pippenger, eds.), pp. 483–495. Raven Press, New York.

Fay, T. (1932). Atypical facial neuralgia, a syndrome of vascular pain. *Ann. Otol. 41:* 1030.

Fromm, G.H. (1969). Pharmacological consideration of anticonvulsants. *Headache 9:* 35.

Fromm, G.H. and S. Landgren (1963). Effect of diphenylhydantoin on single cells in the spinal trigeminal nucleus. *Neurology 13:* 34.

Fromm, G.H., C.F. Terrence, and J.C. Maroon (1984). Trigeminal neuralgia. Current concepts regarding etiology and pathogenesis. *Arch. Neurol. 41:* 1204–1207.

Garcin, R., S. Godlewski, and J. leLapresle (1960). Nevralgie du Trijumeau et Sclerose en Plaques. *Rev. Neurol. 102:* 441.

Gardner-Thorpe, C., J.B. Foster, and D.D. Barwick (1976). Unusual manifestations of herpes zoster: A clinical and eleetrophysiological study. *J. Neurol. Sci. 28:* 427–447.

Gordon, I.R.S. and J.F. Tucker (1945). Lesions of the central nervous system in herpes zoster. *J. Neurol. Neurosurg. Psychiatry 8:* 40–46.

Hakanson, S. (1981). Trigeminal neuralgia treated by injection of glycerol into the trigeminal cistern. *Neurosurgery 9:* 638–646.

Harris, W. (1950). Rare forms of paroxysmal trigeminal neuralgia and the relation to disseminated sclerosis. *Br. Med. J. 1:* 831.

Ignelzi, R.J. and J.K. Nyquist (1976). Direct effect of electrical stimulation on peripheral nerve evoked activity: Implications in pain relief. *J. Neurosurg. 45:* 159–165.

Jannetta, P.J. (1967). Structural mechanisms of trigeminal neuralgia. *J. Neurosurg. 26:* 159.

Jannetta, P.J. (1977). Treatment of trigeminal neuralgia by suboccital and transtentorial cranial operations. *Clin. Neurosurg. 24:* 538–549.

Jannetta, P.J. and R.W. Rand (1967). Gross (mesoscopic) description of the human trigeminal nerve and ganglion. *J. Neurosurg. 26:* 109.

Jannetta, P.J. (1977). Observations on the etiology of trigeminal neuralgia, hemifacial spasm, acoustic nerve dysfunction and glossopharyngeal neuralgia. Definitive microsurgical treatment and results in 117 patients. *Neurochirurgia 20:* 146–154.

Kerr, F.W.L. (1963). The etiology of trigeminal neuralgia. *Arch. Neurol. 8:* 15.

Kugelberg, E. and U. Lindblom (1959). The mechanism of the pain in trigeminal neuralgia. *J. Neurol. Neurosurg. Psychiatry 22:* 36.

Loeser, J.D., R.G. Black, and A. Christman (1975). Electrical stimulation in the nervous system: The current status of electrical stimulation of the nervous system for relief of pain. *Pain 1:* 109–123.

Lovshin, L. (1977). Carotidynia. *Headache 17:* 192–195.

Maroon, J.C. (1978). Hemifacial spasm. *Arch. Neurol. 35:* 481–483.

Matthews, R.J., J.P. DaVanzo, and R.J. Collins (1963). The pharmacology of chlorphenesin carbamate. *Arch. Int. Pharmacodyn. 143:* 574.

Melzack, R. and P.D. Wall (1965). Pain mechanisms: A new theory. *Science 150:* 971–979.

Morley, T.P. (1977). The place of peripheral and subtemporal ablative operations in the treatment of trigeminal neuralgia. *Clin Neurosurg. 24:* 550–556.

Mumenthaler, M. (1976). The pathophysiology of pain. In *Epileptic Seizures—Behavior—Pain* (W. Birkmayer, ed.), pp. 303–305. University Park Press, Baltimore.

Parker, H.L. (1978). Trigeminal neuralgia associated with multiple sclerosis. *Brain 51:* 46.

Raeder, J.G. (1924). Paratrigeminal paralysis of oculopupillary sympathetic. *Brain 47:* 149–158.

Raskin, N.H. and S.P. Prusiner (1977). Carotidynia. *Neurology 27:* 43–46.

Roseman, D.M. (1967). Carotidynia. A distinct syndrome. *Arch. Otolaryngol. 85:* 81.

Rushton, N., P. Goldstein, and J.A. Gibilisco (1969). A psychiatric study of atypical facial pain. *Can. Med. Assoc. J. 100:* 26.

Smith, D.P., L.F. Pilling, J.S. Pearson, and J.G. Rushton, et al. (1969). A psychiatric study of atypical facial pain. *Can. Med. Assoc. J. 100,* 26.

Sternbach, R.A., R.J. Ignelzi, L.M. Deems, and G. Timmermens (1976). Transcutaneous electrical analgesia: A follow-up analysis. *Pain 2:* 35–41.

Sweet, W.H. and J.G. Wepsic (1974). Controlled thermocoagulation of trigeminal ganglion and rootlets for differential destruction of pain fibers. Part 1: Trigeminal neuralgia. *J. Neurosurg. 40:* 143–156.

Sweet, W.H., C.E. Poletti, and J.B. Macon (1981). Treatment of trigeminal neuralgia and other facial pains by retrogasserian injection of glycerol. *Neurosurgery 9:* 647–653.

Tew, J.M. and J.R. Keller (1977). The treatment of trigeminal neuralgia by percutaneous radio frequency technique. *Clin. Neurosurg. 24:* 557–575.

Tomson, T. and L. Bertilsson (1984). Potent therapeutic effect of carbamazepine-10,11-epoxide in trigeminal neuralgia. *Arch. Neurol. 41:* 598–601.

Voorhees, R. and R.H. Patterson (1981). Management of trigeminal neuralgia (tic douloureux). *JAMA 245:* 2521–2523.

Vijayan, N and C. Watson (1978). The pericarotid syndrome. *Headache 18:* 244.

16

Post-Traumatic Headaches

OTTO APPENZELLER

Nowhere is scientific medicine less evident than in the treatment and management of post-traumatic headaches. Great difficulties arise in interpreting and assessing subjective symptoms that usually become overwhelmingly important in the subject's life only some variable time after head injury is sustained. This has led to a proliferation of anecdotal reports that often are contradictory and inconclusive and, despite their extent, leave a fuzzy clinical picture, the description of which causes problems for practitioners who wish to fit their patients into recognizable categories. Many neurologists and neurosurgeons favor their individual pathogenetic mechanisms for post-traumatic headache; however, it should be stressed that probably no one factor is responsible for the ubiquitous occurrence of this vexing symptom, and only a minority of patients can be clearly helped by specific phramacotherapy. Only carefully organized prospective studies of this ever-increasing problem with adequate follow-up and large enough numbers of patients and assessment of the extent of injury and its relation to subsequent symptoms might clarify the picture.

HISTORICAL ASPECTS

Medical records from the earliest times, though limited, describe damage to the head with visible fractures of the skull. In such individuals, the cause of headache was obvious. However, the idea that damage to the brain can occur without obvious external trauma first appeared in a description of a criminal who committed suicide by hitting his head against a wall. At autopsy, the skull was intact and no visible brain damage was seen. In the 19th century, persistent and intractable symptoms after head injury were noted when Rigler (1879) ascribed the increasing incidence of post-traumatic disability after the acceptance of financial compensability for accidental injuries on the Prussian railways. He was skeptical about symptoms in railway workers who demanded compensation and suggested that they may not have a "molecular derangement within the nervous system."

A clear distinction between symptoms due to damage of the brain and those associated with compensation claims was drawn by Strumpell in 1888. He thought that symptoms not obviously due to cerebral damage were widespread and exaggerated and in 1892, Friedmann described a triad of headache, dizziness, and alcohol intolerance. Later, irritability and difficulty in concentration was added, and this quincade was labeled the postconcussion syndrome, headache being the most troublesome and prominent symptom.

This constellation of complaints is common after head injury, but its pathogenesis and management continue to arouse controversy. Many war-injured patients were extensively studied and considerable knowledge about post-traumatic syndromes has accrued, but this has come mainly from severe and penetrating injuries, typical of casualties. However, more and more seemingly superficial or minor closed injuries to the head are even more troublesome to the physician. Even in patients who initially had no obvious evidence of cranial or cerebral trauma, subsequent verifiable atrophic areas in the brain may be demonstrable. And though the headache may not be causally related to the radiographic findings, litiginousness necessitates the admission that *"certo pronunciare non possumus; certum tamen est graves contusiones capitis plerumque molesta sui monumenta post se relinquere"* (I cannot judge; the only certainty is the head injury that continues to trouble)—the opinion of a judge given in 1694 in relation to a patient of Wepfer (1727). This patient, a 26-year-old servant was hit on the head by a staff, with consequent well-described retrograde amnesia, and 6 months later had a continuing headache, dizziness, ringing in the ear, and lassitude.

PATHOGENESIS

A brain concussion imposed on delicate neurotransmitter, neuromodulator, and electrical brain activity interferes with the regulatory capacity of the central, and subsequently the peripheral, autonomic and vasomotor systems. The abnormalities in cerebral blood flow following concussion may lead to very serious consequences. From this alteration in vasomotion arises primary traumatic brain damage and more diffuse secondary disorders of the brain. It is sometimes possible to observe a remarkably rapid post-traumatic atrophy of cerebral tissue attributed to vasomotor disturbances leading to serious impediment of blood flow to the damaged and other parts of the brain (Tonnis, 1956). Courville (1950) and others found diffuse ischemic parenchymatous damage after blunt head trauma and Strich (1956) demonstrated pathologically areas of demyelination years after apparently mild blunt head injuries.

Nevertheless, secondary changes in the brain after trauma and atrophic or demyelinated areas do not seem to be pathogenetically related to post-traumatic headaches, since brain tissue itself is insensitive. These pathologic findings rather demonstrate the relationship between brain concussion and vascular disorders and the serious circulatory disturbance occurring in the peritraumatic period. These derangements of the circulation are characterized by a fall in diastolic blood pressure with orthostasis predisposing to changes in blood flow and changes in blood vessel diameter, including pulsatility of major blood vessels sensitive to pain that are related to the symptomatology of vascular headaches of the migrainous type.

Thus, the immediate postconcussion headache is clinically very similar to migraine. This pulsatile headache increases with Valsalva's maneuver, bending forward, or exertion. The pain, however, is more or less continuous or occurs phasically or in attacks that are diffuse, sometimes frontal. But pain of this nature, if it persists for years after a head injury, can only with difficulty be attributed to the original impact. True post-traumatic migraine is said to be rare.

Cluster headache after a postinjury interval of several months, as reported by Nick (1969), must be unusual for no such case has been observed by Heyck (1975) or others. After reviewing hundreds of head-injured patients with headache, Heyck found post-traumatic migraine to be uncommon in adults, but not in children (Heyck, 1975). Ophthalmic post-traumatic migraine in younger subjects, with flashes of light and scotomatas and unilateral headache, vomiting, sonophobia and photophobia after head trauma, is perhaps related to the excessive reactivity of the autonomic nervous system in children, in whom the head injury may also unmask a latent migrainous diathesis. In older individuals, often those with brain atrophy, continuous nonmigrainous post-traumatic headaches are more frequent. These are attributed to the age-related changes in the cerebral vasculature and impairment of vascular adaption with age. In addition, predisposition to bleeding and numerous microhemorrhages in the meninges and dura after even minor head trauma, with consequent scars and adhesions, play a role in the genesis of the headaches.

INCIDENCE

In assessing incidence, it is necessary to exclude headache resulting from complications of the injury itself, such as subarachnoid hemorrhage, bacterial meningitis, or subdural hematoma. The incidence of headaches without obvious recognizable structural injury varies with the selection of the clinical material and the duration of follow-up. In a number of patients, moreover, analysis of post-traumatic headache is complicated by their development of recurring headaches after a symptom-free interval. The reported incidence varies from 28% (Penfield & Norcross, 1936) to a review of 200 cases of non-war-related head injuries of which 46% complained of headache when consciousness returned and the proportion remained the same at the time of discharge. Three months later, however, only 21% had returned to work, and a further decrease in the number working was found in subsequent months (Guttman, 1943). Surprisingly, headache was a more troublesome symptom in those who were thought to have a less severe injury, but no such relationship was found in patients who had headaches for longer periods of time after the injury. Age was not important in determining the incidence of headache, but those who had an antecedent history of recurrent headache were more prone to develop post-tramatic headache.

In another series (Russell, 1933–34) post-traumatic headache lasting longer than 2 months was found in 100% of patients over the age of 50, which contrasted with an overall incidence of 60% in this series. No relationship was found between the severity of the headache, the duration of residual disabilities, and the severity of injury, but a clear relationship to possible financial compensation was evident.

A different experience was reported by Guttman and Brenner et al. (1944), who were unable to relate the severity and duration of headache to age, neurologic disablement, sex, occupation, circumstances of injury, or intelligence of the subjects. The conclusion that 30 to 50% of patients develop headache after head injury seems to be adequately supported by a variety of authors (Miller, 1968).

The estimated incidence of head injuries ranges from 75,000 to 3 million annually in this country (Caveness, 1979; Jennett & Teasdale, 1981). Injuries sufficiently severe to cause residual disability occur in about 60,000 people annually, and though neurologic sequellae are often overemphasized, those without obvious clinical deficits, but persistent headache and mental symptoms, form the bulk of post-traumatic handicaps and seem to be generally forgotten.

Careful reviews to assess the connection between severity of the injury as evidenced by coma or amnesias or the presence of focal brain damage, subarachnoid bleeding, increased cerebrospinal fluid pressure, or EEG abnormalities and the severity and duration of post-traumatic headache have failed (Friedman & Merritt, 1945; Brenner et al., 1944). Some have even suggested that post-traumatic headache is singularly less troublesome after major cerebral injury and more disabling after minor concussion (Miller, 1961). Nevertheless, scalp lacerations promote headache, whether because of neuroma formation due to injury to cutaneous scalp nerves or other factors remains unclear. Extensive experience (Gurdjian & Webster, 1958) has shown that patients with major cerebral damage and serious parenchymal brain atrophy usually have little in the way of post-traumatic headache. The troublesomeness of headache in those with head injuries without loss of consciousness and those with only momentary impairment of awareness suggests that personality traits play a role in promoting such headaches.

CLINICAL FEATURES

There is no uniform description of the character of the headache. Russell (1933–34) thought they were continuous, but others felt they were mostly intermittent (Simons & Wolff, 1946). The varied and nonspecific nature of post-traumatic headaches were best characterized by Symonds (1960), who showed the variation in the nature of the pain, its location, and the importance of the behavior of the sufferer. The headaches may be throbbing or hammering and occasionally bursting or stabbing in nature. The descriptions given by patients emphasize the distress and are often exaggerated in those with litigation pending.

The best-defined and probably most easily understood post-traumatic headache is associated with injury to the scalp. The origin is visible and the pain is often associated with a sharp, well-localized area of tenderness in the scar or nearby. Percussion may cause a spreading sharp stab of pain. Sometimes head gear cannot be tolerated, or exposure to cold or emotional stress may trigger pain. Compression of a neuroma by contraction of scalp muscles or through release of neurotransmitters and neurohormones might trigger painful afferent stimuli. Sometimes the local pain spreads to cause generalized intermittent headache. Usually, the pain subsides spontaneously within a few months after injury, but repeated injections of local anesthetic in and around painful trigger points often speeds recovery. An associated spreading paresthesia from the injury site is often exaggerated by percussion but usually fades with the disappearance of the pain or after the use of local anesthetic.

Injury to the ligamentous structures of the cervical spine or more serious injury to the spine itself often complicates injury to the head, and this is sometimes overshadowed by extensive head trauma. For variable periods thereafter, such patients may complain of symptoms referable to the cervical spine long after those due to the head injury have disappeared. The injuries to the bony skeleton, disks, or ligaments, and sometimes pressure on spinal nerves, often contribute to the post-traumatic syndrome, including the headache. The cause of the pain may be actual skeletal damage; more often, though, pressure irritation or traction on cervical roots causing irregular and prolonged contraction of neck and scalp muscles is largely responsible for occipital and posterior cervical neck pain and headache. Many patients are relieved by manipulation. However, this is risky, particularly in elderly individuals. Disastrous occlusions of vertebral arteries have been well-documented following such maneuvers. The injection of local anesthetic into tender points in the neck repeated at 2- or 3-day intervals often helps break the vicious circle of muscle spasm and pain. This is usually accompanied by the administration of tricyclics. Physical therapy and traction have advocates, but their effects are unpredictable (Simons & Wolff, 1946).

Generalized post-traumatic headache is difficult to account for and categorize. It is described often not as a pain, but as a fuzziness or dizzy sensation or a feeling of fullness in the head. Such patients are usually able to clearly distinguish between post-traumatic sensations and headache of a different kind, to which they may have been prone before their injury. Similar categorizations are often made by patients whose headache may be a symptom of depression in which, again, inadequate descriptions of abnormal head sensations often distinguish depressive manifestations from headaches due to migraine, increased intracranial pressure, or a hangover.

Generalized headache, which is clearly pain rather than an amorphous head sensation, usually makes its onset with some delay after the injury. This lag has been attributed to post-traumatic amnesia (Symonds, 1942), but it may also appear without an intervening amnestic period. Whether this delay results from a gradual change in neurotransmitters or in perivascular nerve plexus or of the brain itself, which only reaches its pain promoting patterns sometime after injury, is not certain. This type of headache is often unilateral at the onset and may spread from the site of injury. It may be related to exertion or to posture, especially bending forward. When the headache is severe, vomiting may also occur. Stress, fatigue, excitement, bright lights, noise, concentration, or consumption of alcohol often exacerbate the headaches. Rest, quiet, and lying down in a darkened room bring improvement. Analgesics are not universally successful in alleviating the pain, and many patients pass from mild over-the-counter medication to serious polypharmacy dependence.

Within this wide spectrum of post-traumatic headache symptoms, certain patterns are discernible. One pattern is characterized by the features of scalp muscle contraction headaches, usually a tight band around the head or bilateral temple nonthrobbing pain, sometimes occipital. This is often accompanied by tenderness of extracranial structures. It is occasionally relieved by local anesthetic injection, local massage, heat or ice, alcohol or sedatives, and voluntary relaxation and tricyclic antidepressants. This pattern is very similar to an ordinary scalp muscle contraction headache but without antecedent trauma. The second variety of post-traumatic headache is often generalized, occasionally unilateral, and paroxysmal. It may be throbbing and has all the features of migraine, accompanied occasionally by nausea and vomiting, photophobia, and sonophobia. This post-traumatic migraine, though much less common than the former variety of headache, responds to treatment with ergotamine. But, because of its association with trauma, tricyclic antidepressants and resolution of litigation are often helpful in decreasing the frequency of attacks. Nevertheless, many patients become regular migraineurs, with exacerbation and improvement in the frequency and severity of attacks most often related to the usual situational factors. A third variety termed post-traumatic disautonomic cephalalgia (Vijayan & Dreyfus, 1975) is distinct, but rare, and follows injury to the neck. The cause is thought to be trauma to the perivascular sympathetic fibers in the carotid artery sheath. Pain and tenderness of the neck remains for weeks after the injury. Later severe unilateral episodic pulsatile headache occurs, ipsilateral to the injury, in the temporal and frontal areas, and associated with ipsilateral sweating and dilatation of the pupil, blurred vision, photophobia, and nausea. The headaches may last for hours to days and recur at frequent intervals. Sympathetic overactivity (perhaps due to partial injury of sympathetic fibers) with excessive firing, and later sympathetic denervation confirmed by response of the pupil to a weak solution of epinephrine, were found in these patients. Ergotamine is not effective, but propranolol may be useful.

The postconcussion syndrome remains a mystery, and the clinical spectrum is controversial. Psychogenic and organic factors are important in expression of symptoms that include headache, dizziness, impairment of memory, difficulty in concentrating, fatigue, anxiety, irritability, personality changes, and depression (Lindvall, 1974). The occurrence of this syndrome is perhaps even more common after mild trauma to the head (Kay & Derr, 1971; Merrit & McDonald, 1977). Immediately after head injury and for a few days thereafter, the headache and dizziness dominate the symptomatology; its cause is probably multifactorial, including pain at the injury site and diffuse, dull pressure resulting from muscular contraction (Simons & Wolff, 1946), it may be associated with a ''whiplash'' phenomenon arising from the cervical spine from musculoskeletal structures or pressure or tension on nerve roots, or it could be vascular in origin, post-traumatic migraine. Dizziness is common early in the post-traumatic period; abnormal electronystagmographic, audiologic, and vestibular-caloric findings have been reported in such patients (Toglia et al., 1970), but these investigations remain controversial (Lindvall, 1974).

Many neuropsychologic abnormalities, including slowed information processing and difficulty with memory, inability to concentrate, fatigability, irritability, and anxiety, are common features (Rimel, et al., 1982; Gronwall & Wrightson, 1974).

Evidence for brain damage even after minor head injury has been repeatedly presented (Oppenheimer, 1968; Strich, 1956), and the delayed onset of symptoms may be due to difficulties and stressful situations encountered on return to work because of inability to perform previously easy tasks (Gronwall & Wrightson, 1974).

While symptoms continue for months or years after the accident, the perpetuation of disability is not only the result of putative brain damage, usually undetected by present methods of investigation, but also of psychological responses to the accident. Litigation and compensation, though not entirely to blame for persistent disability, certainly promote its continuation (Brooks, 1972). Continued disability after head injury is associated with middle age, married status, social class IV (U.K. classification by Hollingshead) industrial accidents, relatively unskilled occupations, and previous behavioral abnormalities (Kay et al., 1971).

Symptoms persisting for some time after the injury almost invariably involve psychiatric problems. An explanation of the basis of the symptoms, if available, and exploration of life situations, stresses, the occurrence of depression, and alcoholism all may be appropriately addressed by psychotherapy, including the use of pharmacologic intervention. Good responses to tricyclics have been reported (Tyler et al., 1980; Adeloye, 1971). Although many patients eventually recover, this is in large part because of the support of relatives and family, who realize that patients may not be exactly the same after the injury and they may react differently to stresses and emotional stimuli and have difficulty achieving adaptive responses and behaviors.

The relationship of head injury to psychiatric illness is not easily defined by modern techniques, which do not provide an understanding of neuropsychiatric disorders after injury.

Electroencephalography and sleep EEG may be useful in those with closed head injury and the post-traumatic syndrome. Abnormal sleep patterns have been found 5 years after head injury (Prigatano et al., 1982), and a correlation has been reported between the percentage of rapid eye movements (REM sleep and sleep fragmentation) and the development of behavior problems and symptoms of psychopathology after head injury. During the acute recovery period after head injury, a correlation between REM sleep percentage time and cognitive function has also been found. And, a post-traumatic hypersomnia is recognized. This is sometimes prominent 6 months or more after head injury (Association of Sleep Disorders Centers, 1979). The use of electroencephalography for prognostic purposes, however, is not as yet possible.

Schizophrenialike symptoms may follow head injury (Davison & Bagley, 1969; Lishman, 1978). Conversely, 15% of schizophrenics have had head injuries preceding their first psychotic episodes (Lishman, 1978). A variable number ranging from 0.07% to 9.8% of injured patients develop schizophrenialike psychosis (Davison & Bagley, 1969), and there is less genetic predisposition to schizophrenia in those with the disease and antecedent brain injury. Although focal brain lesions have not been clearly related to the subsequent development of schizophrenia, some have suggested that temporal lobe damage or diffuse brain damage is more likely to result in schizophrenia (Davison & Bagley, 1969).

A group of schizophrenics with brain atrophy and CT evidence of ventricular enlargement, together with intellectual deterioration, has been identified. These patients also show intellectual impairment on neuropsychologic tests (Johnstone et al., 1976). But, the distinction between chronic schizophrenics and those who have brain atrophy from other causes is difficult by these methods, and only 54% can be correctly assigned to one or the other group. Chronic schizophrenics also have flattening of affect, retardation, and poverty of speech (Johnstone et al., 1978). Enlargement of ventricles, sometimes a sequela of head trauma, has been correlated with eventual clinical outcome, and the intellectual and memory deficits and social and vocational disabilities seem related to these radiographic findings (Levin et al., (1981). It is tempting to also relate ventricular enlargement to development of schizophrenialike post-traumatic symptoms. In addition, gliosis in the brain of chronic schizophrenics is found in the midbrain, diencephalon, and the limbic system, areas that may show significant damage after head trauma and that are linked to behavioral changes resembling chronic schizophrenia or post-traumatic symptoms (Stevens, 1982).

The posthead-injury depression is frequently associated with headache and is often expressed as discouragement, loss, and demoralization (Rimel, et al., 1982). The severity of the injury, the time after injury of onset of symptoms, and the location of focal neurologic deficits might be related to the development of this post-traumatic affective disturbance. The frontal and temporal lobes are often implicated in those with post-traumatic depression (Robinson & Szetela, 1981). The role of norepinephrine projections to the frontal lobe from the locus ceruleus in the genesis of these depressive disorders remains to be further assessed, but adrenergic agonists have been used in treatment of cognitive deficits (Arnsten & Goldman-Rakic, 1985).

Few neurochemical studies are available to determine the changes in neurotransmitters and neuromodulators that occur after head trauma. An increase in homovanillic acid and 5-hyroxyindoleacetic acid immediately following head injury has, however, been found (Van Woerkom et al., 1977). Moreover, the release of acetylcholine occurring simultaneously with trauma to the brain may be an additional trigger for postconcussive affective disorders (Ward, 1966).

The frequent personality changes after head injury and the accompanying post-traumatic headache have been attributed to diffuse brain damage. Emotional lability, a decrease in control of impulsive actions, apathy, and sometimes indifference associated with intellectual impairment are common (Levin et al., 1982). It is thought that, in a number of such cases, damage to localized brian areas or to neurotransmitter systems responsible for the integration of the personality is the cause of the syndrome, and frontal and temporal lobe personality disorders are frequently found because of the propensity of these areas of the brain to suffer damage. Such patients, particularly those with frontal lobe lesions, may have minimal or no detectable intellectual deficits on testing and show profound personality disorders, but special psychological tests such as the Wisconsin Card Sort and the Stylus Maze tests, may reveal an inability to change behavior in response to verbal signals, a lack of the capacity to follow instructions, and frequent impulsive mistakes (Milner, 1964).

In temporal lobe damage, personality disorders are common and often associated with complex partial seizures. Impulsivity, hyperorality, hypersexuality, visual agnosia, and impairment of memory are the features of more severely brain-injured patients and this, together with somatic complaints of headache and dizziness and the need to treat seizures, leads to polypharmacy and sometimes complicated personality changes resulting more from therapy than from the brain lesions. Sudden violent outbursts with minimal or no provocation in frontal and temporal lobe–damaged patients are often part of the syndrome. These outbursts are facilitated by excessive or immoderate alcohol intake and continued depression, which may perpetuate the aggressive outbursts and persistent psychosocial maladjustments. This, together with the somatization of complaints to the head and persistent headache, makes the management of such patients very difficult (Kwentus et al., 1985).

After head injury, the patient is an expert in this field, and an examination of patient's complaints may give a more complete description of post-traumatic states and generate hypotheses to explain the deficits found in such patients. An endless list of symptoms including headache with varying degrees of post-traumatic amnesia emerges from numerous inquiries; nevertheless, no stable constellation of complaints to satisfy the criteria for a "post-traumatic syndrome" has been found. In a review of 57 patients who sustained a severe closed head injury and who were followed up for 2 years, 84% reported some residual deficits in psychological function, forgetfulness heading the list. In seeking a relationship between post-traumatic amnesia and return to a preinjury work, forgetfulness, slowness, inability to concentrate, and inability to divide attention between two simultaneous activities were found to be positively related to the severity of the injury. Numerous other complaints were not related to severity. A similar pattern emerged when analyses were based on deficits as reported by patients' relatives, but the severity of injury was not related to the number of complaints. In addition, the longer the post-traumatic amnesia persisted, the less likely it was that a patient could resume work at preinjury levels (Van Zomeren & van den Burg, 1985).

Whiplash injury has multiple pathogenetic origins. It results from strain or rupture of paraspinous muscles or ligaments. Cartilage endplates or intervertebral disks may be avulsed and a traumatic arthropathy of the zygapophyseal joints may appear. Cervical spondylosis may predispose to whiplash injury and consequent post-traumatic headache arising from osteoarthritis of the cervical zygapophyseal joints or contraction of muscles resulting from splinting of the cervical spine reflexly and tension myalgia (Edmeads, 1978).

Treatment of these headaches is by heat, neck immobilization, sometimes manipulation and traction, or injection with local anesthetic and steroids. Several injections and the use of anti-inflammatory drugs or tricyclic antidepressants and analgesics are often successful. Some refractory patients may require anterior body fusion of a segment identified as the cause of headache by using distention and analgesic diskography (Pawl, 1977). This should rarely be necessary and should be preceded by a trial of neck immobilization in a collar.

INNERVATION OF CEREBRAL VESSELS—A PATHOGENETIC ROLE?

Patients with head injuries and a definite site of impact often complain of ipsilateral headaches during the post-traumatic period. There is no universally accepted explanation relating ipsilateral headache to symptomatic cerebral hemispheres in migraine, but a trigeminal innervation of the pia and arachnoidal vessels arising from ipsilateral trigeminal structures in the cat has been found. These nerve fibers release substance P, a vasodilator associated with pain perception. Ipsilateral trigeminal sensory responses to cortical stimulation by subdural electrodes in humans have also been reported (Lesser et al., 1985). These responses have been attributed to nerve fibers that accompany pial vessels, which are presumably related to the trigeminal vascular system (Moscowitz, 1984). These findings support the existence of such a perivascular plexus system in the human cerebrovasculature also. It is therefore conceivable that pain perception in those with unilateral head injuries may be ipsilateral to the injury and even be accompanied by visual phenomena sometimes found in patients with post-traumatic headache (Lesser et al., 1985).

The cerebral vessels, like other blood vessels, were until recently thought to be innervated only by sympathetic norepinephrine-containing nerve fibers that mediate constriction and parasympathetic acetylcholine-containing fibers thought to act in a dilatory fashion. This is clearly an incomplete view, since it has become obvious, using selective and sensitive immunohistochemical methods, that neuropeptides are also present in perivascular nerve fibers. Cerebral autoregulation of the vasculature depends in part on sympathetic nerves that modulate cerebral capacitance vessels (Edvinsson, 1982). It is possible, however, that the increasingly larger number of transmitter candidates found in walls of cerebral vessels of animals and humans may play a role as well. It has been suggested that they act by rapidly modifying vessel tone. They are thought to maintain homeostasis in the cerebral circulation, ensuring oxygen and glucose supplies adequate for brain function. The neuropeptides now demonstrated in perivascular nerve plexuses of cerebral vessels include neuropeptide Y (NPY) substance P (SP), calcitonin-gene-related peptide (CGRP), and vasoactive intestinal polypeptide (VIP), all of which probably act as neurotransmitters.

In addition, gastrin-releasing peptide (GRP), cholecystokinin, neurotensin, and somatostatin have also been found, but their role in the control of cerebral vessel tone is less well defined (Edvinsson, 1985).

Physiologic evidence shows that, apart from norepinephrine, vasoconstrictor activity results from cotransmitter-released NPY from sympathetic nerves, and fibers containing this peptide are abundant around major arteries supplying blood to the brain. The additional observation that NPY disappears after superior cervical sympathectomy or after the administration of 6-hydroxy-dopamine, a sympathetic ganglion poison, supports the coexistence of norepinephrine and NPY in sympathetic fibers (Edvinsson, 1985).

Direct neurogenic mechanisms mediating rapid dilatation of cerebral vessels have also been found. Metabolic factors that are released during normal and pathological states (e.g., epilepsy or head injury) are important in maintaining blood flow to the brain, but cholinergic mechanisms arising in central cholinergic neurons are also involved (Bartus et al. 1982). In addition, transmitters distinct from acetylcholine have been shown to cause dilatation of brain vessels. These transmitters are VIP and SP, stored in perivascular nerves in the cerebral vessels (Larsson et al., 1976; Edvinsson et al., 1981). Moreover, nerve fibers showing VIP immunoreactivity are found to a variable extent in the walls of cerebral arteries of laboratory animals and of humans. These fibers are found in the adventitia or at the adventitial medial border of the arteries and are most densely distributed in the rostral part of the circle of Willis. The origin of VIP-containing nerve fibers is not clear, but it has been suggested that they arise from local ganglia or in the brain itself. VIP causes relaxation of isolated cerebral arteries from all animals examined (Edvinsson & Ekman, 1984). Microapplication or superfusion of VIP causes cerebral vasodilatation and an increase in flow, and the experimental injection of VIP into the striaitum or the cortex causes metabolic activation with increases in local glucose consumption in both ipsilateral and contralateral homologous regions (McCulloch & Kelly, 1983). These and many other experimental findings suggest an important role for VIP in cerebral blood flow regulation.

The evidence for sensory nerve endings on intracranial vasculature has recently been strengthened. These endings are of particular importance in the mechanism of vascular head pain. In animals and humans, it is clear that the central portion of intracranial blood vessels are pain sensitive. In addition, meningeal manipulation and distention of dural arteries are all associated with pain. Stimulation of various parts of the vasculature in humans is associated with different types of pain; for example, the pial arteries at the base of the brain, when stimulated, cause a dull and intense ache. Substance P has been demonstrated around these blood vessels and might be a transmitter in some sensory fibers surrounding them. SP is thought to be important in transmission of nociceptor stimuli to the central nervous system through primary sensory neurons (Pernow, 1983). SP-containing fibers around cerebral arteries and veins in mammals and humans are not affected by removal of the superior cervical ganglion or chemical sympathectomy with 6-hydroxy-dopamine, but capsaicin treatment causes a significant loss of these fibers. The major effect of capsaicin is on the sensory system, which implies that SP-containing fibers may be part of the sensory trigeminal system but not part of the sympathetic ganglia (Hokfelt et al., 1980). SP is released from perivascular plexuses by a variety of stimuli, including electrical field stimulation; this suggests a neurotransmitter role for this peptide also.

Calcitonin gene-related peptide (CGRP) may also be involved in nociception and affects the autonomic and endocrine systems. Nerve fibers containing CGRP have been demonstrated by immunohistochemical techniques around cerebral arteries, and this peptide is thought to coexist with SP fibers in perivascular nerve plexuses. CGRP is potentially of great importance in regulating cerebral blood flow. Gastrin-releasing peptide (GRP) is strikingly homologous with the amphibian peptide bombesin. Its presence has been demonstrated around cerebral vessels, but neither GRP nor bombesin are of physiologic importance in experimental cerebral blood flow studies. Low levels of somatostatin have also been found around some cerebral vessels in experimental animals, but the importance of this peptide in the cerebral circulatory regulation is problematic.

Peptides affect cerebral blood flow and, in turn, are influenced by the electrical activity of brain structures, which is clearly deranged at some point in association with cerebral trauma. The effect of trauma on peptides, and consequently on cerebral blood flow and pain, has not been investigated in animals or humans. It is tempting to speculate, however, that the intimate morphologic association of peptide-containing perivascular nerve plexuses, and their partial origin in sympathetic extracranial systems or in the brain itself and effect on the blood–brain barrier subsequent to changes in vasomotor function, may profoundly influence the post-traumatic course of individual patients and their eventual symptomatology.

EFFECTS IN CHILDREN

Prominent symptoms are seen in children sometimes after relatively minor head trauma. Temporary neurologic deficits including post-traumatic blindness (Griffith & Dodge, 1968), hemiparesis (Pickles, 1949), somnolence, irritability, and vomiting (Mealy, 1968) have been reported and associated with the syndrome of post-traumatic migraine. In children, post-traumatic attacks associated with focal neurologic deficits resulting from head trauma are transient in nature and have a tendency to recur. They resemble those described in British soccer players who develop classic migraine after heading the ball or receiving other minor blows to the head (Matthews, 1972).

A study of 25 children with transient post-traumatic neurologic focal deficits pro-duced a constellation of clinical findings. Hemiparetic blindness and somnolent irri-table states were attributed to involvement of the cerebral vasculature. This syndrome resembles classic migraine and presumably has a similar pathogenesis. Head trauma may affect perivascular peptide–containing nerve plexuses and may lead to release of neurotransmitters and neuromodulators, with subsequent migrainous symptoms. In general, patients with this syndrome sustain a blow to the head, which is sufficient to daze momentarily and rarely causes transient unconsciousness. A latent interval between the trauma and the onset of neurologic symptoms is usual and this varies from seconds to hours; but in the majority, the focal neurologic deficits appear within minutes. Many such post-traumatic attacks in children are mistaken for cerebral con-cussion or contusion or acute epidural or subdural hematomas, but it is more likely that they are migrainous in nature.

Some patients with this syndrome studied by angiography showed occlusion of branches of the middle cerebral arteries after transient focal neurologic deficits. Such attacks might, therefore, reliably be attributed to vascular spasms (Haas et al., 1975). Evidence of spasm of vessels triggered by trauma supports the similarity of this post-traumatic syndrome to classic migraine. It suggests that neurogenic mechanisms are primarily responsible for vascular phenomena and consequent focal neurologic defi-cits superimposed and complicated by dysfunction of the brain and of the nerve supply to its blood vessels.

LATE EFFECTS

Good recovery after closed head injury is not always assurance that deficits may not appear and be measurable at a later date. Twenty patients with good recovery from closed head injury, according to the Glasgow head injury scale, matched with a group of similar intelligence, language capacity, age, sex, and handedness, under-went intensive neuropsychologic examination. The results showed that, despite good immediate recovery, poorly defined symptoms including difficulties in concentration, irritability and fatigue, and problems with tasks comparable to those carried out prior to injury persisted. The previous history of these patients was unremarkable and did not include psychiatric, neurologic, medical, other behavioral disorders, or alcohol-ism. Results of verbal or performance vigilance tests, the Wechsler Memory Quo-tient, the trailmaking test, Wisconsin Card Sorting, and the Stroop Test including word list generating or indexes of aphasia and apraxia were no different from those of controls. Patients were, however, significantly worse on consonant trigram tests, which require the recall of three consonants after varying intervals of counting back-wards by threes, and on the Wechsler memory scale. The speed of tapping of the dominant finger was difficult for patients to assess, and the Stroop color time story delay reproduction, of the Wechsler memory scale, and perseverative errors were all abnormal.

The two groups were best distinguished from each other by the trigram consonant test and the delay in the Wechsler memory scale. Both of these could correctly clas-sify 85% of participants in this study. Subtle deficiencies may remain even after good recovery, and the most important impairment involves the amount of information that can simultaneously be handled by postinjured patients (Stuss et al., 1985).

REFERENCES

Adeloye, A. (1971). Clinic trial of fluphenazine in the post-concussional syndrome. *Practitioner 206:*517–518.

Arnsten, A.F.T. and P.S. Goldman-Rakic (1985). α2-adrenergic mechanisms in prefrontal cortex associated with cognitive decline in aged non-human primates. *Science 230:*1273–1276.

Association of Sleep Disorders Centers (1979). Diagnostic classification of sleep-wake disorders. *Sleep 2:*5–119.

Bartus, R.T., R.L. Dean III, B. Beer, and A.S. Lippa (1982). The cholinergic hypothesis of geriatric memory dysfunction. *Science 217:*408–417.

Brenner, C., A.P. Friedman, H.H. Merritt, and D.E. Denny-Brown (1944). Post-traumatic headache. *J. Neurosurg. 1:*379–391.

Brooks, D.N. (1972). Memory and head injury. *J. Nerv. Ment. Dis. 155:*350–355.

Caveness, W.F. (1979). Incidence of craniocerebral trauma in the United States in 1976 and trends from 1970–1975. In *Advances in Neurology,* Vol. 22 (R.A. Thompson and J. R. Green, eds.), pp. 1–3.

Courville, C.B. (1950). Contributions to the study of cerebral anoxia. *Bull. Los Angeles Neurol. Soc. 15:*99–103.

Davison, K. and C.R. Bagley (1969). Schizophrenia-like psychosis associated with organic disorders of the central nervous system. *Br. J. Psychiatry 4 (Suppl.):*113–184.

de Morsier G. (1943) Les encéphalopathies traumatiques. Étude neurologique. *Schweiz. Arch. Neurol. Neurochir. Psychiat. 50:*161–169.

Edmeads, J. (1978). Headaches and head pains associated with diseases of the cervical spine. *Med. Clin. North Am. 62:*533–544.

Edvinsson, L. (1982) Sympathetic control of cerebral circulation. *Trends Neurosci. 5:*425–429.

Edvinsson, L. (1985). Functional role of perivascular peptides in the control of cerebral circulation. Trends Neurosci. 8: 126–131.

Edvinsson, L. and R. Ekman (1984). Distribution and dilatory effect of vasoactive intestinal polypeptide (VIP) in human cerebral arteries. *Peptides 5:*329–331.

Edvinsson L., J. McCulloch, and R. Uddman (1981). Substance P: Immunohistochemical localization and effect upon cat pial arteries in vitro and in situ. *J. Physiol. (London) 318:*251–258.

Friedman, A.P. and H.H. Merritt (1945). Relationship of intracranial pressure and presence of blood in the cerebrospinal fluid to the occurrence of headaches in patients with injuries to the head. *J. Nerv. Ment. Dis. 102:*1–7.

Friedmann, M. (1892). Über eine besondere schwere From von Folgezustanden nach Gehirnerschutterung und über den vasomotorischen Symptomenkomplex bei der selben in Allgemeinen. *Arch. Psychiat. 23:*230–267.

Griffith D.F. and P.R. Dodge (1968). Transient blindness following head injury in children. *N. Engl. J. Med. 278:*648–651.

Gronwall, D. and P. Wrightson (1974). Delayed recovery of intellectual function after minor head injury. *Lancet II:*605–609.

Gurdjian, E.S. and J.E. Webster (1958). *Head Injuries, Mechanisms, Diagnosis and Management.* Little, Brown, Boston.

Guttman, L. (1943). Post-contusional headache. *Lancet I:*10–12.

Haas D.C., G.S. Pineda, and H. Lourie (1975). Juvenile head trauma syndromes and their relationship to migraine. *Arch. Neurol. 32:*727–730.

Heyck, H. (1975). *Der Kopfschmerz,* 4th ed., p. 218. Georg Thieme Verlag, Stuttgart.

Hokfelt T., O. Johansson, A. Ljungdahl et al. (1980). Peptidergic neurones. *Nature (London) 284:*515–521.

Jennett, B. and G. Teasdale (1981). *Management of Head Injuries.* F.A. Davis, Philadelphia.

Johnstone, E.C., T.J. Crow, C.D. Frith et al. (1976). Cerebral ventricular size and cognitive impairment in chronic schizophrenia. *Lancet II:*924–926.

Johnstone, E.C., T.J. Crow, C.D. Frith et al. (1978). The dementia of dementia praecox. *Acta Psychiat. Scand. 57:*305–324.

Kay, D.W.K., T.A. Derr, and L.P. Lassman (1971). Brain trauma and the postconcussion syndrome. *Lancet II:*1052–1055.

Kwentus, J.A., R.P. Hart, E.T. Peck et al. (1985). Psychiatric complications of closed head trauma. *Psychosomatics 26:*8–17.

Larsson, L.I., L. Edvinsson, J. Fahrenkrug et al. (1976). Immunohistochemical localization of a vasodilatory polypeptide (VIP) in cerebrovascular nerves. *Brain Res. 113:*400–404.

Lesser, R.P., H. Luders, G. Klem et al. (1985). Ipsilateral trigeminal sensory responses to cortical stimulation by subdural electrodes. *Neurology 35:*1760–1763.

Levin, H.S., A.L. Benton, and R.G. Grossman (1982). *Neurobehavioral Consequences of Closed Head Injury.* Oxford University Press, New York.

Levin, H.S., C.A. Meyers, R.C. Crossman et al. (1981). Ventricular enlargement after closed head injury. *Arch. Neurol. 38:*623–629.

Lindvall, F. (1974). Causes of postconcussional syndrome. *Acta Neurol. Scand. 56 (Suppl.):*1–145.

Lishman, W.A. (1978). *Organic Psychiatry.* Blackwell Scientific Publications, London.

Matthews, W.B. (1972). Footballer's migraine. *Br. Med. J. 2:*326–327.

McCulloch, J. and P.A.T. Kelly (1983). A functional role for vasoactive intestinal polypeptide in anterior cingulate cortex. *Nature (London) 304:*438–440.

Mealy, J., Jr. (1968). *Pediatric Head Injuries,* pp. 56–57. Charles C Thomas, Springfield, Ill.

Merrett, J.D., and J.R. McDonald (1977). Sequellae of concussion caused by minor head injury. *Lancet 1:*1–4.

Miller, H. (1961). Accident neurosis. *Br. Med. J. 1:*919–925, 992–998.

Miller, H. (1968). Post-traumatic headache. In *Handbook of Clinical Neurology,* Vol 5 (P.J. Vinken and G.W. Bruyn eds.), pp. 178–184. North-Holland Publishing, Amsterdam.

Milner, B. (1964). Some effects of frontal lobectomy in man. In *The Frontal Granular Cortex and Behavior* (J.M. Warren and K. Akert, eds.), pp. 313–334. McGraw-Hill, New York.

Moskowitz, M.A. (1984). The neurology of vascular head pain. *Ann Neurol. 16:*157–168.

Nick, J. and C. Sicard-Nick (1969). Chronic post-tramatic headache. In *Research and Clinical Studies in Headache,* Vol. II (A.P. Friedman, ed.), pp. 115–168. Karger, Basel.

Oppenheimer, D.R. (1968). Microscopic lesions in the brain following head injury. *J. Neurol. Neurosurg. Psychiat. 31:*299–306.

Pawl, R.P. (1977). Headache, cervical spondylosis and anterior cervical fusion. *Surg. Ann. 9:*391–408.

Penfield, W. and N. Norcross (1936) Subdural traction and post-traumatic headache. Study of pathology and therapeusis. *Arch. Neurol. Psychiatry 36:*75–94.

Pernow, B. (1983). Substance P. *Pharmacol. Rev. 35:*85–141.

Pickles, W. (1949). Acute focal edema of the brain in children with head injuries. *N. Engl. J. Med. 240:*92–95.

Prigatano, G., M. Stahl, W. Orr et al. (1982). Sleep and dreaming disturbances in closed head injury patients. *J. Neurol. Neurosurg. Psychiatry 45:*78–80.

Rigler, J. (1879). *Über die Folgen der Verletzungen auf Eisenbahnen, insbesondere der Verletzungen des Ruckenmarks.* G. Reimer, Berlin.

Rimel, R., B. Giordani, J. Barth et al. (1982). Moderate head injury: Completing the clinical spectrum of brain trauma. *Neurosurgery 11:*344–351.

Robinson, R.C. and B. Szetela (1981). Mood change following left hemisphere brain injury. *Ann. Neurol. 9:*447–453.

Russell, W.R. (1933–34). The after-effects of head injury. *Trans. Med. Chir. Soc. Edinb. 113:*129–141.

Simons, D.J. and H. G. Wolff (1946). Studies on headache; mechanisms of chronic post-traumatic headache. *Psychosom. Med. 8:*227–242.

Stevens, J.R. (1982). Neuropathology of schizophrenia. *Arch. Gen. Psychiatry 39:*1121–1129.

Strich, S.J. (1956) Diffuse degeneration of the cerebral white matter in severe dementia following head injury. *J. Neurol. Neurosurg Psychiatry 19:*163–185.

Strumpell, A. (1888). *Über die traumatische Neurosen.* Gustav Fischer, Berlin.

Stuss, D.T., P. Ely, H. Hugenholtz et al. (1985). Subtle neuropsychological deficits in patients with good recovery after closed head injury. *Neurosurgery 17:*41–47.

Symonds, C.P. (1942). Discussion on differential diagnosis and treatment of post-contusional states. *Proc. Roy. Soc. Med. 35:*601–607.

Symonds, C.P. (1960). Post-traumatic headache. In *Injuries to the Brain and Spinal Cord* (S. Brock, ed.). Cassell, London.

Toglia, J.V., E. Rozenberg, and M. Ronis (1970). Post-traumatic dizziness. *Arch. Otolaryngol. 92:*485–492.

Tonnis, W. (1956). Beobachtungen an frischen gedeckten Hirnschadigungen. In *Das Hirntrauma* (R. Rehwald, ed.), pp. 77–111. Thieme, Stuttgart.

Tyler, S., H. McNelly, and L. Dick (1980) Treatment of post-traumatic headache with amitriptyline. *Headache 20:*213–216.

Van Woerkom, T.C.A.M., A.W. Teelken, and J. M. Minderhound (1977). Difference in neurotransmitter metabolism in frontotemporal-lobe contusion and diffuse cerebral contusion. *Lancet I:*812–813.

Van Zomeren, A.H., and W. van den Burg (1985). Residual complaints of patients two years after severe head injury. *J. Neurol. Neurosurg. Psychiatry 48:*21–28.

Vijayan, N., and P.M. Dreyfus (1975). Post-traumatic dysautonomic cephalalgia. *Arch. Neurol. 32:*649–652.

Ward, A.A. (1966). The physiology of concussion. In *Head Injury Conference Proceedings* (W.F. Caveness and A.E. Walker, eds.), pp. 203–208. J.B. Lippincott, Philadelphia.

Wepfer, J.J. (1727). Observationes medicopracticae de affectibus capitis internis et externis. Observation 10, Schaffhausen.

17

Headache and the Eye

THOMAS J. CARLOW

Headache is commonly localized to the eye and periorbital region. Without obvious ocular pathology, the eye itself is rarely responsible for the pain and discomfort (Chamlin, 1962; Lance, 1973; Cameron, 1976; Carlow & Appenzeller, 1976; Behrens, 1978; Newman & Burde, 1979; Worthen, 1980). The main topics discussed in this chapter are the neuroanatomy of eye pain, refractive and muscle imbalance headache, disease of the eye and orbit, referred eye pain, and photophobia.

NEUROANATOMY OF EYE PAIN

The ophthalmic division of the trigeminal nerve carries afferent pain fibers from the orbit and periorbital region. Painful sensation is carried in this division from the cornea, ciliary body, iris, lacrimal gland, conjunctiva, nasal mucous membrane, eyelid, eyebrow, forehead, and scalp anterior to a coronal plane bisecting the head at the ears. In the cavernous sinus (Whitnall, 1932; Penfield & McNaughton, 1940; Ray & Wolff, 1940; Feindel et al., 1960), the trigeminal nerve branches to innervate the major vessels at the base of the brain, the cerebellar tentorium, falx cerebri, and cranial nerves 3, 4, and 6. The anterior fossa and sphenoid wing (McNaughton, 1937) are sparsely supplied by a few small ophthalmic nerve branches. The nasociliary nerve separates from the ophthalmic division at the level of the anterior cavernous sinus. After entering the orbit, it divides into multiple long ciliary nerves that course with the optic nerve to the base of the globe, then traverses the eye between the sclera and choroid to supply the ciliary body, iris, and cornea. Two other major ophthalmic branches enter the orbit at the superior orbital fissure. The frontal nerve hugs the orbit roof, then splits into the supratrochlear and supraorbital nerve supplying the forehead near the midline, the upper eyelid, and the superior lateral nose. The lacrimal nerve passes laterally in the orbit to innervate the lacrimal gland and a small area of the upper outer eyelid (Chapter 3).

REFRACTIVE DISORDERS AND MUSCLE IMBALANCE

Refractive disorders and muscle imbalance have been overemphasized as a source of ocular headache. Despite symptomatic relief achieved with correction of a refractive error or ocular motor imbalance, the etiologic site for "eye-strain" headache (Mitchell, 1876) may be quite distant from the eye. Excessive accommodation and/or prolonged sustained extraocular muscle contraction have been formulated as explanations for this type of headache (Worthen, 1980). Bilateral orbital heaviness with a steady, dull, frontal, bitemporal headache typically manifests when school work or other activity requires prolonged close work. Sleep or simply eye closure commonly relieves this afternoon or evening headache that is temporally related to sustained eye use. It is never associated with other systemic symptomatology, such as nausea or vomiting.

Refractive Disorders

Myopia, hypermetropia, astigmatism, and presbyopia are common refractive errors. Myopia is the only refractive disorder unrelated to "ocular" headache. Hypermetropia, astigmatism, and presbyopia can be partially corrected by either excessive accommodation or sustained extraocular muscle contraction, supporting the theories explaining refractive headache. Eckardt and associates (1943) experimentally induced refractive errors resulting in bilateral periorbital heaviness and occasional frontal and bitemporal or even occipital headache in hyperopia and astigmatism but not in myopia.

When two retinal images fail to fuse, a marked difference in image size or aniseikonia may be responsible, secondary to a pronounced asymmetry in ocular refractive power or anisometropia. Eye strain headaches have been attributed to aniseikonia and anisometropia and have been alleviated with refractive lenses designed to equalize the retinal image size disparity. This form of "ocular" headache may be primarily psychogenic.

Strabismus

Strabismus, or muscle imbalance, very rarely produces headache following prolonged, sustained extraocular muscle effort to maintain monocular vision. Simultaneous contraction of neck and scalp muscles may contribute to the cephalgia, however, cervical electromyography in tension headache and migraine has not shown a difference between the headache and headache-free states (Pozniak-Patewicz, 1976). Hyperphoria is the only statistically significant muscle imbalance related to ocular headache (Waters, 1970). A full medical and neurologic examination should be performed before prescribing prisms for muscle imbalance headache, particularly for a vertical dissociation, to oviate missing a posterior fossa or orbital lesion.

Convergence Insufficiency

Convergence insufficiency, in contradistinction to other heterophorias, can be responsible for ocular headache and is frequently overlooked. Generalized headache maximal in the periorbital region, blurred near vision, and horizontal diplopia with prolonged close work are common complaints. Reading will typically be unimpaired for a short period, followed by the preceding symptomatology; complaints resolve with nonconvergent tasks and recur with repeated attempts at close work. Occasionally, an initial presbyopic correction can uncover convergence insufficiency; accommodation relaxes, resulting in an increased need for convergence with any near activity.

Two simple bedside tests are useful (Burian & Van Noorden, 1974). First, determine the point where a fixation target moving toward the nasion blurs or appears double and/or one eye breaks fixation and drifts outward. The distance from this point to the outer orbital rim is the objective near point of convergence (NPC)—normal is 5 to 10 cm. If the NPC is 20 to 30 cm from the orbital rim, convergence insufficiency can be diagnosed. A second method uses a red glass placed before one eye and determines the point where a white fixation light, again moving toward the nasion, splits or is perceived as a red and white light. The distance from this break point to the outer orbital rim is the subjective NPC. The subjective and objective NPC have the same significance. Orthoptic exercises to strengthen convergence can be beneficial. A fixation target held at arms length is followed in to the tip of the nose as the arm is flexed and then out again as the arm is extended. This can be combined with jump exercises, a near point is fixated alternately with a distant target. These orthoptic exercises should be performed for 5 to 10 minutes, two to three times daily. Base-in prisms in a bilateral bifocal distribution can relieve the ocular symptomatology in those refractory to orthoptic exercises, such as Parkinson's disease. This subjective discomfort can also be ameliorated by occluding one eye during periods of extensive near work.

Ocular Neurosis

Headache and "eye strain" beginning abruptly and coincident with any attempt to read or use the eyes, in the presence of a normal ophthalmologic examination should be considered an ocular neurosis (Derby, 1930). Despite reassurance, these patients are frequently convinced that their symptoms are secondary to their glasses or an ocular muscle weakness. Psychotherapy should be instituted; recalcitrant cases may require psychiatric consultation.

DISEASE OF THE EYE AND ORBIT

Conjunctiva, Cornea

Conjunctivitis causes minimal orbital discomfort with diffuse vascular injection and mild photophobia. The conjunctiva contains relatively few pain fibers, which ac-

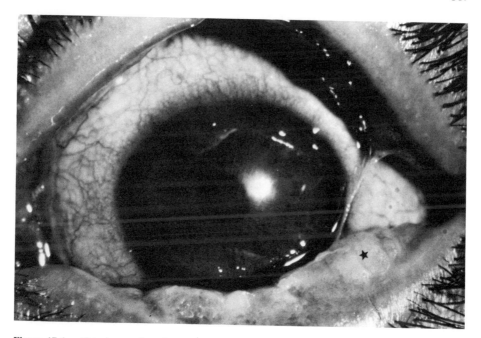

Figure 17-1. Chronic vernal conjunctivitis with an edematous, boggy palpebral conjunctiva (star) and diffusely injected bulbar conjunctiva.

counts for the marked inflammatory response (Figure 17-1) without severe pain. Tearing and itching are evident, it can be separated from other causes of a red or injected eye by a normal visual acuity, pupil, and cornea exam. Treatment depends on the underlying etiology.

Severe pain and tenderness will result from either trauma to or a foreign body on or in the cornea. Intense photophobia is combined with diffuse conjunctival injection, lacrimation, and blepharospasm. Corneal edema may cause minimally impaired visual acuity, but the pupillary examination will be normal. If untreated, a mild iritis may result, with miosis and anterior chamber inflammation. Once the offending agent has been removed, pain can be relieved with a cycloplegic drug and a pressure patch. Antibiotics should be added under the direction of an ophthalmologist.

Recurrent corneal erosion syndrome can resemble cluster or other forms of episodic headache. It can follow corneal injury or infection, is unilateral, involving the forehead and periorbital region, and is associated with marked blepharospasm and photophobia. The pain frequently occurs upon awakening or after sustained eye closure. Slit lamp examination will document a corneal epithelial break. Pressure patching during the period of reepithelialization can give substantial pain relief.

Iris, Ciliary Body

Uveitis includes inflammation of the iris, ciliary body, and/or choroid. It can be subdivided into anterior uveitis involving the iris (iritis), or ciliary body (cyclitis), or both (iridocyclitis), and posterior uveitis involving the choroid (choroiditis), or retina and choroid (chorioretinitis). Two major types of uveitis, nongranulomatous and granulomatous, may be distinguished both clinically and pathologically. Anterior uveitis is typically nongranulomatous; it can be an autoimmune or collagen vascular disorder, and in the majority of cases has no clear etiology. Granulomatous uveitis is more diffuse with pathologic signs in the posterior and anterior uvea. Both a slit lamp examination and indirect ophthalmoscopy are required to identify and localize uveitis. Anterior uveitis or iritis is an important source of orbital pain. Eye discomfort is moderately severe in the distribution of the trigeminal ophthalmic division. Vision is blurred with marked photophobia, lacrimation, a clear cornea, and miotic pupil. Marked limbal injection, corneal and scleral junction, is a hallmark of anterior uveitis. The eye is tender, with periorbital discomfort worse at night and in the early morning hours. Pain may be referred to the ear, teeth, or sinuses. Marked reduction of headache intensity and orbital discomfort can follow the instillation of mydriatics. A definitive diagnosis can be elusive, requiring topical or systemic antibiotics and/or steroids.

Glaucoma is responsible for 15% of all blindness in the United States (Scheie & Albert, 1969). It is clinically useful to classify glaucoma as angle closure, open-angle, a combination of angle closure and open angle, or congenital (Kolker & Hetherington, 1970).

Severe ocular pain that spreads to involve the entire head characterizes acute-angle closure glaucoma. Blurred vision and marked photophobia with nausea and vomiting, can be intense enough to suggest laparotomy. Examination reveals a mid-dilated pupil, a steamy edematous cornea (Figure 17-2), and an exquisitely tender eye. Minimal ocular compression demonstrates a hard rigid globe and intensifies the ocular and periocular pain. The normal flow of aqueous fluid from the posterior chamber into the anterior chamber, to be absorbed by the trabecular meshwork and canal of Schlemm, is blocked at the pupil and at the angle formed by the iris and the cornea by a forward iris displacement. Intensive miotic therapy, carbonic anhydrase inhibitors, glycerol, and intravenous urea or mannitol can lower intraocular pressure and relieve the headache and eye discomfort. Angle closure glaucoma can be a surgical emergency and should be referred to an ophthalmic surgeon.

A low-grade diffuse headache can be present for years before open-angle glaucoma is diagnosed and decreased visual acuity noted. Examination documents a pale optic nerve head with a large vertically aligned optic cup (Figure 17-3), retinal nerve fiber layer drop out, and the corresponding visual field deficit. Intraocular pressures range between 30 and 45 mm Hg, presumably from decreased trabecular meshwork porosity. Open-angle glaucoma is an urgent ophthalmologic problem and should be referred to an opthalmologist.

Optic Neuritis

Pain with eye movement is encountered in optic neuritis, influenza, orbital cellulitis, orbital periostitis, and myositis (Roy, 1975). Retro-orbital pain has been reported in 60% of patients with optic neuritis; one third have ocular pain with eye movement. Pain commonly commences when the eyes are moved in one direction and may

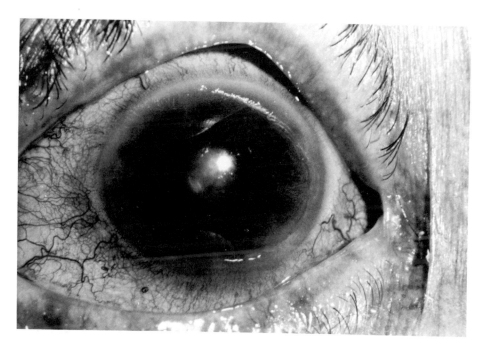

Figure 17-2. Acute angle closure glaucoma with a mid-dilated fixed pupil, steamy cornea, and diffusely injected bulbar conjunctiva.

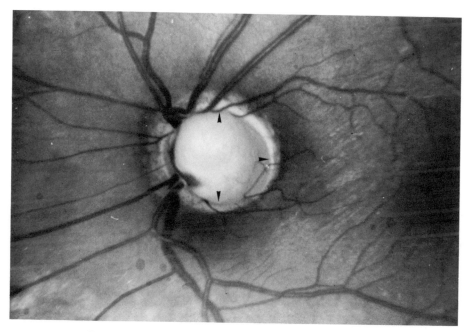

Figure 17-3. Severely cupped (arrows) glaucomatous optic nerve.

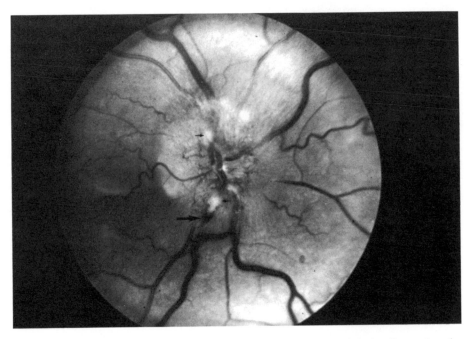

Figure 17-4. Papillitis is seen with a swollen optic nerve, dilated veins, exudates (small arrows), and a hemorrhage off the nerve head (large arrow).

proceed or follow the onset of visual dysfunction. The eye and periorbital region may be tender to mild pressure. Long ciliary nerve irritation coursing adjacent to the swollen optic nerve sheath is the theoretical source for the ocular discomfort. Visual loss deteriorates over days to weeks, plateaus for several weeks, then slowly improves to normal or near-normal visual acuity in 85 to 90% of cases within 6 months (Nikoskelainen & Riekkinen, 1973). The majority of patients with retrobulbar optic neuritis will have a normal-appearing optic nerve head; 20% will have a papillitis or swollen optic nerve head (Figure 17-4) clinically indistinquishable from unilateral papilledema without an assessment of visual function. Color vision and brightness comparison will be depressed and an afferent pupillary defect, Marcus Gunn pupil, will be observed on the involved side. If the ocular discomfort and eye pain are intense, prompt relief can be achieved with a burst of oral corticosteroids, whether or not this treatment preserves vision and reduces visual loss is unclear and controversial. Because the majority of isolated optic neuritis cases are idiopathic, the workup should be directed to the treatable causes, such as inflammation and infection.

Orbital Tumor

Primary orbital neoplasms are usually not associated with headache and eye pain. Metastatic orbital tumors and neoplasms that erode the orbital bony vault—for example, nasopharyngeal carcinoma—can cause severe frontal head pain when the trigeminal ophthalmic division is compromised.

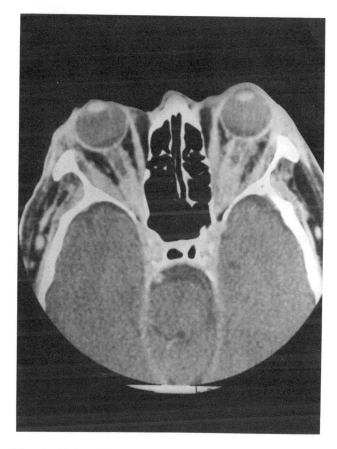

Figure 17-5. Bilateral orbital pseudotumor with enlarged extraocular muscles and swollen optic nerve sheaths.

Orbital Pseudotumor

Orbital pseudotumor is responsible for approximately 10% of all exophthalmus (Ingalls, 1953; Henderson & Farrow, 1973) and is the only orbital lesion that consistently demonstrates both proptosis and orbital pain. This nonspecific inflammatory process will cause abrupt orbital pain, unilateral and sometimes bilateral proptosis, conjunctival chemosis, and ophthalmoplegia with diplopia. Idiopathic orbital pseudotumor may have an elevated erythrocyte sedimentation rate while all other laboratory studies are normal. A CT scan (Figure 17-5) can help to separate this orbital process from disorders that mimic it clinically. A reactive adjacent sinus inflammation and a swollen, enlarged optic nerve may complicate CT scan interpretation. Dramatic resolution of proptosis, ophthalmoplegia, orbital pain, and visual loss can be seen 24 to 48 hours after initiating high-dose oral corticosteroids. Orbital cellulitis with lid and conjunctival edema, proptosis, and tenderness of the globe on retropulsion can give a similar clinical picture. Fever, prostration, an elevated white blood count with an abnormal differential, tenderness over the sinuses, radiographic studies, and otolaryngologic consultation can help to separate these two entities.

Thyroid Orbitopathy

Thyroid orbitopathy does not cause severe orbital pain, however, patients can complain of relatively intolerable pain with eye movement, particularly with upgaze. High-dose corticosteroids can provide remarkable pain relief; however, the pain frequently returns with any attempt to taper or discontinue treatment.

Orbital Trauma

Orbital pain may follow significant orbital trauma (Sutula & Weiter, 1980) or surgery. Removal of a neuroma formed from the end of a severed nerve may resolve the ocular discomfort (Wolter & Benz, 1964; Folberg et al., 1981).

Superior Orbital Fissuritis—Tolosa–Hunt Syndrome

Multiple cranial nerves and blood vessels enter the orbit through the superior orbital fissure. Nongranulomatous or granulomatous disease of this bony aperture can result in a severe, boring, retro-orbital pain with involvement of cranial nerves 2 through 6, a superior orbital fissuritis, or Tolosa–Hunt syndrome (Smith & Taxdal, 1966). Retro-orbital pain commonly precedes a third nerve paresis, with subsequent involvement of the fourth, fifth, sixth, and second cranial nerves. Pupil sparing is seen in approximately 50% of cases, and 10% show signs of impaired vision (Schatz & Farmer, 1972). Because this syndrome can be produced with tumor, aneurysm, or an inflammatory disease such as systemic lupus erythrohematosis or syphilis, a complete laboratory and neuroradiologic evaluation is mandatory. Magnetic resonance imaging (MRI) may prove to be the only study needed to permit a therapeutic trial of corticosteroids. This boring retro-orbital pain can be totally relieved within 24 hours after beginning systemic corticosteroids. The ophthalmoplegia can require weeks or months to resolve. Without treatment, symptoms can persist for months only to remit spontaneously and then recur at irregular intervals. The superior orbital fissure syndrome and pseudotumor of the orbit may be a pathologic continuum delineated only by locale.

Herpetic and Postherpetic Trigeminal Neuralgia

Herpetic and postherpetic involvement of the trigeminal ophthalmic division results in a steady, uncomfortable, irritating temporal and periorbital pain that can precede the herpetic rash by several days. Rash regression requires 2 to 3 weeks, with either total resolution or a postherpetic neuralgia. Corneal infiltrates and an iritis are frequently observed when the rash involves the nose; the nasociliary nerve supplies both areas. Herpetic trigeminal neuralgia can be differentiated from tic douloureaux by its steady, sustained, burning, nonstaccato character. Treatment of the acute and post-herpetic rash phases can be extremely discouraging. Levodopa (Kernbaum & Hauche-corne, 1981) begun during the acute phase can decrease the intensity of the pain and the incidence of postherpetic neuralgia. Postherpetic neuralgia can be intractable to all current treatment; however, high-dose amitriptyline (Taub, 1973), baclofen (Fromm et al., 1984), narcotics, and a trancutaneous stimulator may be tried.

REFERRED EYE PAIN

Pathologic involvement of structures innervated by the trigeminal ophthalmic nerve in the cavernous sinus (Thomas & Yoss, 1970) and meningial ophthalmic division branches that supply the cerebellar tentorium, falx cerebri, cribiform plate, and sphenoid wing can cause pain referrable to the eye and periorbital region. Detailed discussions of many of these disorders can be found in the appropriate chapter—for example, aneurysm, temporal arteritis, cluster headache, ophthalmoplegic migraine, temporal mandibular joint syndrome, and nasopharyngeal carcinoma.

Isolated Painful Oculomotor Palsy

A supraclinoid aneurysm (Green et al., 1964; Rucker, 1966; Rush & Younge, 1981) is the most common cause of an isolated third-nerve palsy or paralysis. Thirty percent of all intracranial aneurysms lie at the junction of the internal carotid and posterior communicating artery. Of those with intracranial aneurysms, 50% will develop a third-nerve paresis, with women predominating. Retro-orbital pain (Soni, 1974) can precede the third-nerve paresis, by up to 2 weeks, in the trigeminal ophthalmic nerve distribution. When the pupil is dilated and fixed to a *bright* light a supraclinoid aneurysm at the junction of the internal carotid and posterior communicating artery compressing the third nerve as it enters the posterior aspect of the cavernous sinus must be a primary consideration.

The next most common etiology for an isolated third-nerve paresis is vascular disease which includes hypertension and diabetes mellitus. Similar to supraclinoid aneurysm, eye pain may antedate the onset of diplopia and the third-nerve paresis by days to weeks; however, the pupil is spared (Goldstein & Cogan, 1960; Nadeau & Trobe, 1983). This oculomotor paresis is not dependent on the degree of diabetic or hypertensive control. The diplopia may disappear within weeks or persist for several months. Without definite subjective and objective signs of improvement at 3 months, other etiologies should be considered.

The diagnostic evaluation of an isolated painful oculomotor paresis or paralysis is somewhat controversial; primarily it depends on pupillary involvement. If the pupil is fixed to a bright light, a cerebral angiogram (possibly only an MRI) is mandatory, particularly with evidence of subarachnoid hemorrhage (SAH). If the pupil responds to light, a minimum of two fasting blood sugars, a hypertensive workup, and com-plete neurologic examination are suggested. Rarely, an internal carotid–posterior communicating artery aneurysm may present without pupillary involvement or SAH, with pupillary dysfunction delayed for 7 days (Kissel et al., 1983). Close observation with a reevaluation at 7 days is required. If the oculomotor paresis is not resolving by the third month or if no evidence of diabetes of hypertension can be documented, a complete clinical and laboratory evaluation including CBC, sedimentation rate, FTA, ANA, thyroid screen, Tensilon test, forced ductions, possible lumbar puncture, CT scan, MRI, and cerebral angiography should be considered.

Raeder's Paratrigeminal Syndrome

Raeder's paratrigeminal syndrome (Grimson & Thompson, 1980) can be divided into migrainous and symptomatic varieties. In the migrainous form, an edematous intra-cavernous carotid artery underlies the ocular discomfort and sympathetic signs, whereas in the symptomatic form the etiology is a well-defined structural lesion with involvement of multiple parasellar cranial nerves. The migrainous form can be distinguished from cluster headache by the character and nature of the pain, it is continuous over weeks to months, and it is not grouped in clusters. Sympathetic signs of miosis, ptosis, and decreased supraorbital sweating are seen on the involved side. Oculosympathetic forehead sweat gland fibers follow the internal carotid artery, while the majority of the facial sudomotor fibers course with the external carotid artery. This "suicidal" pain has been relieved with ergotamine tartrate, methysergide, corticosteroids, lithium, and calcium-channel blockers.

Carotid Cavernous Fistula

Carotid cavernous fistulas may be congenital, atherosclerotic, or traumatic and become manifest when a carotid artery or one of its branches ruptures into the cavernous sinus. Ocular bruit, pulsating proptosis, conjunctival chemosis (Figure 17-6) and injection, diplopia, blurred vision, and periorbital pain and headache are all secondary to the raised orbital venous pressure. The pain can be moderately severe, constant, boring, and retro-orbital in character. Preservation of visual function and periorbital pain relief may require either a direct surgical or invasive neuroradiologic procedure.

Pituitary Apoplexy

Two thirds of pituitary adenoma patients have a chronic headache history, either mild or severe. Rarely, spontaneous hemorrhage into a pituitary adenoma causes severe headache, partial or complete ophthalmoplegia, and sudden bilateral blindness. Craniotomy or transphenoidal decompression combined with corticosteroid replacement can be life-saving.

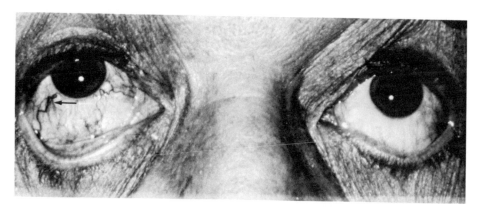

Figure 17-6. Carotid cavernous fistula with dilated bulbar conjunctival vessels (arrow).

Nasopharyngeal Carcinoma

Godtfredsen (1965) found that 25% of nasopharyngeal carcinoma patients presented with ocular signs alone, primarily pain or numbness in the first or second trigeminal nerve division. Seventy percent of his entire series had first and second trigeminal division neuralgias, 65% had ophthalmoplegia, 17% had exophthalmus, and 16% had a Horner's syndrome. Otolaryngologic evaluation combined with a CT or MRI are required, particularly in a male in his seventh or eighth decade with unexplained chronic periorbital pain.

Vascular Disease

Ocular pain and headache (Andrell, 1943; Fisher, 1951; Currier et al., 1961; Fisher, 1968) have been documented with internal carotid, middle cerebral, posterior cerebral, and vertebrobasilar artery disease. The pain can be excrutiating, precede the stroke, and resolve or persist after the stroke ends. Acute or chronic carotid artery obstruction with insufficient collateralization can produce an injected painful globe, corneal edema, anterior chamber cells, a middilated pupil, cataract, rubeosis, abnormal intraocular pressure, retinal microaneurysms, neovascularization, and nerve fiber infarcts (Knox, 1969). Acute eye pain has resolved following endarterectomy for high-grade internal carotid artery stenosis (Cohen & McNamara, 1980).

Spontaneous internal carotid artery dissection (Figure 17-7) (Mokri et al., 1979) can result in ipsilateral periorbital head pain at the angle of the jaw and an ipsilateral Horner's syndrome. Anticoagulants may prevent further cerebral embarrassment from a subsequent distal thrombosis, and corticosteroids in high doses (Fisher, 1981) may dramatically relieve pain.

Severe orbital and supraorbital pain can occur ipsilateral to infarction in the vertebrobasilar artery distribution. It is usually described as a burning or soreness, which is transient or permanent. Currier et al. (1961) have postulated that this orbital pain

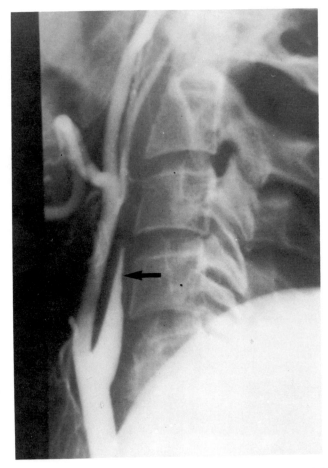

Figure 17-7. Internal carotid artery dissection is seen with a tapered (arrow) occluded internal carotid artery.

manifests when both the trigeminal descending and the brain-stem reticular pathways are involved simultaneously.

GREATER OCCIPITAL NEURALGIA

A frequently overlooked cause of isolated periorbital pain is an inflammation of the greater occipital nerve as it exits between the occiput and the first cervical vertebra to pierce the large cervical muscle tendinous insertions (Knox & Mustonene, 1975). Pain can begin in the occipital region, radiate over the scalp to the eye, or simply be isolated to the orbit (Bode, 1979; Lieppman, 1980). The periorbital referred pain is believed secondary to dysfunction in the descending brain-stem trigeminal pathways and greater occipital nerve fiber interconnections. A soft cervical collar at bedtime to prevent neck extension, hot packs, analgesics, physical therapy, and local anesthetic injection at a point halfway between the mastoid and greater occipital protuberance have all found advocates.

Photophobia

Photophobia, or intense painful intolerance to light exposure, has not been fully explained, especially without obvious ocular disease (Lebensohn, 1951). With iris irritation or inflammation, a light reflex inducing a miosis and iris traction can partially explain local or orbital photophobia. Severe photophobia can be evident in the absence of ocular pathology such as meningitis, SAH, migraine, and retrobulbar optic neuritis; this suggests a combined disturbance at the brain stem and cortical levels. (Worthen, 1980).

SUMMARY

- The eye is rarely responsible for headache and periorbital discomfort if ophthalmic signs are not obvious.
- Correction of refractive and strabismus disorders seldom relieves headache. Convergence insufficiency is an exception.
- "Eye-strain" headache commencing abruptly with any eye use is commonly the result of an ocular neurosis.
- Conjunctivitis and corneal lesions are treatable causes of headache. The recurrent corneal erosion syndrome can mimic cluster and other episodic headache disorders.
- Anterior uveitis and angle closure glaucoma are important treatable causes of headache that are best treated by an ophthalmologist.
- Periorbital pain and tenderness seen with optic neuritis is usually transient; however, when severe, responds to oral corticosteroids.
- Metastatic orbital tumors cause ocular pain whereas primary orbital tumors rarely cause headache.
- Orbital pseudotumor and the Tolosa–Hunt syndrome fall on a continuum of the same pathologic process. Both respond to corticosteroids, recur at irregular intervals, and simulate other pathologic processes.
- Any structure innervated by the ophthalmic division of the trigeminal nerve can be a source for referred eye pain.
- Oculomotor nerve palsy can be preceded by severe orbital and periorbital eye pain, commonly secondary to aneurysm or vascular disease. The pupillary examination usually separates these two entities.
- Cavernous sinus lesions are frequently responsible for referred eye pain, for example, Raeder's paratrigeminal syndrome, pituitary apoplexy, carotid cavernous fistula, and nasopharyngeal carcinoma.
- Disease of the anterior and posterior cerebral circulation can present with eye pain. Spontaneous internal carotid artery dissection pain can be treated with corticosteroids.

- Greater occipital neuralgia is a common treatable cause of ocular and head pain that is not well recognized.
- Photophobia may have an obvious orbital etiology or be unexplained and have both a central trigeminal and cortical substrate.

ACKNOWLEDGEMENTS

I would like to thank Michelle Thompson, medical transcriber, and Buddy Crofton, photographer, for their help in preparing this chapter.

REFERENCES

Andrell, P. (1943). Thrombosis of the internal carotid artery: A clinical study of nine cases diagnosed by arteriography. *Acta Med. Scand. 114:*336–372.

Behrens, M.M. (1978). Headaches associated with disorders of the eye. *Med. Clin. North Am.* 62:507.

Bode, D.D., Jr. (1979). Ocular pain secondary to occipital neuritis. *Ann. Ophthalmol. 11:*589–594.

Burian, H.M., and G.K. Van Noorden (1974). *Binocular Vision and Ocular Motility.* C.V. Mosby, St. Louis.

Cameron, M.E. (1976). Headaches in relation to the eyes. *Med. J. Aust. 1:*292–294.

Carlow, T.J. and O. Appenzeller (1976). Ophthalmic causes of headache. In *Pathogenesis and Treatment of Headache,* pp. 187–195. Spectrum Publications, New York.

Chamlin, M. (1962). Headache of ocular origin. *Int. J. Neurol. 31:*360–367.

Cohen, M.M., and M.F. McNamara (1980). Eye pain due to carotid stenosis. *Ann. Ophthalmol. 12:*1056–1057.

Currier, R.D., C.L. Giles and R.N. DeJong (1961). Some comments on Wallenberg's lateral medullary syndrome. *Neurology 11:*778–791.

Derby, G.S. (1930). Ocular neuroses: An important cause of so-called eyestrain. *JAMA 95:*913–917.

Eckardt, L.B., J.M. McLean, and H. Goodell (1943). Experimental studies on headache: The genesis of pain from the eye. *Proceedings of the Association for Research in Nervous Mental Diseases,* Vol. 23, pp. 209–227. Baltimore, Williams & Wilkins.

Feindel, W., W. Penfield, and F. McNaughton (1960). The tentorial nerves and localization of intracranial pain in man. *Neurology 14:*555–563.

Fisher, C.M. (1951). Occlusion of the internal carotid artery. *Arch. Neurol. Psychiatry 65:*346–377.

Fisher, C.M. (1968). Headache in cerebrovascular disease. In *Handbook of Clinical Neurology* (P.J. Vinken and G.W. Bruyn, eds.) Vol. 5, pp. 124–156. North Holland Publishing, Amsterdam.

Fisher, C.M. (1981). The headache and pain of spontaneous carotid dissection. *Headache* 22:60–65.

Folberg, R., V.B. Bernardino, G.L. Aguilar, and G.M. Shannon (1981). Amputation neuroma mistaken for recurrent melanoma in the orbit. *Ophthalmic Surg. 12:*275–278.

Fromm, G.H., C.F. Terrence, and A.S. Chattha (1984). Baclofen in the treatment of trigeminal neuralgia: Double-blind study and long-term follow-up. *Ann. Neurol. 15:*240–244.

Godsfredsen, E. (1965). Diagnostic and prognostic roles of ophthalmoneurologic signs and symptoms in malignant nasopharyngeal tumors. *Am. J. Ophthalmol. 59*:1063.

Goldstein, J.E., and D.G. Cogan (1960). Diabetic ophthalmoplegia with special reference to the pupil. *Arch. Ophthalmol. 64*:592.

Green, W.R., E.R. Hackett, and N.E. Schlezinger (1964). Neuro-ophthalmologic evaluation of oculomotor nerve paralysis. *Arch. Ophthalmol. 72*:154.

Grimson, B.S., and H.S. Thompson (1980). Raeder's syndrome: A clinical review. *Surv. Ophthalmol. 24*:199–210.

Henderson, J.W., and G.M. Farrow (1973). *Orbital Tumors*. W.B. Saunders, Philadelphia.

Ingalls, R.G. (1953). *Tumors of the Orbit and Allied Pseudotumors*. Charles C. Thomas, Springfield, Ill.

Kernbaum, S., and J. Hauchecorne (1981). Administration of levadopa for relief of herpes zoster pain. *JAMA 246*:132–134.

Kissel, J.T., R.M. Burde, T.G. Klingele, and H.E. Zieger (1983). Pupil-sparing oculomotor palsies with internal carotid posterior communicating artery aneurysms. *Ann. Neurol. 13*:149–154.

Knox, D.L. (1969). Ocular aspects of cervical vascular disease. *Surv.* Ophthalmol. *13*:245.

Knox, D.L., and E. Mustonene (1975). Greater occipital neuralgia: An ocular pain syndrome with multiple etiologies. *Trans. Am. Acad. Ophthalmol. Otolaryngol. 79*:513–519.

Kolker, A.E., and J. Hetherington (1970). *Diagnosis and Therapy of the Glaucomas;* 3rd ed. C.V. Mosby, St. Louis.

Lance, J.W. (1973). *The Mechanism and Management of Headache;* 2nd ed. Butterworth, London.

Lebensohn, J.E. (1951). Photophobia: Mechanism and implications. *Am. J. Ophthalmol. 34*:1294–1300.

Lieppman, M.E. (1980). Occipital neuralgia: The ophthalmic entity and its treatment. *Ophthalmology 87*:94.

McNaughton, F.L. (1937). The innervation of the intracranial blood vessels and dural sinuses. *Arch. Res. Neur. Ment. Dis. 8*:178.

Mitchell, S.W. (1876). Headaches from eye strain.*Am. J. Med. Sci. 71*:363–375.

Mokri, B., T. Sundt, and O. Houser (1979). Spontaneous internal carotid dissection, hemicrania, and Horner's syndrome. *Arch. Neurol. 36*:677–680.

Nadeau, S.E., and J.D. Trobe (1983). Pupil-sparing in oculomotor palsy: A brief review. *Ann. Neurol. 13*:143–148.

Newman, S., and R.M. Burde (1979). Headache and the ophthalmologist. *Sight Sav. Rev. 49* (3):99.

Nikoskelainen, E., and P. Riekkinen (1973). Retrospective study of 117 patients with optic neuritis. *Acta Ophthalmol. Scand. 50*:690–718.

Penfield, W., and F. McNaughton (1940). Dural headache and innervation of the dura mater. *Arch. Neurol. Psychiatry 44*:43–75.

Pozniak-Patewicz, E. (1976). "Cephalic" spasm of head and neck muscles. *Headache 15*:261–267.

Ray, B.S., and H.G. Wolff (1940). Experimental studies on headache: Pain-sensitive structures in the head and their significance in headache. *Arch. Surg. 41*:813–856.

Roy, F.H. (1975). *Practical Management of Eye Problems: Glaucoma, Strabismus, Visual Fields*. Philadelphia, Lea & Febiger.

Rucker, C.W. (1966). The causes of paralysis of the third, fourth, and sixth cranial nerves. *Am. J. Ophthalmol. 61*:1293.

Rush, J.A., and B.R. Younge (1981). Paralysis of cranial nerves III, IV, and VI. *Arch. Ophthalmol. 99*:76–79.

Schatz, N.J., and P. Farmer (1972). Tolosa–Hunt syndrome. The pathology of painful ophthalmoplegia. In *Neuro-ophthalmology*. (J.L. Smith, ed.), Vol. 6, pp. 102–112. C.V. Mosby, St. Louis.

Scheie, H.G., and D.M. Albert (1969). *Adler's Textbook of Ophthalmology*, 8th ed. W.B. Saunders, Philadelphia.

Smith, J.L., and D.S.R. Taxdal (1966). Painful ophthalmoplegia: The Tolosa-Hunt syndrome. *Am. J. Ophthalomol. 61:*146–147.

Soni, S.R. (1974). Aneurysms of the posterior communicating artery and oculomotor paresis. *J. Neurol. Neurosurg. Psychiatry 37:* 475–484.

Sutula, F.C., and J.J. Weiter (1980). Orbital socket pain after injury. *Am. J. Ophthalmol. 90:*692–696.

Taub, A. (1973). Relief of post-herpetic neuralgia with psychotrophic drugs. *J. Neurosurg. 39:*235–239.

Thomas, J.E., and R.E. Yoss (1970). The parasellar syndrome: Problems in determining etiology. *Mayo Clin. Proc. 45:*617–623.

Trobe, J.D., J.S. Glaser, and J.D. Post (1978). Meningiomas and aneurysms of the cavernous sinus. *Arch. Ophthalmol. 96:*457–467.

Waters, W.E. (1970). Headache and the eye. *Lancet 2:*1–12.

Whitnall, S.E. (1932). *The Anatomy of the Human Orbit and Accessory Organ of Vision,* 2nd ed. Oxford University Press, New York.

Wolter, J.R., and C.A. Benz (1964). Bilateral amputation neuromas of eye muscles. *Am. J. Ophthalmol. 57:*287–289.

Worthen, D. (1980). The eyes as a source of headache. In *Wolff's Headache and Other Head Pain* (D.J. Dalessio, ed.) 4th ed., pp. 388–402. Oxford University Press, New York.

18

The Radiologic Investigation
of Headaches

JACK ZYROFF
STANLEY G. SEAT

Since headache may be a symptom of many different diseases, its radiographic investigation traditionally involved all of the neuroradiologic procedures. Such investigations, however, were dramatically altered by computerized tomography (CT), which was introduced to the medical community by Godfrey N. Hounsfield in 1973. CT revolutionized neurologic diagnosis through its sensitivity, specificity, and simplicity. Except for the intravenous injection of iodinated contrast material, with its occasional adverse reactions, CT is a noninvasive procedure that can be performed on outpatients. Technical improvements in CT have provided better spatial resolution for the consistent demonstration of lesions less than 1 cm in diameter. These high-resolution units are faster, thus allowing diagnosis in uncooperative or moribund patients. New software allows image reformation in coronal, sagittal, or oblique planes to provide additional spatial orientation of lesions, thus aiding in surgical therapy. CT has become so dominant that modern neurologic diagnosis cannot be practiced without it.

Magnetic resonance (MR) imaging is a diagnostic technique that has recently entered clinical practice. This technique demonstrates exquisite anatomic detail in brain imaging and, in many areas, has surpassed CT in its sensitivity to pathologic alterations. MR is based on the effects of radiofrequency waves on protons in a magnetic field. It is a low-energy technique that, to date, has shown none of the known biohazards associated with x-rays. Although nuclear magnetic resonance has been used by chemists for *in vitro* analysis since 1947, its application to imaging was possible only as a result of advances in computer technology in the 1970s and, in many respects, can be considered a by-product of CT.

Although skull radiography, plain film tomography, angiography, and radionuclide brain imaging still have roles to play and, in some instances, are still the procedures of choice, their use is diminishing and their indications are being redefined. A trend toward less invasive examinations has been witnessed, reducing the risk and cost to the patient. Pneumoencephalography has essentially been eliminated. Arteriography,

Table 18-1 Changes in length of hospitalization, costs, and radiologic studies over a 6-year period in patients with pituitary adenomas

	1976	1978	1980
No. of patients	20	20	20
Average length of hospitalization (days):			
Preoperative	6.8	3.9	1.9
Postoperative	8.1	6.5	6.2
Totals	14.9	10.4	8.1
Average costs/patient adjusted to 1980 levels (in $):			
Total hospital bill	$10,092	$6,829	$4,899
Diagnostic radiology (% of total)	$ 1,747(17)	$1,045(15)	$ 585(12)
Types of studies (No.):			
Plain skull radiography	5	0	1
Sellar tomography	10	15	16
Pneumoencephalography	20	20	0
Carotid arteriography	17	4	0
CT	2	3	20

in most centers, is now confined to diagnosing specific vascular disorders (e.g., aneurysms, vascular malformations, vascular occlusive disease, etc.). Vascular disease is often suspected from screening noninvasive tests, such as CT, MR, Doppler ultrasonography, or radioisotope studies. Selective cerebral arteriography is mandatory for treatment planning, particularly where demonstration of vascular anatomy is of utmost importance.

Skull radiography and plain film tomography, though noninvasive and low in cost, provide only limited information about the calvarial vault or intracranial calcifications and no direct information about the brain itself. They are, therefore, poor screening tools and are relegated to an occasional supplementary role.

The trend toward noninvasive neurodiagnostic procedures has been cost-effective in spite of the high cost of modern equipment. Reduction in the number of tests and in the length of hospitalization has had a significant and favorable economic impact (Wortzman, 1975; Newton et al., 1983) (Table 18-1).

TUMORS

In patients with intracranial tumors, headache may be an early and prominent symptom. The frequency of headaches appears to be the same in rapidly growing or slowly growing neoplasms. A review of various neoplasms indicates the following incidences of headaches: meningioma (46%), pituitary adenoma (51%), glioblastoma (57%), and metastases (65%) (Heyk, 1968). In patients with nonlocalizing intracranial pressure, 20% had lateralizing supratentorial neoplasms, and 10% had midline and intraventricular neoplasms (Huckman et al., 1976).

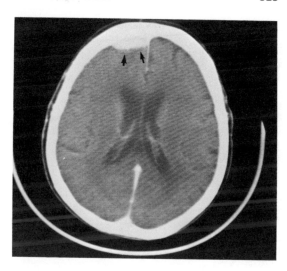

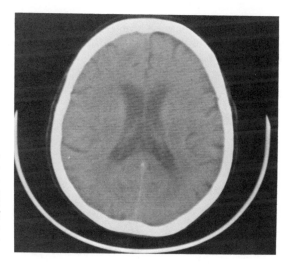

Figure 18-1. Meningioma: *(A)* Precontrast CT scan shows no abnormalities. *(B)* Postcontrast CT scan. Homogeneously enhancing mass that has a broad base of attachment to the frontal dura *(arrows).* Typical appearance of meningioma. The importance of intravenous contrast material in tumor visualization is illustrated.

CT has been reported to have an accuracy rate as high as 90 to 98% in detecting brain tumors (Christie et al., 1976). The routine use of intravenous iodinated contrast material has been extremely important in enhancing brain tumor visualization, defining tumor extension, and even characterizing the degree of malignancy (Salazar et al., 1981).

CT examination in patients with suspected meningiomas demonstrated 95 to 100% accuracy in tumor detection, with 85% specificity for meningiomas. Many meningiomas have been discovered in patients with no neurologic findings, some as tiny as 7 mm in diameter (Weisberg, 1979; New et al., 1980). Meningiomas typically appear as homogeneously dense or isodense masses on precontrast CT scans, with uniform enhancement following intravenous contrast administration. The presence of a broad base of dural attachment is highly specific (Figure 18-1).

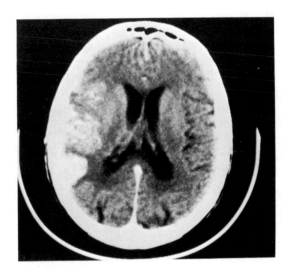

Figure 18-2. Carcinomatous meningitis. A 56-year-old male with recent onset of headache and disorientation. Diagnosis of oat-cell carcinoma of the lung was made several years earlier. A postcontrast CT scan shows enhancement along the right temporal cortical sulci.

Gliomas and metastases can have a varied appearance on CT scan, depending on tumor type and location (Figure 18-2). Calcification, cyst formation, and necrosis are variable features that can be identified. Most lesions are intracerebral and exhibit some degree of mass effect and/or edema. In malignancies, CT allows clear separation of tumor mass from surrounding edema with the use of intravenous contrast material, thus making possible a safe means of following the therapeutic response. The presence of associated obstructive hydrocephalus and the necessity for shunt placement can be easily determined. Stereotactic frames have been developed that, combined with CT localization, allow needle biopsies of deep neoplasms through a simple burr hole. This procedure can be safely performed on selected malignant tumors for purposes of histologic diagnosis and staging, thus obviating the necessity for a more extensive craniotomy (Brown et al., 1981).

MR has shown superiority to CT in the demonstration of many brain tumors. Because of superior contrast resolution, MR has demonstrated infiltrative gliomas not apparent or less confidently visualized by high-resolution CT (Figure 18-3). Tumors of the posterior fossa, which may be concealed by bone artifacts on CT, are clearly displayed by MR (Brant-Zawadski et al., 1984) (Figure 18-4). Zimmerman et al. (1983) have reported a 13% improvement in tumor detection by MR over CT and a significant improvement in the demonstration of tumor extension. The configuration of brain tumors and their relationship to adjacent structures is better displayed on MR, since direct coronal and sagittal views are routinely possible without image degradation. At this time, MR seems to be less sensitive than contrast CT in demonstrating calcification and some benign neoplasms, as well as in separating tumors from surrounding edema (Bradley et al., 1984). These limitations may be circumvented with intravenous paramagnetic contrast agents and/or appropriate imaging protocols.

The role of angiography in tumor evaluation has steadily diminished as neurosurgeons develop greater confidence in CT and MR. Although the risk of angiography

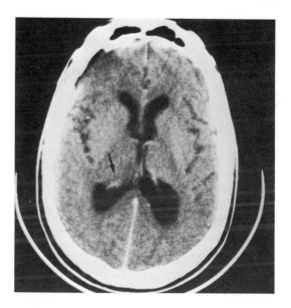

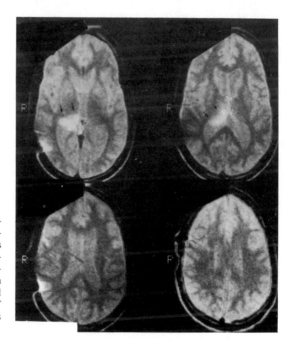

Figure 18-3. Infiltrative glioma. A 45-year-old male with headache and tremulousness: *(A)* Contrast CT scan shows very subtle posterior bulging of the pulvinar of the thalamus *(arrow)*. No density change is evident. *(B)* MR scan demonstrates tumor with subependymal extension more obviously than the CT scan *(arrows)*. Grade IV astrocytoma was confirmed on biopsy.

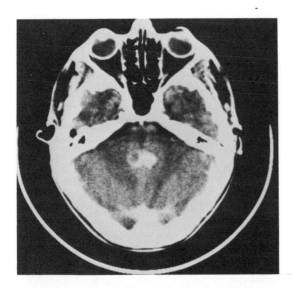

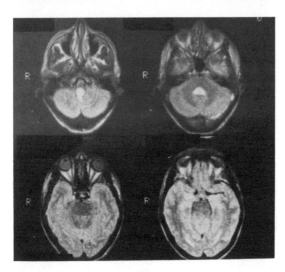

Figure 18-4. Ependymoma, fourth ventricle. A 69-year-old female with headache, tinnitus, and balance disturbance: *(A)* Contrast high-resolution CT scan shows an enhancing tumor in the region of the fourth ventricle. The inferior extent of the tumor could not be assessed because of bone artifact. *(B)* MR scan in the axial projections also clearly documents a tumor. No bone artifact is present.

has decreased with improved techniques, various authors have reported an incidence of serious complications from catheter angiography ranging from 0.5 to 10%, depending on patient risk factors, angiographer experience, and method of data collection (Mani et al., 1978). Digital subtraction angiography (DSA) frequently provides adequate imaging with further risk reduction because of reduced contrast volumes and catheter sizes. Angiography is helpful in surgical planning and preoperative embolization of highly vascular neoplasms. The angiographic demonstration of venous thrombosis by some tumors may alter the surgical approach. Intracarotid chemotherapy of malignant neoplasms through angiographic catheters has some proponents (Bonstelle et al., 1983).

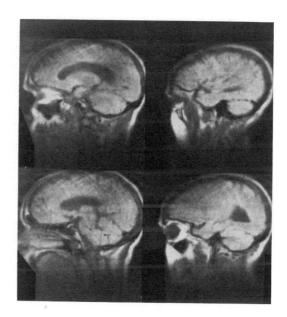

Figure 18-4. (cont.) *(C)* MR scan in the sagittal projection establishes an intraventricular location, an important factor in surgical planning *(arrows).*

INTRACEREBRAL HEMORRHAGE

Subarachnoid and intracerebral hemorrhage are well-known causes of sudden headaches that represent neurologic emergencies. Although the diagnosis is often made by clinical examination or lumbar puncture, the etiology is usually established by radiologic investigation. The potential causes of intracerebral bleeding are numerous, including aneurysms, vascular malformations, tumors, trauma, infarction, and bleeding disorders (Figure 18-5).

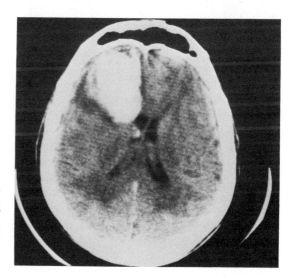

Figure 18-5. Intracerebral hemorrhage. An elderly male with sudden onset of frontal headache. Noncontrast CT scan shows high-density characteristics of acute hemorrhage in the right frontal lobe. Biopsy documented amyloid angiopathy.

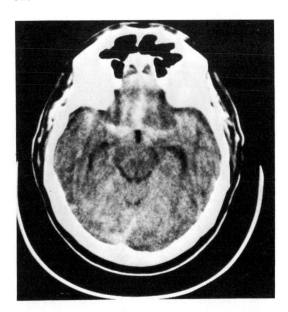

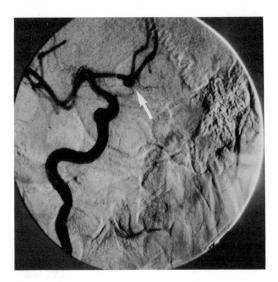

Figure 18-6. Subarachnoid hemorrhage, aneurysm. A 47-year-old male with abrupt onset of headache and photophobia: *(A)* Noncontrast CT scan shows high-density acute bleeding in basal cisterns and interhemispheric fissure. *(B)* Angiogram documents aneurysm of anterior communicating artery on an oblique view of the right carotid artery injection *(arrow).*

The sensitivity of high-resolution contrast CT in the demonstration of intracranial aneurysms is directly related to the size and location of the aneurysms. Because most aneurysms tend to be located near the skull base and are less than 1 cm in diameter, they may be confused with bone, normal looping, or ectatic blood vessels, or they may simply be too small to see. The larger aneurysms are usually identified but may be confused with tumors unless they are clotted, calcified around the rim, or clearly associated with a hematoma. Although a localized intracerebral hematoma is clearly seen by CT, a small bleed in the subarachnoid space may dissipate quickly and not be readily identified. Lumbar puncture continues to be a more sensitive test for blood

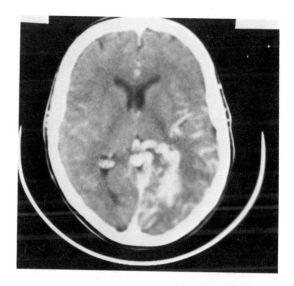

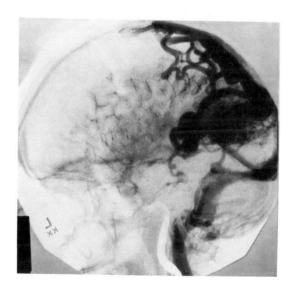

Figure 18-7. Arteriovenous malformation. A 43-year-old female with headaches: *(A)* Contrast CT scan shows characteristic serpentine and linear enhancement of enlarged blood vessels. *(B)* Arteriography confirms the location of the AVM as well as the arterial supply and venous drainage, critical information for therapeutic planning.

in the subarachnoid space. None of these observations, however, minimizes the role of CT in aneurysm evaluation. The presence of a local intracerebral hematoma is extremely important in localizing the potential bleeding site and in aiding the arteriographer in the search for a bleeding source (Inoue et al., 1981) (Figure 18-6). Areas of ischemia may be identified that suggest severe arterial spasm, a fact that has prognostic implications and may alter angiographic and surgical timing (Davis et al., 1982).

Vascular malformations can often be suspected from their CT appearance alone. A collection of serpentine or linear enhancing structures is usually specific enough for diagnosis (Figure 18-7). However, a small AVM may be atypical in its CT pre-

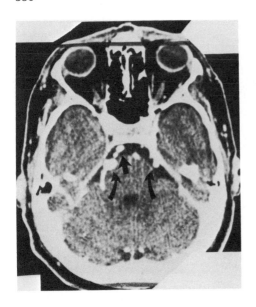

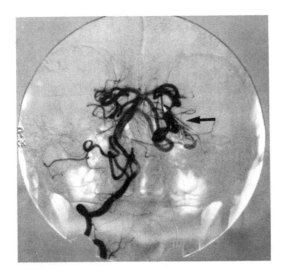

Figure 18-8. Dural AVM, tentorial. A 53-year-old male with nonlocalized headaches and dysesthesias: *(A)* Thin-section high-resolution postcontrast CT scan raises the suspicion of too many vessels in the perimesencephalic cistern *(arrows). (B)* Vertebral angiography shows an obvious arteriovenous malformation, arising from the inferior surface of the tentorium, with associated venous aneurysms *(arrow).* Arteriography was necessary in this case for diagnosis as well as therapeutic planning.

sentation and simulate a small neoplasm. Because of their proximity to bone, dural AVMs are infrequently identified by CT unless large or hemorrhagic; angiography is required instead for demonstration (Figure 18-8). Conversely, some so-called cryptic AVMs may be seen with CT and not with angiography (Kramer & Wing, 1977; LeBlanc et al., 1979).

MR has been particularly encouraging in vascular disease. Because rapid blood flow in arteries produces signal "dropout," arterial anatomy is conspicuously visualized and separable from adjacent tissues on MR. AVMs and aneurysms can often be clearly identified and specifically diagnosed (Figures 18-9 and 18-10). The signal

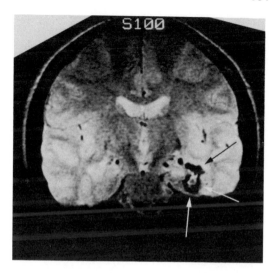

Figure 18-9. Arteriovenous malformation, MR. Coronal MR scan of a temporal AVM demonstrates conspicuity of vascular anatomy. The blood vessels appear black because of blood flow *(arrows)*. No additional contrast material was necessary. (Courtesy of Dr. John H. Hesselink, UCSD Medical Center, San Diego, Calif.)

characteristics may also allow for quantification of blood flow in major intracranial vessels (Mills et al., 1984).

Any candidate for interventional therapy of aneurysms or AVMs requires selective multivessel arteriography for diagnosis and evaluation. No other procedure provides the vascular detail necessary for determining and planning operative or embolic therapy (Figure 18-11).

EXTRACEREBRAL HEMORRHAGE

Extracerebral hemorrhage may occur as a sequel to trauma, bleeding disorders, or CSF hypotension and is often an occult cause for headache, sometimes presenting in

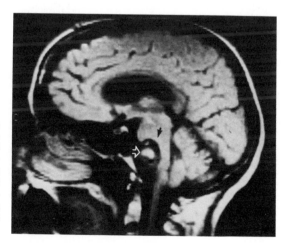

Figure 18-10. Thrombosed aneurysm, MR. Sagittal MR scan shows a large, round, discrete mass adjacent to the pons *(black arrow)*. The high-intensity contents are compatible with thrombus *(white arrow)*. The surrounding low intensity was believed to represent either calcification or flow. Surgery confirmed a thrombosed aneurysm arising from the vetebrobasilar junction.

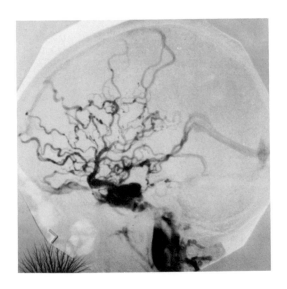

Figure 18-11. Carotid-cavernous fistula. A 50-year-old female with headaches and chemosis of right eye. Arteriography shows direct communication between the cavernous carotid artery and the cavernous venous sinus, subsequently treated by balloon occlusion. The cortical venous system fills extensively under arterial pressure. No history of trauma was present. Conventional head CT scan was unrevealing.

the absence of other compelling neurologic findings. Both CT and MR are sensitive and specific in the diagnosis of subdural or epidural hematoma. Because blood composition changes with age, the appearance of hematomas on CT and MR also changes, creating pitfalls and the potential for missed diagnoses. In acute hemorrhage, the CT density of blood is greater than that of normal brain tissue, probably secondary to the high protein concentration of red cells. As clot lysis takes place, the CT density diminishes with time. Careful examination of the ventricular system and white matter for mass effect is mandatory in situations in which the hematoma is isodense to brain on CT (Dolinskas et al., 1977) (Figure 18-12). In MR, a hyperacute hematoma may produce little change in T1 signal but a low T2 signal. With time, hemoglobin changes

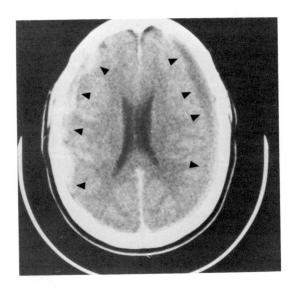

Figure 18-12. Bilateral subdural hematomas. Noncontrast CT scan demonstrates ventricular compression without midline shift. Extracerebral collections are evident bilaterally *(arrows)*. The density of the hematomas ranges from white to black, depending on their age and stage of clot lysis.

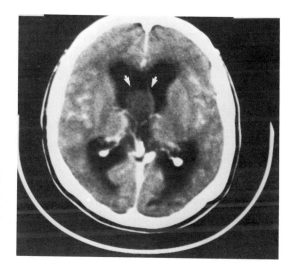

Figure 18-13. Colloid cyst. A 43-year-old female with headache and memory loss. CT scan shows a low-density midline lesion with associated hydrocephalus *(arrows)*. Surgery confirmed a colloid cyst arising from a cavum septum pellucidum with obstruction bilaterally of the foramina of Monroe.

to methemoglobin, which is paramagnetic, thereby increasing the signal intensity of the clot in relation to surrounding brain tissue. The presence of a surrounding membrane or edema can confuse the MR picture. The selection of an appropriate imaging sequence is critical in demonstrating hematomas on MR (Gomori et al., 1985).

OBSTRUCTIVE HYDROCEPHALUS

Headache may follow ventricular obstruction, especially if the obstruction is acute. The diagnosis of hydrocephalus is obvious on either CT or MR. Intravenous iodinated contrast material is important in CT for excluding possible causes of obstruction, especially tumors. In addition to strategically located malignant neoplasms, many benign lesions such as colloid cysts, choroid plexus papillomas, craniopharyngiomas, and intraventricular meningiomas can produce ventricular obstruction. Headaches in these cases may be chronic or positional and unassociated with other neurologic findings (Figure 18-13). Stenosis at the aqueduct of Sylvius or foramen of Monroe can be partial and intermittent, often presenting in adult life with intermittent headaches. Relative ventricular size can aid in pinpointing the site of ventricular obstruction, but sometimes ventriculography with water-soluble contrast material may be necessary. MR affords the advantage of direct sagittal and coronal imaging, which reproducibly demonstrates the foramina of Monroe, the aqueduct of Sylvius, and the inferior fourth ventricle, all common sites of obstruction not easily seen on CT (Figure 18-14). MR also sensitively demonstrates periventricular CSF extravasation, which may aid in separating hydrocephalus from cerebral atrophy (Bradley et al., 1984).

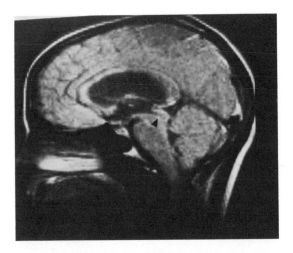

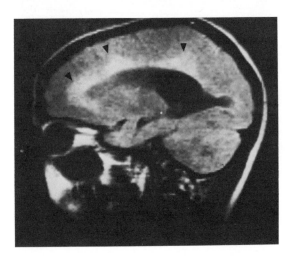

Figure 18-14. Aqueductal stenosis. A middle-aged female with a longstanding history of intermittent headaches: *(A)* Sagittal MR scan best demonstrates narrowing of the aqueduct of Sylvius *(arrow)* with enlargement of the third and lateral ventricles. *(B)* A more lateral MR section shows periventricular high signal areas, suspicious for transependymal CSF migration *(arrows)*.

INFLAMMATORY DISEASE

Although meningitis and encephalitis are clinical diagnoses, recognition of their radiographic manifestations, especially their sequelae, is useful in patient management (Figure 18-15). MR is extremely sensitive to brain edema and is useful in localizing encephalitic areas for brain biopsy. Subdural empyemas have been clearly localized and diagnosed by MR, even when very thin (Bydder, 1982). Granulomatous, fungal, and parasitic infestations have all been seen on CT and MR when they are present in a localized form (Figure 18-16). Vascular occlusions, vasculitis, and mycotic aneurysms are sequelae of CNS infections that are best documented by arteriography.

Cerebral abscesses have been diagnosed earlier, since the advent of CT. Their response to antibiotic therapy can be easily followed. The appearance of abscesses

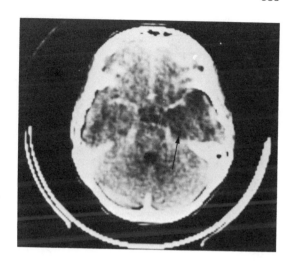

Figure 18-15. Herpes encephalitis. A 14-year-old female with acute onset of headaches and fever. CT scan shows unilateral temporal lobe edema *(arrow)*. Biopsy confirmed herpes simplex encephalitis.

in different phases of evolution can be characterized to provide greater precision in the timing of surgical intervention (Whelan & Hilal, 1980).

MISCELLANEOUS HEAD AND FACE PAIN

Because headache is such a nonspecific symptom, the yield of radiologic investigation in patients with headache alone is expectedly low in the absence of neurologic symptoms (Baker, 1983). In patients with "chronic recurrent" headache who had a normal neurologic examination, Weisberg (1982) found that the CT was abnormal in fewer than 0.5% of cases. The presence of an abnormal EEG increased the yield on

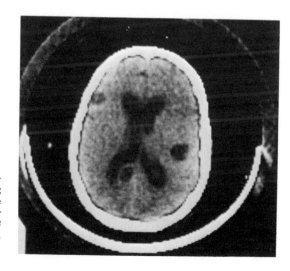

Figure 18-16. Cysticercosis. A 70-year-old female from Mexico with increasing headaches. CT scan shows multiple nonenhancing parenchymal cysts. Other CT sections showed calcifications. CSF studies supported the radiologic impression of cysticercosis.

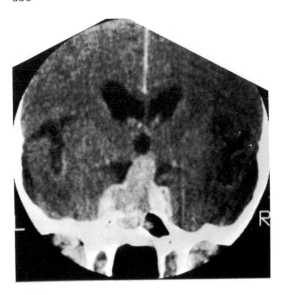

Figure 18-17. Pituitary adenoma. A 76-year-old male with headaches. High-resolution CT scan in the coronal plane with contrast material demonstrates a large intrasellar and suprasellar mass compatible with a pituitary adenoma, confirmed at transphenoidal surgery. No endocrine activity was documented.

CT. The patients with CT lesions had been symptomatic for 6 months to 17 years. Furthermore, removal of the lesion in those patients in whom it was felt to be a probable cause for headaches produced no relief following surgery. This led investigators to conclude that the lesions were probably unrelated to the patients' headaches and evidently represented incidental findings. Routine necropsy studies have shown a high incidence of asymptomatic pituitary adenomas and meningiomas (Wood, 1957; Weisberg, 1975)(Figure 18-17).

Benign intracranial hypertension (BIH), also known as pseudotumor cerebri, presents with headache and papilledema. CT findings in these patients are usually nonspecific, but occasionally demonstrate small ventricles, cisterns, and sulci (Hahn & Schapiro, 1976). Because of anatomic variability, the significance of these findings is made more apparent when sequential CT scans demonstrate a change. The primary purpose of radiographic investigation in these patients is to exclude a mass lesion.

Patients with classic migraine are rarely investigated radiologically. Of 200 patients with the clinical diagnosis of migraine who underwent CT, only two clinically unsuspected lesions were detected in the occipital lobe—a glioma and an angioma; four others showed evidence of ischemia in the occipital cortex (Weisberg et al., 1984). Angiography and cerebral blood flow studies performed during acute migraine attacks have shown arterial spasm (Figure 18-18). This is consistent with reports of neurologic complication in patients studied by angiography during acute attacks (Dukes & Vieth, 1964). Holzner et al. (1985) recently reported a 4.2% incidence of vascular malformations by arteriography in patients with complicated migraine. When migraine is associated with third-nerve paresis, arteriography may be indicated to exclude a posterior communicating artery aneurysm.

Patients with cluster headaches, temporal arteritis, or tic douloureux do not merit radiologic investigation unless atypical neurologic features are present. Atypical trigeminal neuralgia has been reported with posterior fossa and middle fossa tumors, aneurysms, and vascular malformations (Dandy, 1934)(Figures 18-19 and 18-20).

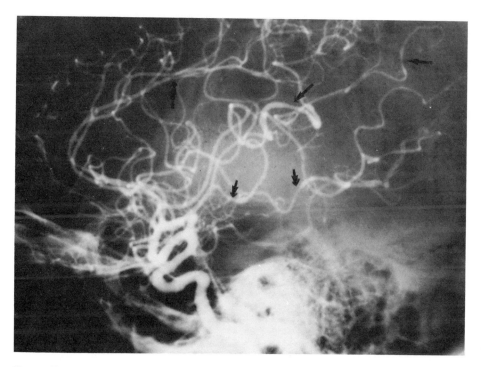

Figure 18-18. A 35-year-old female with migrainous headaches. Arteriogram during acute attack of migraine shows multiple areas of segmental arterial narrowing, compatible with vasospasm *(arrows)*. A similar appearance can be seen with vasculitis. The patient was not restudied to document reversibility.

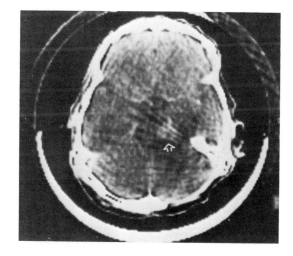

Figure 18-19. Metastasis, cranial nerve V. A 58-year-old male with atypical trigeminal neuralgia. Contrast CT scan shows an enhancing mass in the upper cerebellopontine angle *(arrow)*. The fifth cranial nerve was encased by tumor at surgery. The pathology was squamous cell carcinoma. A primary carcinoma of the lip had been resected 12 years earlier. No other metastases are known.

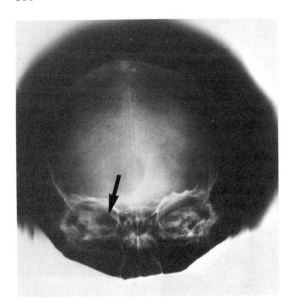

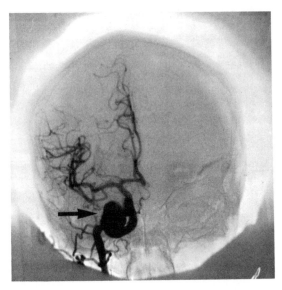

Figure 18-20. Aneurysm, petrous carotid artery. A 73-year-old female with a 4-year history of facial pain: *(A)* Skull x-ray (AP view) shows erosion of the right petrous apex *(arrow)*. *(B)* Angiogram shows a large aneurysm arising from the petrous segment of the right internal carotid artery *(arrow)*.

High-resolution CT or MR are the procedures of choice in these instances. Visualization of the basal cisterns and cranial nerves can be aided by introducing small amounts of air or water-soluble contrast material intrathecally. Arteriography may be considered in selected cases if evidence suggests a vascular lesion.

Diseases of the paranasal sinuses, pharynx, and infratemporal fossa occasionally present with headache or facial pain. Plain films of the paranasal sinuses are the most useful screening test for sinus disease; CT is more accurate, however, in visualization of the sphenoid and ethmoid sinuses. Both CT and MR have proven useful in discovering and staging tumors of the nasopharynx and parapharyngeal spaces, although

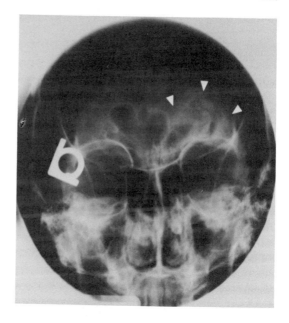

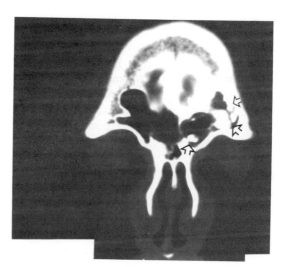

Figure 18-21. Frontal osteomyelitis: *(A)* Sinus x-ray (Caldwell view) shows sclerosis and poor delineation of the frontal sinus wall *(arrows)*. A bony density is identified within the sinus. *(B)* CT scan in coronal view shows sinus wall erosion with multiple sequestered bony fragments within the sinus *(arrows)*, compatible with chronic osteomyelitis.

CT is more useful in demonstrating bone destruction of the skull base and sinus walls (Hasso, 1984)(Figures 18-21, 18-22, and 18-23).

SUMMARY

Many organic causes of headache can be diagnosed or excluded by radiographic procedures. Computerized tomography (CT) and magnetic resonance (MR) imaging

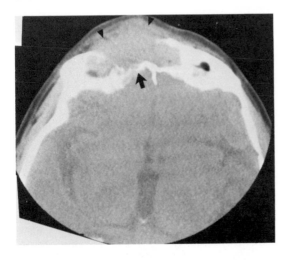

Figure 18-22. Carcinoma, frontal sinus. An 83-year-old male with frontal head pain and a history of chronic polypoid sinusitis. CT scan best demonstrated a mass in the frontal sinus with destruction of the sinus walls *(arrows)*. The histologic diagnosis was squamous cell carcinoma.

have dramatically altered neurologic diagnosis, having largely replaced more invasive and expensive, and less accurate, procedures. With the few exceptions noted, all other radiographic procedures have been confirmatory or additive in diagnosing intracranial disease. CT has also facilitated patient therapy and management, provided earlier diagnoses, and contributed to reduced hospital costs. MR has numerous advantages that make it a superb neurodiagnostic imaging tool, and many feel that it will ultimately become the screening procedure of choice in neuroradiology. Imaging technology is currently expanding so rapidly that close cooperation between clinician and neuroradiologist is more mandatory than ever to ensure that each patient receives the proper procedures in the proper sequence.

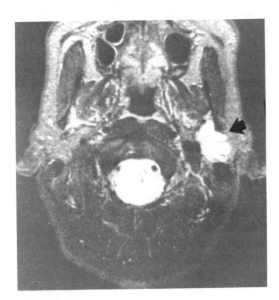

Figure 18-23. Parotid tumor. A 33-year-old male with atypical left facial and temporal pain. MR scan shows an enlargement of the deep lobe of the parotid gland with increased signal intensity compatible with tumor *(arrow)*.

REFERENCES

Baker, H.L., Jr. (1983). Cranial CT in the investigation of headache: Cost-effectiveness for brain tumors. *J. Neuroradiol. 10:*112–116.

Bonstelle, C.T., S.H. Kori, and H. Rekate (1983). Intracarotid chemotherapy for glioblastoma after induced blood–brain barrier disruption. *Am J. Neuroradiol. 4:*810.

Bradley, W.G., Jr. V. Waluch, R.A. Yadley et al. (1984). Comparison of CT and MR in 400 patients with disease of the brain and cervical spinal cord. *Radiology 152:*695.

Brant-Zawadski, M., J.P. Badami, C.M. Mills et al. (1984). Primary intracranial tumor imaging: A comparison of magnetic resonance and CT. *Radiology 150:*435.

Brown, R.A., T. Roberts, and A.G. Osborn (1981). Simplified CT-guided stereotaxic biopsy. *Am. J. Neuroradiol. 2:*115.

Bydder, G.M., R.E. Steiner, I.P. Young et al. (1982). Clinical NMR imaging of the brain: 140 cases. *Am. J. Roentgenol. 139:*215.

Christie, J.H., M. Hirofumi, T.G. Raymundo et al. (1976). Computed tomography and radionuclide studies in the diagnosis of intracranial disease. *Am. J. Roentgenol. 127:*171–174.

Dandy, W.E. (1934). Concerning the cause of trigeminal neuralgia. *Am. J. Surg. 24:*447.

Davis, K.R., J.P. Kistler, R.C. Heros et al. (1982). Neuroradiologic approach to the patient with a diagnosis of subarachnoid hemorrhage. *Radiol. Clin. North Am. 20:*87.

Dolinskas, C.A., L.T. Bilaniuk, R.A. Zimmerman, and D.E. Kuhl (1977). Computed tomography of intracerebral hematomas. I. Transmission CT observations on hematoma resolution. *Am. J. Roentgenol. 129:*681–688.

Dukes H.T. and R.G. Vieth (1964). Cerebral angiography during migraine prodrome and headache. *Neurology 14:*636.

Gomori, J.M., R.I. Grossman, H.I. Goldberg et al. (1985). Intracranial hematomas: Imaging by high-field MR. *Radiology 157:*87–93.

Hahn, F.J.Y. and A.L. Schapiro (1976). The excessively small ventricle on CAT of the brain. *Neuroradiology 12:*137.

Hasso, A.N. (1984). CT of tumors and tumor-like conditions of the paranasal sinuses. *Radiol. Clin. North Am. 22:*119.

Heyck, H. (1968). Examination and differential diagnosis of headache. In *Handbook of Neurology,* (P.J. Vinken, G.W. Bouyn, eds.) Vol. 5, pp. 25–36. North Holland Publishing, Amsterdam.

Holzner, F., P. Wessely, K. Zeiler, et al. (1985). Zerebrale Angiographie bei komplizierter Migraine—Reaktionen, Zwischenfalle. *Klin. Wochenschr. 63:*116–122.

Hounsfield, G.N. (1973). Computerized transverse axial scanning (tomography); Part 1. Description of system. *Br. J. Radiol. 46:*1016–1022.

Huckman, M.S., J.S. Fox, and R.G. Ramsey (1976). Computed tomography in the diagnosis of pseudotumor cerebri. *Radiology 119:*593.

Inoue, Y., S. Saiwai, T. Miyamoto, et al. (1981). Post contrast computed tomography in subarachnoid hemorrhage from ruptured aneurysm. *J. Comput. Assist. Tomogr. 5:*341.

Kramer, R.A. and S.D. Wing (1977). Computed tomography of angiographically occult cerebral vascular malformations. *Radiology 123:*649–652.

Le Blanc, R., R. Ethier, and J.R. Little (1979). Computerized tomography findings in arteriovenous malformation of the brain. *J. Neurosurg. 51:*765–772.

Mani, R.L., R.L. Eisenberg, E.J. McDonald, Jr., et al. (1978). Complications of catheter cerebral arteriography: Analysis of 5,000 procedures. *Am. J. Roentgenol. 131:*861.

Mills, C.M., M. Brant-Zawadski, L. Crooks et al. (1984). Nuclear magnetic resonance: Principles of blood flow imaging. *Am. J. Roentgenol. 142:*165.

New, P.F.J., S. Aranow, and J.R. Hesselink (1980). National Cancer Institute Study: Evaluation of computed tomography in diagnosis of intracranial neoplasms: IV. Meningiomas. *Radiology 136:*665.

Newton, D.R., S. Witz, D. Norman et al. (1983). Economic impact of CT scanning on the evaluation of pituitary adenomas. *Am. J. Roentgenol. 140:*573.

Salazar, O.M., P. Van Houtte, W.M. Plassche, Jr. et al. (1981). The role of computed tomography in the diagnosis and management of brain tumors. *Comput. Tomogr. 5:*256–267.

Weisberg, L.A. (1979). Computed tomography in the diagnosis of intracranial meningioma. *Comput. Tomogr. 3:*115–126.

Weisberg, L.A. (1975). Asymptomatic enlargement of the sella turcica. *Arch. Neurol. 33:*483.

Weisberg, L.A. (1982). Incidental CT findings. *J. Neurol. Neurosurg. Psychiatry 45:*715.

Weisberg, L.L., C. Nice, and M. Katz (1984). Head and face pain. In *Cerebral Computed Tomography: A Text-Atlas,* 2nd ed., p. 279. W.B. Saunders, Philadelphia.

Whelan, M.A. and S.K. Hilal (1980). Computed tomography as a guide in the diagnosis and follow-up of brain abscesses. *Radiology 135:*663.

Wood, M.W., R.J. White, and J.W. Kernchan (1957). One hundred intracranial meningiomas found incidentally at necropsy. *J. Neuropathol. Exp. Neurol. 16:*337.

Wortzman, G., R.C. Holgate, and P.P. Morgan (1975). Cranial computed tomography: An evaluation of cost effectiveness. *Radiology 117:*75.

Zimmerman, R.A., L.T. Bilaniuk, R.J. Packer et al. (1983). Cerebral NMR imaging: Early results with a 0.12 T resistive system. *Am. J. Roentgenol. 141:*1187.

19

Headache Associated with Brain Tumor

MICHAEL H. LAVYNE
R.H. PATTERSON, JR.

When considering the relationship of headache to an underlying intracranial mass lesion, one must realize that no single headache pattern is typical of brain tumor. However, headache is a symptom noted by approximately 60% of patients with brain tumor, and the recent onset of headaches or a change in the nature of chronic headache in patients over 40 years of age suggests the possibility of a brain tumor. Such patients should undergo either magnetic resonance scanning or computerized cranial scanning with and without intravenous injection of contrast to rule out an otherwise occult neoplasm.

On the basis of a careful review of 72 patients with primary brain tumor undertaken 40 years ago (Kunkle et al., 1942), and a general review of the literature since that time, we can attempt to (1) define the quality and intensity of brain tumor headache, (2) outline the common mechanism of brain tumor headache as it relates to the location of the tumor, and (3) define what patterns of headache may be of value in the diagnosis and localization of brain tumor before confirming the diagnosis with a radiographic study.

THE QUALITY AND INTENSITY OF BRAIN TUMOR HEADACHE

Headache that is of a dull nature, not rhythmic and throbbing, is typical of patients with supratentorial tumor. This type of headache is sometimes severe but rarely as intense as that observed in patients seen with migraine or ruptured cerebral aneurysm, meningitis, or headache induced by reaction to certain foods or drugs (Henderson & Raskin, 1972). Brain tumor headache rarely interferes with sleep and is worsened by maneuvers that increase intracranial pressure, such as coughing, straining at stool, or altering one's position from erect to recumbent or vice versa. It is also commonly aggravated by fever. Thus, a patient with a brain tumor who contracts a minor upper respiratory tract infection will experience increased headache while febrile. If the headache varies in intensity at all during the day, it is likely to be worse in the early morning. Even when the tumor directly invades or compresses cranial nerves containing afferent pain fibers, the pain is usually not as severe as that seen with trigeminal neuralgia. Severe pain is often accompanied by nausea and vomiting and generally is due to brain shift with compression of the brain stem. Of 132 patients with headache and brain tumor reported by the Mayo Clinic (Rushton & Rooke, 1962), 46% experienced nausea and vomiting. These two symptoms seem not to be related to increased intracranial pressure, since one third of patients with nausea and vomiting had no clinical evidence of raised intracranial pressure. Furthermore, in a group of patients with brain tumor but without headache, none had nausea or vomiting; yet five of these patients did have papilledema. Occipital or suboccipital headache was sometimes associated with "stiffness" or aching in the muscles in the neck and tilting of the head toward the side of the tumor. These contracted neck muscles may become a source of additional pain and tenderness (Simons et al., 1943). It was not at all uncommon for patients with episodic headache caused by brain tumor to manifest cervical muscle spasm and tenderness; however, the intensity of the headache did not correlate with the degree of neck pain. Thus, the association of headache and cervical muscle spasm raises the question of brain tumor, and this possibility needs to be investigated by further studies.

THE PATHOPHYSIOLOGY OF BRAIN TUMOR HEADACHE

Two clinical observations bearing on the mechanism of brain tumor headache introduce this section. The first observation involves data obtained during the operative exposure of intracranial contents that are pain-sensitive to mechanical stimulation. Intracranial pain-sensitive structures include the great venous sinuses and their tributaries from the surfaces of the brain, the dural arteries, the cerebral arteries at the base such as the carotids, basilar and vertebral arteries and their major branches near their sites of origin, parts of the dura at the base, and the intracranial portions of the trigeminal, glossopharyngeal, vagus, and upper cervical nerves. Stimulation of the pain-sensitive structures on or above the superior surface of the tentorium cerebelli results in pain transmitted by the trigeminal nerve and is referred in specific regions to the anterior half of the head. Stimulation of the pain-sensitive intracranial structures on or below the inferior surface of the tentorium results in pain over the posterior half of the head and appears to be transmitted by pain fibers in the 9th, 10th, and upper three cervical nerves (Ray & Wolf, 1940).

A second important fact in understanding the pathophysiology of brain tumor headache is that raised intracranial pressure is not essential to its production (Kunkle et al., 1943). Thus, elevating the intracranial pressure in normal human subjects to levels as high as 510 mm of saline by intrathecal injection of mock CSF consistently failed to cause headache.

In one series of 72 patients with brain tumor from The New York Hospital, the symptom of headache occurred almost as commonly in those patients without increased intracranial pressure as it did in those with increased intracranial pressure (19

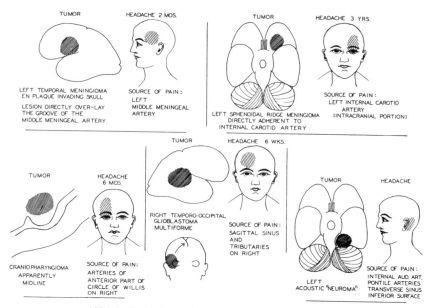

LOCAL TRACTION HEADACHE IN PATIENTS WITH NORMAL INTRACRANIAL PRESSURE

Figure 19-1. Five examples of patients with tumor headache produced by local traction. Intracranial pressure was normal in all. The structures that were the probable sources of the pain are listed in each case.

of 23 versus 46 of 49) (Kunkle et al., 1942). Of the 23 patients without raised intracranial pressure, 19 had headache as a primary symptom. In all the patients, the existence and location of headache could be explained by traction on or distortion of the directly neighboring pain-sensitive structures, and in some at operation performed under local anesthesia the headache was reproduced by touching pain-sensitive cranial structures (Ray & Wolff, 1940). In these cases the following structures were thought to be pain-sensitive: (1) for the four supratentorial meningiomas, the superior sagittal sinus and its tributaries, the middle meningeal artery, or the arteries at the skull base; (2) for the one glioma, the superior sagittal sinus and its tributaries; (3) for the three craniopharyngiomas, the arteries at the base; (4) for the pituitary tumors, the large arteries at the base and, in one patient, the lining of the sphenoid sinus; and (5) for the four cerebellopontine angle tumors, the internal auditory artery, the pontine arteries, the dura adjacent to the internal auditory meatus, and the transverse sinus. Figure 19-1 shows examples of this group. Three patients with pituitary tumor in whom local traction did not entirely account for the headache had pain in the occiput or suboccipital region in addition to frontotemporal headache. The pain in the back of the head in these three of seven patients with pituitary tumors is unexplained.

Headache in patients with raised intracranial pressure and brain tumor does not usually result from traction on pain-sensitive structures neighboring the tumor. In the New York Hospital series cited earlier, fewer than 50% of the patients with headache and elevated intracranial pressure harbored mass lesions to explain their headaches on the basis of local traction. The majority suffered either from occipital headache in association with supratentorial tumor or from a frontal headache in association with a posterior fossa tumor. An analysis of this group of patients illuminates this paradox.

DISTANT TRACTION THROUGH EXTENSIVE DISPLACEMENT OF THE BRAIN

Approximately one half of the patients with supratentorial tumor had headache in the posterior half of the head—that is, the occipital, suboccipital, and postauricular regions. In seven patients, the pain was bilateral. In the seven patients with unilateral headache, the pain was ipsilateral to the tumor in all but one. In each instance, these patients had pain at other head regions. Headache in these locations cannot be explained by local traction, for there is no evidence that any supratentorial structure can be the direct source of occipital headache. Downward pressure on the tentorium cerebellum causes only frontal orbital pain, probably through traction on the upper surfaces of the transverse sinus (Ray & Wolff, 1940). It is known, however, that when the supratentorial mass lesions cause generalized, increased intracranial pressure, there is often a shift of the brain, producing distortion of the supra- and infratentorial structures, and thus traction or pressure on the transverse and occipital sinuses, the basilar and vertebral arteries, as well as the lower cranial and upper cervical nerves. The latter probably accounts for the posterior occipital headache in those patients with supratentorial tumor and raised intracranial pressure.

Herniation of the hippocampal gyrus through the incisura tentorium may also be responsible for occipital head pain from supratentorial tumor. In a 1941 review of autopsied cases of supratentorial tumor, such a complication was found in 80% of the series (Schwarz & Rosner, 1941). It is presumed that the uncal herniation compresses the adjacent brain stem and presumably the posterior cerebral artery. This mechanism is probably of minor importance, since posterior head pain was no more common in patients with transtentorial herniation than in those without it.

To summarize, occipital head pain in patients with supratentorial tumor probably occurs because the mass expands to such an extent that traction is produced on pain-sensitive structures in the posterior fossa by displaced brain tissue. In contrast with the local traction phenomenon, this may be conveniently termed distant traction, and in patients with extensive brain shift, traction can affect structures on the same side as the tumor or on both sides, thus referring pain to both sides of the head.

Headache from distant traction may develop through obstruction of the CSF pathways causing hydrocephalus. Bifrontal headache was a symptom in 2 out of 3 (10 out of 14) of the patients with infratentorial tumor and raised intracranial pressure. All of these patients harbored tumors—two cerebellopontine angle tumors and seven cerebellar or fourth ventricular tumors—that obstructed the outflow of cerebral spinal fluid at the aqueduct or fourth ventricle, producing hydrocephalus. The frontal headache was bilateral in all but one patient.

The association of obstructive hydrocephalus with frontal headache in patients with posterior fossa tumor has been noted by many (Cushing, 1931; Dandy, 1945). There is direct evidence that hydrocephalus is causally related to headache. Distention of one lateral ventricle with a balloon at operation induces homolateral frontal headache, and traction on the veins draining into the superior sagittal sinus can also produce unilateral headache (Ray & Wolff, 1940). Experimental distention of the third ventricle has been found to cause diffuse headache arising from traction on the large vessels at the base of the brain.

Occasionally patients are encountered with tumor headache unexplained by local or distant traction. In the New York Hospital series two patients with raised intracranial pressure experienced headache not clearly explained by either of these two mechanisms. The first was a 24-year-old woman who had had a left temporal headache for 5 months. She harbored a right acoustic schwannoma that raised the intracranial pressure and produced hydrocephalus. The other was a 44-year-old woman with right occipital headache of 6 months' duration. She had a left cerebellar hemangioblastoma with hydrocephalus and raised intracranial pressure. The surprising pattern of headache referred to the opposite side of the head could not be explained. In 44 of 46 patients with headache and raised intracranial pressure, however, the existence and location of the headache could be accounted for on the basis of the mechanisms outlined above. It should be emphasized that the association of raised intracranial pressure with headache due to distant traction does not assume that raised intracranial pressure in and of itself causes headache. Rather, it indicates that those factors that bring about distant traction—that is, displacement of the brain structures directly by tumor or indirectly by hydrocephalus—also are a common cause of generalized intracranial pressure elevation.

In contradistinction to patients with intermittent headache associated with brain tumor, there is a small group of patients who have continuous headache or no headache in association with their lesions. In the New York Hospital series, seven cases, or about a tenth of the patient group, experienced persistent headache. All the patients had supratentorial tumors and all had evidence of raised intracranial pressure. An additional seven patients denied headache at any time during their illness. Two of the seven patients had glioblastomas, one in the corpus callosum and the second in the left frontal lobe, and two others had meningiomas, the first a left parasagittal parietal tumor causing seizures, and the second in the right frontotemporal convexity. The other three cases were low-grade mixed gliomas of the temporal lobe and a craniopharyngioma. When tumors grow slowly, the adjacent structures may adapt sufficiently to prevent production of pain. Perhaps this accounts for the absence of pain in the two patients with meningioma. However, in common with all of these cases was the fact that the patients did not have significantly elevated intracranial pressure and were investigated for the occurrence of personality change or the recent onset of seizure due to tumor growth in an epileptogenic brain region.

THE VALUE OF HEADACHE IN THE LOCALIZATION OF BRAIN TUMOR

We noted that headache in brain tumor patients without raised intracranial pressure could be explained entirely in terms of local traction. However, if intracranial pressure is raised and distant traction is involved, the tumor cannot be localized by the character of the headache because bilateral pain-sensitive structures are commonly distorted. If intracranial pressure is very high and extensive shift to the brain is present, headache may be referred to the opposite side from the tumor or even from front to back or vice versa. The combination of frontal and occipital headache was noted in 25% of the patients in the New York Hospital series. The group with fronto-occipital headaches included patients with meningioma, glioblastoma, third ventricular tumor, pituitary tumor, cerebellopontine angle, cerebellar, and fourth ventricular tumors. Except for the two patients with pituitary tumors, all the tumors were accompanied by raised intracranial pressure. Although obstructive hydrocephalus was present in only one of the supratentorial tumors, the third ventricular cyst and all five infratentorial tumors produced hydrocephalus. These data indicate that fronto-occipital headache occurs almost as frequently with supratentorial tumors as with those occurring below the tentorium. In addition, the presence of fronto-occipital headache does not necessarily indicate that obstructive hydrocephalus is present.

Headache over the vertex was noted infrequently in this series. Only five patients experienced it, and these were patients with pituitary tumor, craniopharyngioma, and a midline olfactory groove meningioma. In the latter two, intracranial pressure was elevated. In two other patients who reported vertex headaches, the tumors were found in the midline of the cerebellum and the parasagittal parietal meninges. Both of these patients had raised intracranial pressure.

Headache from midline tumors is not always bilateral. In The New York Hospital, 23 patients with midline tumors had headache—bilateral in 17 and unilateral in 6. Local traction apparently was the mechanism for the headache when it was unilateral, probably because tumor growth was asymmetrical. Whatever the cause, it is clear that unilateral headache may occur with midline tumor.

Although headache is often of limited value in localizing brain tumor, it can sometimes be helpful. If headache is caused solely by local traction, it is likely to be of direct value in localizing the lesion. Even then, the headache does not overlie the tumor in about 40% of the patients. In this series, patients with supratentorial meningioma of glioma experienced headache above the tumor approximately 50% of the time. With infratentorial tumors, headache occurred overlying the tumor 66% of the time with cerebellar or fourth ventricular tumors and 100% of the time in the few patients with cerebellopontine angle tumors.

Headache was the first symptom of brain tumor in most patients with posterior fossa tumors, except for those with cerebellopontine angle tumors. The tumors above the tentorium were more likely to present with other symptoms, including visual disturbances, paresthesias, seizures, or personality changes. Other authors have reported similar observations, as the data of Northfield (1938) and Rushton and Rooke (1962) demonstrate (Table 19-1). The frequent occurrence of headache as the first symptom in patients with cerebellar or fourth ventricular tumor reflects the early appearance of obstructive hydrocephalus in the presence of these lesions. Cerebellopontine angle tumors are less frequently associated with hydrocephalus in the early stages, and since they press on adjacent cranial nerves, early symptoms are more likely to be vertigo, deafness, or tinnitus. Whether or not supratentorial tumors cause focal symptoms or signs before headache appears depends on the region of the brain involved.

Pain in the back of the head, occipital or posterior auricular, was present alone or in part in 50% of the patients. As described in the preceding section, such pain was

Table 19-1 Headache as the first symptom of brain tumor

Location of tumor	Frequency of headache as first symptom (%)		
	Kunkle, Ray, & Wolff (1942)	Northfield (1938)	Rushton & Rooke (1962)
Supratentorial Tumor			
Meningioma	33	36	
Glioma	50	36	
Third ventricle tumor	50		48
Pituitary tumor	13		
Craniopharyngioma	28		
Intratentorial Tumor			
Cerebellopontine angle tumor	14	0	
Cerebellar and fourth ventricular tumors	82	83	52

present in 17 of 47 patients with supertentorial tumor, and in each of these patients, headache was also present in one of several areas in the anterior half of the head. Except for the patients with pituitary tumors, all had headache accompanied by increased intracranial pressure. In contrast, posterior pain was present in almost all the patients with infratentorial tumor. Of the 18 patients, 16, or almost 90%, had posterior headache. The two without such headache had an acoustic tumor and a cerebellar astrocytoma, both accompanied by raised intracranial pressure. It seems that posterior headache did not identify tumor as being above or below the tentorium. On the other hand, there is evidence that when posterior headache was absent, the tumor was rarely infratentorial.

HEADACHE IN RELATION TO VARIOUS TUMOR TYPES

Headache as an initial symptom in patients with craniopharyngioma was rare and its location unpredictable. Similarly, pituitary tumors also rarely produced headache as the initial symptom, with the site of headache presenting nothing of specific value. Patients with cerebellopontine angle tumors rarely experienced headache as an early symptom. But when headache occurred, it was generally behind the ear over the mastoid. Headache occurred as a first symptom in about a third of the patients with meningiomas. In approximately 50% of the 14 patients with headache, the pain was predominantly unilateral on the same side as the tumor, and in all but 2 of the 14 cases, the headache was due to local traction. One might expect that because meningiomas are in contact with pain-sensitive structures at the base and over the cerebral convexities, headache as an initial symptom might occur in a higher proportion of patients than the one third of the patients in this series. However, it is probable that the slow growth allowed the pain-sensitive structures to adjust to displacement. Gliomas, although they usually lack direct contact with pain-sensitive structures, presented with headache as the first symptom in half of the cases when they occurred above the tentorium and even more frequently when they occurred below the tentorium. Such tumors produce headache as a result of their rapid rate of growth, with consequent elevated intracranial pressure and brain shift.

SUMMARY

From the studies in the literature, a few generalizations concerning brain tumor headache as an aid to localization are justified:

- The headache of a brain tumor overlies the tumor in approximately one third of all patients.
- Tumor headache, in the absence of raised intracranial pressure causing papilledema, is of great value in localizing the tumor. In about two thirds of such patients, the headache overlies or is near the tumor, and when the pain is unilateral it is usually on the same side as the tumor.
- Headache may be absent with any of the common types of supertentorial tumors.
- Although the headache of posterior fossa tumors is almost always suboccipital, it may occur elsewhere as well.
- Headache is usually the first symptom of posterior fossa tumor, except in cerebellopontine angle tumors.
- The headache associated with a cerebellopontine angle tumor is frequently, and sometimes solely, postauricular.
- Headache from supratentorial tumor is rarely occipital except when associated with papilledema and raised intracranial pressure.
- When supertentorial tumors cause pain in the back of the head, headache in the front of the head is usually also present; when headache is both frontal and occipital, it indicates extensive displacement of the brain.
- When brain tumor headache is continuous, its value in localizing the lesion is greatly enhanced.

REFERENCES

Cushing, H. (1931). Experiences with the cerebellar astrocytomas. *Surg. Gynecol. Obstet.* 52:129.

Dandy, W.E. (1945). *Surgery of the Brain.* Prior, Hagerstown.

Henderson, W.R. and N. H. Raskin (1972). "Hot dog" headache: Individual susceptibility to nitrite. *Lancet* 2:654.

Kunkle, E.C., B.S. Ray, and H.G. Wolff (1942). Studies on headache: The mechanisms and significance of headache associated with brain tumor. *Bull. N.Y. Acad. Med. 18*:400.

Kunkle, E.C., B.S. Ray and H.G. Wolff (1943). Experimental studies on headache: Analysis of the headache associated with changes in intracranial pressure. *Arch. Neurol. Psychiatry 49:*323.

Northfield, D.W.C. (1938). Some observations on headache. *Brain 61:*133.

Ray, B.S. and H.G. Wolff (1940). Experimental studies on headache. Pain sensitive structures of the head and their significance in headache. *Arch. Surg. 41:*813.

Rushton, J.G. and E.D. Rooke (1962). Brain tumor headache. *Headache 2:*147.

Schwarz, G.A. and A.A. Rosner (1941). Displacement and herniation of the hippocampal gyrus through the incisura tentorii. *Arch. Neurol. Psychiatry 46:*297.

Simons, D.J., E. Day, H. Goodell, and H.G. Wolff (1943). Experimental studies on headache; Muscles of the scalp and neck are sources of pain. *Assoc. Res. Nerv. Ment. Dis. 23:*228.

20

Headache Associated with Alterations in Intracranial Pressure

FRANCIS W. GAMACHE, JR.
R.H. PATTERSON, JR.

Fay in 1937 and shortly later Ray and Wolff (1940) stimulated the tentorium, the meninges, the major intracranial vessels at the skull base, and the cranial nerves of patients undergoing cranial surgery under local anesthesia. They found that stretching or distorting these structures produced headache. Stimulation of the supratentorial compartment caused the sensation of pain in the forehead, which suggested that these structures were innervated by the trigeminal nerve. Pain brought on by stimulating structures in the posterior fossa was probably transmitted by the 9th and 10th cranial nerves and the upper three cervical nerves because the pain was referred to the posterior half of the head.

These observations formed an early basis for the understanding that one cause of headache is traction of major intracranial structures such as the large arteries and veins. Other investigators observed when the same structures were inflamed they became even more sensitive to pain. Studies performed on volunteers in the 1940s and 1950s documented the fact that the infusion of mock spinal fluid at pressures as high as 850 mm of water did not usually produce headache (Ray and Wolff, 1940). This suggests that elevation of intracranial pressure by itself does not produce headache.

Years of clinical experience have documented that if large volumes of either ventricular or lumbar CSF are removed, headache often follows. Presumably this is due to loss of support for the brain, which then sags and stretches pain-sensitive structures. Since these experiments, little additional data have been compiled to shed light on the mechanism of headache accompanying changes in intracranial pressure.

Traction on pain-sensitive structures, though it is a probable mechanism for headache in patients with conditions such as brain tumor, is an unlikely cause of migraine or other chronic recurrent headaches that affect so much of the population.

A review of our understanding of intracranial dynamics is appropriate to assist in a better understanding of headache related to changes in intracranial pressure and brain shift. If lumbar puncture is performed in the sitting position, pressure at the cisterna magna averages O mm of water, with a range of -85 to $+40$ mm of water (Loman et al., 1935). Pollock and Boshes (1936) postulated that the skull is an imperfectly closed container with atmospheric pressure able to contribute to changes in intracranial pressure by applying itself to intracranial blood vessels, especially veins. Evidence to support this theory was provided by the work of O'Connell (1970), who found that if lumbar puncture pressure was measured in the lateral decubitus position and then the patient was turned to the supine position, the pressure would increase by 80 mm of water. On the other hand, if the patient turned to the prone position, the pressure fell by the same amount. The 80-mm difference correlated with the distance between the plane of the needle and the level of the right side of the heart. Changing the patient from prone to supine changed the position of the column of venous blood with respect to the needle, and thus affected measurements of intracranial pressure.

Total intracranial volume is actually occupied by a combination of brain, spinal fluid, blood, and any lesion that might exist. Work by Nylin et al. (1961) demonstrated that approximately 7% of the total intracranial volume was blood and 10% was spinal fluid. Because the volume of brain is generally fixed, blood and spinal fluid volume thus represent buffers against changes in intracranial volume and pressure. Since spinal fluid envelopes the brain and blood vessels, it also helps to distribute changes in intracranial pressure evenly. Spinal fluid also damps venous outflow in arterial-induced brain pulsations. In addition, when spinal fluid leaves the intracranial compartment, more intracranial volume becomes available for capillary bed filling. An increase in the velocity of blood flow might otherwise be necessary to achieve similar increases in capillary perfusion, that is, blood volume per unit of time.

In 1948 Foldes and Arrowood demonstrated the factors important in governing alterations in intracranial pressure: changes in volume (i.e., brain, blood, CSF) and the time over which the volume change took place. In 1967 Langfitt extended those findings by demonstrating that intracranial pressure changes were also related to acid–base metabolism, mean arterial blood pressure, and temperature. These factors appear to affect intracranial pressure through interrelated changes in cerebral autoregulation (Langfitt, 1982, Miller, 1975).

In 1960 Lundberg demonstrated transient increases in intracranial pressure as high as 50 to 100 mm Hg in patients with cerebral lesions, which he termed "plateau waves." These periods of elevated intracranial pressure occasionally lasted for hours and were most commonly associated with increases in mean arterial blood pressure and blood volume. The pressure elevations were not reversed by altering pco_2 or po_2 alone. Headache was frequently, but not invariably, observed at the peak pressure achieved during the plateau waves.

Papilledema is the only reliable clinical sign of elevated intracranial pressure (Langfitt 1982). However, headache is rarely seen with elevation of intracranial pressure alone. Headache reflects stretching of pain-sensitive structures such as the middle meningeal artery, large arteries, or the dura at the base of the brain, venous sinuses, and bridging veins. Headache upon awakening early in the morning is commonly associated with brain tumors; it likely results from vascular congestion due to retention of carbon dioxide during sleep and clears on hyperventilation. Nausea, vomiting, and various cranial nerve palsies may result from displacement or traction of the brain stem.

Intracranial pressures are now being recorded by international convention in millimeters of mercury (mm Hg) rather than millimeters of water. Upper limits of normal are considered to be 15 to 20 mm Hg. Any pressures equal to or greater than 20 mm Hg are frankly elevated. Hence, the level of pressures measured by Lundberg sustained for 5 minutes or more were clearly elevated. Interestingly, most of the patients who experienced plateau waves also demonstrated papilledema and headache with only minimal neurologic dysfunction. The extent of the rise in intracranial pressure depends on the volume of the mass lesion, the rate at which it expands, the total intracranial volume available to the mass, the relative volumes of blood and spinal fluid available for displacement, and the anatomic configuration of the tentorial hiatus. This combination of factors determines the "pressure–volume" relationship, or the so-called intracranial compliance. Abrupt increases in volume are less well tolerated than volumetric changes that develop slowly. For example, patients with a seemingly large meningioma may present with the insidious onset of headache, whereas a patient experiencing a rapid but small increase in brain volume as produced by a sudden hemorrhage may experience severe headache and neurologic dysfunction. The pathophysiology of such changes is well summarized by Miller (1975).

Alterations in blood pressure, pulse, breathing, and consciousness considered by clinicians as evidence of increased intracranial pressure reflect brain shift and subsequent dysfunction of the reticular activating system. Primary injury to the brain stem can produce neurologic abnormalities without any increase in intracranial pressure (Johnston & Jennett, 1973). This explains why Lundberg among others (1968) has observed large numbers of patients with elevated baseline ventricular pressures in whom changes in neurologic status did not correlate with increased pressures. Neurologic symptoms occurred most frequently at pressure peaks (e.g., 80 mm Hg) that were superimposed on elevated baseline pressures. Some patients have experienced only headache in association with these peak pressures. Thus, neurologic symptoms and headache correlate directly with absolute intracranial pressure measurements in only a general way. Headache may also be augmented by increased sensitivity of the pain-sensitive intracranial structures, for example, by inflammation from meningitis.

Lumbar puncture headaches have been shown to be associated with a lowered cerebrospinal fluid pressure, also referred to as intracranial hypotension. Clinical evidence suggests that total spinal fluid volume must be decreased by approximately 10% or more before headache will occur in the upright position (Merritt & Fremont-Smith, 1938; Targowla & Lamache, 1928). Thus, measures to reduce losses, such as placing the patient in a recumbent position, aid in overcoming the headache associated with lumbar puncture. Larger holes are likely to leak more fluid than smaller ones, and many holes leak more than a single hole. Methods employing hormonal substances such as vasopressin generally produce no significant difference in the resolution of postlumbar puncture headache (Aziz et al., 1968). Low-pressure headaches have also been observed in patients who leak spinal fluid from the nose or ears or in patients who drain an excess of fluid through a ventricular shunt. Correction of the headache in these situations requires correcting the CSF leak or replacing the shunt valve with one that opens at a higher pressure.

In the case of an acute elevation of intracranial pressure such as occurs in acute hydrocephalus, a severe headache may occur, attributed to a sudden increase in the intracranial fluid volume. Another clinical condition, known as "benign" intracranial hypertension or pseudotumor cerebri, occurs primarily in young, obese females who typically present with papilledema and generalized headaches. These headaches frequently develop insidiously. The exact etiology of the disorder remains unknown, but elevated spinal fluid pressure is its principle feature. A recent study demonstrated an inverse relationship between CSF pressure and CSF protein, and the authors postulated abnormalities in CSF absorption as the mechanism responsible for the elevated pressure (Chandra et al., 1986).

SUMMARY

Simple elevation of intracranial pressure in an otherwise healthy patient does not produce headache. Headache is more commonly the reflection of traction on pain-sensitive structures in and around the base of the brain such as the large arteries and veins, which surround and anchor the brain. Metabolic conditions, blood pressure, blood volume, and the temporal pattern of changes in these parameters more likely account for the development of headache. Sudden shifts in intracranial homeostasis associated with marked rises or falls in intracranial pressure are more likely to produce headache than moderate changes in the intracranial environment or changes that develop slowly.

REFERENCES

Aziz, H., J. Pearce, and E. Miller (1968). Vasopressin in the prevention of lumbar puncture headache. *Br. Med. J. 4*:677–680.

Chandra, V., S. Bellur, and R. Anderson (1986) Low CSF protein concentration in idopathic pseudotumor cerebri. *Ann. Neurol. 19*:80–82.

Fay, T. (1937). Mechanism of headache. *Arch. Neurol. Psychiatry 37*:471–473.

Foldes, F.F. and J.G. Arrowood (1948). Changes in cerebrospinal fluid pressure under the influence of continuous subarachnoid infusion of normal saline. *J. Clin. Invest. 27*:346–351.

Johnston, I.H. and W.B. Jennett (1973). The place of continuous intracranial pressure monitoring in neurosurgical practice. *Acta Neurochir. 29*:53–63.

Kunkle, E.C., B.S. Ray, and H.G. Wolff (1943). Experimental studies on headache. Analysis of the headache associated with changes in intracranial pressure. *Arch Neurol Psychiatry 49*:323–358.

Langfitt, T., J.D. Weinstein, N.F. Kassell et al. (1967). Contributions of trauma, anoxia, and arterial hypertension to experimental acute brain swelling. *Trans. Am. Neurol Assoc. 92*:257–259.

Langfitt, T.W. (1982). Increased intracranial pressure and the cerebral circulation in *Neurological Surgery* (J.R. Youmans, ed.), p. 878. W.B. Saunders, Philadelphia.

Loman, J.A., A. Myerson, and D. Goldman (1935). Effects of alterations in posture on cerebrospinal fluid pressure. *Arch Neurol. Psychiatry 33*:1279–1284.

Lundberg, N. (1960). Continuous recording and control of ventricular fluid pressure in neu-
    rosurgical practice. *Acta Psychiatr. Scan. 36:*. (Suppl. 149) 1–113.

Lundberg, N., S. Cronquist, and A. Kjallquist (1968). Clinical investigations on interrelations
    between intracranial pressure and intracranial hemodynamics. *Prog. Br. Res. 30:*69–
    75.

Merritt, H.H. and F. Fremont-Smith (1938). The Cerebrospinal Fluid, p. 224–226. W.B.
    Saunders, Philadelphia.

Miller, J.D. (1975). Volume and pressure in the craniospinal axis. *Clin. Neurosurg. 22:*76–
    105.

Nylin, G., S. Hedlund, and O. Regnstrom (1961). Studies of the cerebral circulation with
    labeled erythrocytes in man. *Circ. Res. 9:*664–674.

O'Connell, J.E. (1970). Cerebrospinal fluid mechanics. *Proc. Roy. Soc. Med. 63:*507–518.

Pollock, L.J. and B. Boshes (1936). Cerebrospinal fluid pressure. *Arch. Neurol. Psychiatry
    36:*931–974.

Ray, B.S. and H.G. Wolff (1940). Experimental studies on headache. Pain sensitive structures
    of the head and their significance in headache. *Arch. Surg. 41:*813–853.

Targowla, R. and A. Lamache (1928). Les Accidents d'intolerance a la ponction lombaire.
    *Presec. Med. 36:*1111.

21

The Surgical Treatment
of Head and Neck Pain

DENNIS E. BULLARD
BLAINE S. NASHOLD, JR.

Head and neck pain represents an extremely complex and difficult set of problems for the clinician. This region has a multitude of crucial structures that are extensively innervated. The complexity and extent of this innervation present difficulties for both accurate diagnosis of the cause of the pain and its subsequent treatment. Moreover, craniofacial pain is often associated with an extremely strong emotional component. This is clearly seen in the cephalic neuralgias and in the degree of agony associated with cancers of the head and neck. This chapter provides an overview of currently available surgical approaches to the treatment of several of the most common head and neck pain syndromes.

TRIGEMINAL NEURALGIA

Although John Locke first described trigeminal neuralgia (tic douloureux) in 1677, this characteristic syndrome of lancinating facial pain is still poorly understood. The prototypic patient is a middle-aged female with pain in the right lower portion of her face, which usually occurs suddenly, lasts for a matter of seconds, and is brought about by touching a facial or oral trigger spot, exposure to cold or heat, eating, speaking, or smiling. The pain is frequently cyclic with asymptomatic periods. The neurologic examination is unremarkable unless there is an underlying disease entity, such as multiple sclerosis. Although relationships between trigeminal neuralgia and the subsequent development of facial herpetic lesions (Stookey & Ransohoff, 1959) or the discovery of lesions adjacent to the gasserian ganglion and to the nerve root entry zone have been seen, the definitive etiology of this syndrome is not known.

The first approach to his problem is medical. In many cases, phenytoin or carbamazepine can provide satisfactory treatment. Other agents, such as baclofen and clonazepam, have also been reported to be of some limited benefit. In a significant number of patients, however, surgical intervention is necessary. The types of procedures available can be broadly divided into destructive and nondestructive procedures.

Destructive Procedures

Peripheral Nerve

Interruption of the sensory input from the face to the cortex has been attempted at multiple points including the peripheral nerves, the ganglion, the root, and the trigeminal tract in the medulla oblongata. The peripheral branches of the trigeminal nerve including the supraorbital, infraorbital, lingual, and mental nerves and the second and third trigeminal divisions may be injected, divided, or avulsed. With peripheral nerve procedures, it is important that the nerve treated involve the trigger point rather than the area into which the pain radiates. Stookey and Ransohoff summarize their results with alcohol injections of the peripheral nerves and división in more than 1500 patients treated between 1912 and 1952 (Stookey & Ransohoff, 1959). For alcohol injections of the major trigeminal nerve branches and divisions, the average pain relief ranged from 8.5 to 16 months. Associated complications included sensory loss on the face, paresthesias, and weakness in the muscles of mastication. Other authors have reported similar success rates and have stressed the value of this procedure in establishing the diagnosis before other, more destructive procedures are used (White & Sweet, 1969; Pennybacker, 1961). Attempts to inject other noxious substances, such as phenol, have not resulted in any significant improvement in this basic procedure (White & Sweet, 1969).

An alternative is direct surgical division or avulsion of the peripheral branches of the nerve. In general, the anatomic distribution of the pain relief and facial numbness is better defined and the pain relief is more prolonged than with injections, ranging from 2 to 3 years (Grantham & Segerberg, 1952; Quinn, 1965). For all peripheral procedures, the major limitations are the obligatory loss of facial sensation and the high likelihood that the pain will return. Both of these procedures appear to have definite places as means of providing temporary relief to individuals with well-circumscribed pain in whom other procedures are not acceptable.

Ganglion

The ganglion or the root immediately proximal to the ganglion may also be approached surgically. Unfortunately, most large trials using alcohol have had an unacceptable incidence of morbidity including cranial nerve palsies, keratitis, transient paralysis of the masseter, and paresthesias (White & Sweet, 1969; Stookey & Ransohoff, 1959). Others have attempted to obtain responses utilizing phenol (Putnam & Hampton, 1936) or boiling water (Jaeger, 1957), without a significant improvement in response or morbidity. Most recently, glycerol has been used for injection into the retrogasserian cistern of Meckel's cave (Lunsford, 1985; Hakanson, 1981). Hakanson originally described this technique and reported that 96 out of 100 patients were pain free after the initial injection, with a recurrence rate of 31% 1 to 6 years following injection. Although other authors have not had this same degree of success

(Lunsford, 1985; Sweet et al., 1981), the overall response rates appear to be equivalent to the alcohol injections with the advantage of a significant reduction in postoperative sensory loss and cranial nerve deficits.

At the present time, one of the most frequently employed surgical techniques for the treatment of trigeminal neuralgia is modification of the percutaneous electrocoagulation of the gasserian ganglion, first introduced by Kirschner (Kirschner, 1932). The popularity of this procedure has increased since 1970, when Sweet and Wespic introduced the use of a radiofrequency generator to produce a more controlled thermocoagulation, thereby allowing selective destruction of the c and A delta pain fibers. In 1974, these authors reported that 91% of their 214 patients with trigeminal neuralgia had initial pain relief with a recurrence rate of only 22% between 2.5 and 6 years after surgery (Sweet & Wespic, 1974). Subsequent authors, using various modifications of this technique, have reported satisfactory initial pain relief in 78 to 99% of patients with recurrence rates ranging from 11 to 64%, depending on the length of follow-up (Burchiel et al., 1981; Nugent & Berry, 1974; Onofrio, 1975; Tew, 1979; Nugent, 1985). In general, this technique appears to provide satisfactory pain relief in the majority of patients with a relatively low morbidity and mortality and with the ability to repeat the procedure as needed (Nugent, 1985).

Retrogasserian Neurotomy

The trigeminal nerve root may be approached surgically either through the subtemporal or the suboccipital approach. Wilkins has summarized the early results from the subtemporal approach series, reporting significant relief of pain in 95 to 99% of patients with a recurrence rate of 5 to 20% and an operative mortality of 1 to 3% (Wilkins, 1985). The alternative suboccipital approach, which was developed by Dandy, allowed selective partial division of the sensory root of the fifth nerve near its entrance into the pons. By this approach, surgeons reported satisfactory pain relief with recurrence rates of only 18 to 30% and a major morbidity of 1 to 10% (Wilkins, 1985).

Trigeminal Tractotomy

Sjoquist proposed the surgical disruption of the descending trigeminal tract in the medulla oblongata in 1938 (Sjoquist, 1938). The advantage of this approach was in the potential for preserving facial touch sensation and motor function for the trigeminal distribution. Limited studies using this procedure with various modifications, however, have shown variable results with associated deficits including analgesia in the ipsilateral 9th and 10th cranial nerve, and 2nd cervical nerve distribution and mixed sensory losses with ipsilateral ataxia, and proprioceptive dysfunction, and/or contralateral pain and temperature loss (Stookey & Ransohoff, 1959; McKenzie, 1954; Crue et al., 1967; Hosobuchi & Rutkin 1971).

Nondestructive Procedures

In 1920, Cushing suggested that trigeminal neuralgia could be caused by compression of the posterior trigeminal root (Cushing, 1920). Dandy subsequently noted abnormal vessels or other lesions in approximately 60% of patients who were operated on for trigeminal neuralgia using the posterior fossa approach (Dandy, 1929, 1934). Then, in 1959, Gardner and Miklos reported the successful treatment of trigeminal neuralgia by decompressing the trigeminal root at the brain stem, inserting a sponge between an arterial loop and the nerve (Gardner & Miklos, 1959). Subsequently, Gardner found vascular compression in 7 out of 18 cases (Gardner, 1962).

Jannetta has since expanded and popularized this approach to the treatment of trigeminal neuralgia. In his extensive experience, 79.8% of patients had good results after one microvascular decompression. With a second or third procedure, this increases to 83.2% and, with additional medical therapy, reaches 96.5% (Jannetta, 1985). This procedure involves a suboccipital craniectomy with exposure of the trigeminal root at the brain stem. If an offending vascular lesion is found, this is carefully dissected away from the root and the root entry zone and is separated by a small sponge, muscle plug, or Teflon pledget. In Jannetta's experience with 414 patients who did not have multiple sclerosis, 244 had arterial compression, 54 had venous compression, 96 had mixed arteriovenous compression, 15 had tumors, and single patients had an aneurysm, an arteriovenous malformation, or no pathologic lesion. His morbidity rate in more than 800 microvascular decompressions has included two operative deaths, two postoperative deaths after tumor excision, an incidence of permanent cranial nerve deficit of less than 3%, and major complications such as infections or hemorrhages of less than 0.5% (Jannetta, 1985). Rarely, a patient with trigeminal neuralgia will also have hemifacial spasms, the syndrome of tic convulsive. In general, this responds to vascular decompression of the root entry zone for the seventh cranial nerve in the nervus intermedius.

Selection of Therapeutic Modality

From the previous discussion, it can be concluded that multiple surgical procedures are available for the treatment of trigeminal neuralgia. It is best in selecting which to employ to try to tailor the success rate and potential morbidity to best fit the patient's need. The scheme outlined by Wilkins (1985), well demonstrates such an approach. If the patient is more than 70 years of age or has major medical problems, limited surgical procedures are preferable. With tic restricted to the forehead, supraorbital–supratrochlear nerve avulsion is the initial surgical treatment of choice. If the tic is restricted to the cheek, alcohol injection or avulsion of the infraorbital nerve is recommended. For these patients with tic involving the eye, the third division, or multiple divisions, or in patients with multiple sclerosis, percutaneous trigeminal radio frequency coagulation or percutaneous retrogasserian glycerol infection is recommended. For younger patients, or those older than 70 years who are in good health, microvascular decompression is the initial treatment recommended. If a vascular lesion or other pathologic entity is not recognized at the time of surgery, the caudal half or two thirds of the main sensory root of the trigeminal nerve is divided adjacent to the pons. For patients who decline this, a percutaneous radiofrequency thermocoagulation or retrogasserian glycerol injection is recommended. For recurrence of symptoms following surgical intervention, most procedures can be safely repeated with a decreased but generally reasonable response rate.

GLOSSOPHARYNGEAL NEURALGIA

The first clinical observations on glossopharyngeal neuralgia were made in 1910 by Weisenburg (Weisenburg, 1910). This was followed 10 years later when Sicard and Robineau characterized the clinical syndrome of glossopharyngeal neuralgia and developed a cure by cervical section of the nerve with excision of the superior cervical ganglion and the pharyngeal branch of the vagus nerve (Sicard & Robineau, 1920). Dandy, in 1927, introduced the intracranial section of the ninth nerve in the posterior fossa, which has been the standard neurosurgical treatment until a recent development using a percutaneous technique for coagulation of the nerve in its foramen (Dandy, 1927; Tew, 1982).

The clinical syndrome closely resembles trigeminal neuralgia in its presentation. The syndrome can be divided into two types: (1) primary spontaneous neuralgia and (2) secondary neuralgia resulting from direct compression of the glossopharyngeal nerve by a specific pathologic condition.

Primary Spontaneous Neuralgia

The onset of the syndrome occurs in the fourth decade and beyond, with older persons predominating and equal distribution of male and female.

The neuralgia occurs suddenly and in paroxysms, with the patient experiencing agonizing pain originating from the throat in the region of the posterior pharynx. The attacks occur in bursts of pain that totally incapacitate the patient. The attacks may last for long periods of time or suddenly stop to reappear months or years later if no treatment is instituted. The painful paroxysms may be spontaneously aggravated or triggered by swallowing, talking, or movement of the tongue, and the examining physician must be careful to avoid touching the back of the throat, which might trigger an attack. Daily activity, such as eating, swallowing and talking, become difficult, if not impossible, for the patient. Even a sneeze or cough may set off a painful paroxysm, and the patient begins to dread the pain. The diagnosis is not difficult because the typical history can be confirmed by anesthetizing the posterior pharyngeal region, resulting in a temporary cessation of the attacks and relief of pain for which the patient is grateful. The patient seeks medical help early because of the severity of the pain. Medical treatment using Tegretol and/or Dilantin should be tried initially, but if rapid control of pain does not occur, surgical relief is necessary because finding a cure is very important to the patient. Intracranial section of the pharyngeal nerve, as advocated by Dandy, has a low risk with today's microneurosurgical techniques, and it offers a high rate of cure. If, for some reason, the patient cannot tolerate a neurosurgical operation and medication fails, a percutaneous coagulation technique for the nerve in its foramen appears to be as effective for pain relief (Tew, 1982). The pain experienced in glossopharyngeal neuralgia is among the most severe pain. The patient who suffers from it requires rapid and decisive treatment.

Secondary Glossopharyngeal Neuralgia

Pathologic conditions such as tumors, inflammation, and infection may involve the base of the skull and secondarily compress the ninth nerve, producing intractable pain. Tumors, both malignant and benign, directly involving the pharyngeal wall, tonsil, and tongue may also be a source of the pain.

The onset of the pain may be similar to primary glossopharyngeal neuralgia with sudden, intermittent attacks, but in general the pain is more insidious in its onset and constant in its intensity over a longer period of time, and increasing as the pathologic process progresses. The development of neurologic signs, such as motor and sensory deficits, should always alert the examiner to a secondary cause of the pain; it is not usually seen in primary glossopharyngeal neuralgia. The pain may precede the overt development of the motor and sensory dysfunction by some months, but it becomes evident that the ninth nerve and adjacent cranial nerves are involved as the disease process spreads. The diagnosis may be more difficult in secondary neuralgia until the pathologic process is evident. However, the use of the CT scans and magnetic resonance imaging (MRI) to visualize the base of the skull greatly improves the diagnosis of these difficult lesions. Medical treatment is less successful in this group of patients, and neurosurgical intervention should be considered early before narcotic addiction becomes a problem. The intracranial section or the percutaneous coagulation of the ninth nerve may be more difficult because of the nature of the pathologic condition involving the peripheral nerves at the base of the skull. The trigeminal nerve is also occasionally involved, and the best surgical approach is the percutaneous coagulation of both the fifth and ninth nerves. When direct intervention involving the ninth nerve is not possible because of the pathologic process, a unilateral stereotaxic mesencephalotomy with coagulation of the periaqueductal gray contralateral to the pain will often result in good pain relief along with cessation of paroxysmal pain, which is often activated by pharyngeal or tongue movements. Stereotaxic mesencephalotomy is performed under local anesthesia and has a low risk with effective pain relief.

GENICULATE NEURALGIA

IN 1907, Hunt described herpetic vesicular rashes in the mucocutaneous distribution of the nervus intermedius portion of the seventh nerve and coined the term geniculate neuralgia to describe the associated paroxysmal pain (Hunt, 1907). Subsequently, the term Ramsey Hunt syndrome has been used to describe geniculate neuralgia in association with a herpetic infection of the geniculate ganglion. Geniculate ganglion neuralgia is also seen without associated herpetic infections. Although the Ramsay Hunt syndrome is often self-limited, the idiopathic variety may be associated with cyclic episodes of excruciating pain. In this latter case, carbamazepine is the initial drug of choice and is often effective. In contrast, postherpetic neuralgia is often refractory to carbamazepine. Should this be the case, a secondary trial of sodium valproate is in order. If these fail to provide satisfactory relief, or if unacceptable side effects occur, surgical section of the nervus intermedius or the geniculate ganglion can be performed. Clark and Taylor first reported suboccipital craniectomy for section of the nervus intermedius for the treatment of geniculate neuralgia (Clark & Taylor, 1909). Furlow also reported satisfactory results with a similar approach (Furlow, 1942). Pulec later emphasized the need for further subtotal sectioning of the geniculate ganglion because of the additional afferent fibers that passed through the main motor trunk of the facial nerve rather than the nervus intermedius (Pulec, 1976). In his series, he was able to relieve ostalgia in all 15 of his patients without any corresponding facial paralysis. For this procedure, he used microsurgical technique and approached the geniculate ganglion through the middle cranial fossa.

POSTHERPETIC FACIAL PAIN

Intractable pain occurs in 10% of patients after an herpetic attack; the incidence of facial pain is probably less, but its occurrence is a difficult therapeutic challenge. The pain follows a dermatomal pattern, and its distribution is evident from the chronic skin changes associated with the herpetic infection. In 10% of patients with herpes zoster, the face is involved with a predilection for the opthalmic division. The patient complains of severe pain deep in or around the eye radiating into the forehead. The pain may be triggered by touching the region of the first division of the trigeminal nerve, but in some patients the entire face may be involved in the herpetic infection, with pain involving all three divisions of the trigeminal nerve. The pain is usually constant, with sharp electric shocks occurring spontaneously or activated by minimal afferent stimulation such as air blowing on the involved skin.

Once the pain is chronic, medical treatment is of no benefit. Some evidence, however, suggests a role for sympathetic blocks in the early management of this problem (Tenicela et al., 1985). Neurosurgical intervention that involves the peripheral portion of the trigeminal nerve has been unsuccessful. In 1984, Friedman, Nashold, and Ovelmen-Levitt reported significant relief of pain in patients with postherpetic pain after lesions on the dorsal root entry zone of the spinal cord (Friedman et al., 1984). Sixty percent of the patients were relieved for a 2-year period. The pain afferents from the trigeminal dorsal root are organized in the nucleus caudalis at the spinomedullary junction. The anatomic and physiologic characteristics of the nucleus caudalis of the trigeminal closely resemble the organization of the dorsal horn in the spinal cord. In 1984, Nashold made electrolytic lesions in the trigeminal nucleus caudalis for intractable facial pain of herpes. In six of the eight patients who underwent the caudalis nucleus DREZ operation, there was good sustained pain relief for a period of 2 years. Although a longer follow-up is necessary to fully evaluate this new neurosurgical operation, its initial results have been encouraging, especially in view of the intractability of postherpetic facial pain, which has been unresponsive to a variety of treatments.

PAIN OF HEAD AND NECK DUE TO INVASIVE TUMORS

Invasive tumors of the head and neck often result in widespread intractable pain. Unilateral head and neck pain is easier to treat than midline or diffuse pain, and different surgical strategies are needed. The invasive nature of the head and neck tumors often involve multiple cranial nerves including V, VII nervus intermedius, IX, X, and the upper cervical dorsal roots. Direct section of the involved roots using a dorsal rhizotomy may be complicated by sepsis, lower tissue resistance as a result of radiation, and difficulty with breathing and swallowing; general debilitation of the patient further complicates the treatment.

Four types of neurosurgical procedures can be used to control pain. The selection of the appropriate neurosurgical operation depends on the extent and degree of the tumor involvement of the head and neck. These procedures include surgical rhizotomy, DREZ, and stereotaxic mesencephalic tractotomy.

Percutaneous trigeminal and/or glossopharyngeal coagulation can be useful in relief of unilateral pain involving these two cranial nerves only. Contraindication for the percutaneous technique would be localized involvement of the neural foramen of the fifth and ninth nerves by the tumor. The percutaneous operation has the advantage of low risk since it is performed under local anesthesia.

Dorsal rhizotomy or intracranial section of the cranial nerves involved in the pain process is a much older neurosurgical procedure. The risks are greater, however, and it is now only an operation of historical interest.

Pain from wider regions of the head and neck, including the ear, primarily involve the trigeminal, glossopharyngeal, and cervical nerves and can be more effectively treated by dorsal root entry zone lesions combined with lesions of the upper dorsal cervical roots. The suboccipital area is rarely involved by the primary tumor; however, general anesthesia must be used and this does add to the risk. When more extensive regions of the head and neck are involved, the patient may develop both pain and suffering. A stereotaxic midbrain lesion involving the periaqueductal gray is effective in reducing both of these components. Nashold, in 1972, reported on eight patients suffering from head and neck pain due to carcinoma of the larynx, tongue, and tonsil. The pain was often triggered by talking, eating, and swallowing. The patient can experience painful spasm of coughing and trismus, and because of the fear of respiratory obstruction or choking, these patients often become very anxious and suffer with their pain. A stereotaxic midbrain lesion reduces not only the primary pain but the suffering and anxiety as well. The operation is low risk because it can be done under local anesthesia through a small cranial burr hole, despite the extensive involvement of the tumor. The effectiveness of the lesion is further controlled by the use of electrical stimulation at the time of the operation to control its location. Pain relief was experienced by these eight patients for up to 9 months. The treatment has subsequently been used in a larger group of patients with head and neck tumors, with similar improvement in the pain and suffering. The major side effect of a midbrain tractotomy is alteration of ocular function due to the nearness of the lesion to the brain-stem ocular nuclei that control ocular movements. With careful localization of the lesion probe in the midbrain in the awake patient, the only major ocular defect is the loss of upward gaze, which subjectively the patient is often unaware of.

Tumors of the head and neck result in some of the most complex pain syndromes treated by the surgeon. Each patient's problem must be carefully analyzed to select the proper neurosurgical operation; if this is done, significant pain relief can be accomplished.

CENTRAL PAIN

Central facial pain syndromes based on thalamic infarctions, central deafferentation, and postoperative anesthesia dolorosa are an extremely difficult group of problems to treat. In the past, ablative procedures such as thalamotomies, mesencephalotomies, trigeminal medullary tractotomies or stereotaxic prefrontal leukotomies were often employed with variable success (White & Sweet, 1969). The concept of sectioning the spinothalamic tract by means of medullary spinothalamic tractotomy for neck and shoulder pain has proven beneficial in some patients with neck and shoulder pain too high for either percutaneous or open spinal cordotomies (White & Sweet, 1969). The usefulness of this procedure has proved limited because of the technical difficulty and the associated postoperative ataxia. Medullary trigeminal tractotomy has also been employed in the treatment of lateral facial pain (Walker, 1942; Sjoquist, 1938). In general, however, these procedures are associated with unacceptably high levels of morbidity. One modification is the stereotaxic percutaneous trigeminal tractotomy, developed by Crue and his associates (1967); others include the modifications developed by Fox (1971) and Hitchcock (1970). Although these procedures appear to be reasonably effective in limited situations, they have not been widely used. At the present time, the ablative procedure of choice for deafferentation pain in the face appears to be the caudalis nucleus DREZ, developed by Nashold.

More recently, the evolution of the conceptual distinction between nociceptive and deafferentation pain and their differential response to ablative surgery has stimulated further exploration for alternative approaches to pain control. One of these is the electrical stimulation of brain-stem structures (Turnbull, 1984). Sites for insertion of implantable electrodes have included the medial lemniscus of the midbrain, the somatosensory relay nuclei of the thalamus, the posterior limb of the internal capsule, and the periventricular and periaqueductal gray regions in the brain stem. In a wide variety of pain problems, variable results have been obtained (Adams et al., 1974). Mazar et al. (1979) reported their results with the insertion of stimulating electrodes into the sensory thalamic nuclei. In 83 of 93 patients with deafferentation pain, satisfactory relief was obtained, whereas none of 17 patients with nociceptive cancer pain had any relief. In contrast, Meyerson et al. (1979) reported satisfactory pain relief in 7 of 13 patients with cancer pain in whom periventricular electrodes were inserted. Hosobuchi (1980) has reported significant peripheral pain relief in 16 of 22 patients by indwelling stimulation of the periaqueductal gray matter. Other investigators have had varying responses with both periventricular and periaqueductal stimulation for a variety of pain syndromes (Richardson & Akil, 1977; Hosobuchi et al., 1974; Schvarcz, 1980). Unfortunately, these studies are difficult to compare. The nature of the pain treated, whether nociceptive or deafferentated, and the anatomic distributions vary considerably. Moreover, evidence suggests that the exact site of the electrode insertion and the frequency and pattern of electrical stimulation may be crucial in the responses obtained (Boivie & Meyerson, 1982; Hosobuchi et al., 1974; Mundinger & Neumuller, 1982).

An alternative is the insertion of catheters and infusion pumps, which allow intermittent or continuous delivery of narcotic analgesics to the central nervous system through the ventricles or subarachnoid space. For patients with cancer, this appears to be a satisfactory form of therapy (Leavens et al., 1982; Onofrio et al., 1981). Its use for nonmalignant facial pain syndromes has not been established.

OCCIPITAL NEURALGIA

The physician frequently encounters individuals with pain radiating into the posterior occipital region. There is often an associated history of a flexion–extension injury or direct trauma. The differential diagnosis includes C2 or 3 root lesions, degenerative cervical disease, congenital craniovertebral anomalies and myofascial disease. In the presence of a careful normal examination and detailed skull and cervical spine films, a diagnosis of occipital neuralgia can be made, although in general ill-defined syndromes like this should be avoided. The presence of any associated neurologic deficits requires more extensive evaluation, including myelography, CT scanning, or NMR evaluation. If a bruit is present, vertebral angiography is also in order.

Initial therapy should consist of reassurance to the patient, deep heat, restriction of activities, a mild analgesic, and nonsteroidal anti-inflammatory agents, cervical collars should be avoided. With refractory pain and a focal trigger point, a local block with 1% xylocaine and/or steroids often results in significant temporary or even permanent relief of this problem. If the relief is temporary, with persistent return of the syndrome, consideration can be given to an alcohol block, nerve section, or avulsion. If selectively used, these techniques may provide permanent pain relief for a small portion of the patients. Of the operative procedures, the avulsion of the greater occipital nerve as it penetrates the deep cervical fascia under local anesthesia provides the best opportunity for permanent relief. At the time of surgical exploration, identification of focal entrapment may preclude the necessity for avulsing the nerve. In a small number of cases, the lesser occipital nerve, which penetrates the deep cervical fascia at the apex of the posterior cervical triangle, is the cause of the syndrome.

SUMMARY

Because of the complexity of the innervation of the head and neck, it is crucial that an exact diagnosis be made before surgical therapy is instituted. For certain syndromes, a general set of surgical recommendations can be made:

- For trigeminal neuralgia, surgical intervention is warranted only after a failure of medical management. In elderly or debilitated patients, avulsion or injection of the distal branch of the nerve, retrogasserian injection with glycerol, and percutaneous radiofrequency lesion are the procedures of choice. In younger patients, microvascular decompression appears to be the reasonable initial procedure.
- For primary spontaneous glossopharyngeal glossopharyngeal neuralgia, intracranial section of the 9th and 10th nerves should be considered. In debilitated

patients, percutaneous coagulation is an alternative. For secondary glosso-pharyngeal neuralgia, treatment of the primary problem and either section of the 9th and 10th cranial nerves or a unilateral stereotaxic mesencephalotomy should be considered.

- For the rare problem of geniculate neuralgia, section of the nervus intermedius and/or the peripheral 20% of the geniculate ganglion can be used.
- For postherpetic facial pain, the caudalis nucleus DREZ operation appears to have a great deal of potential, although it is still a relatively untried procedure.
- The treatment of facial pain due to invasive tumors of the head and neck depend on the extent and degree of the tumor involvement. These include percutaneous rhizotomy, dorsal rhizotomy, DREZ, and stereotaxic mesence-phalic tractotomy. An additional option is the insertion of a reservoir for the direct instillation of opiates into the lateral ventricles.
- For central deafferentation pain, ablative procedures such as DREZ of the caudalis nucleus or trigeminal medullary tractotomies may have a role in certain cases. Periventricular or periaqueductal gray stimulation appears promising, but only limited data are available at this time to evaluate this new technique.
- For occipital neuralgia, surgical decompression or avulsion should be considered only in patients with a definitive diagnosis of occipital neuralgia, a reproducible trigger point, and in whom prolonged intensive medical management has failed.

REFERENCES

Adams, J.E., Y. Hosobuchi, and H.L. Field (1974). Stimulation of internal capsule for relief of chronic pain. *J. Neurosurg. 41:*741–744.

Boivie, J. and B.A. Meyerson (1982). A correlative anatomical and clinical study of pain suppression by deep brain stimulation. *Pain 13:*113–126.

Burchiel, K.J., T.D. Steege, J.F. Howe, and J.D. Loeser (1981). Comparison of percutaneous radiofrequency gangliolysis and microvascular decompression for the surgical management of tic douloureux. *Neurosurgery 9:*111–119.

Clark, L.P. and A.S. Taylor (1909). True tic douloureux of the sensory filaments of the facial nerve. *JAMA 53:*2144–2146.

Crue, B.L., E.M. Todd, E.J.A. Carregal, and O. Kilham (1967). Percutaneous trigeminal tractotomy—case report—utilizing stereotactic radiofrequency lesion. *Bull. Los Angeles Neurol. Soc. 32:*86–92.

Cushing, H. (1920). The major trigeminal neuralgia and their surgical treatment based on experience with 332 gasserian operations. First Paper. The varieties of facial neuralgia. *Am. J. Med. Sciences 160:*157–184.

Dandy, W.E. (1927). Glossopharyngeal neuralgia (tic douloureux). Its diagnosis and treatment. *Arch. Surg. 15:*198–214.

Dandy, W.E. (1929). An operation for the cure of tic douloureux. Partial section of the sensory root at the pons. *Arch. Surg. 18:*687–734.

Dandy, W.E. (1934). Concerning the cause of trigeminal neuralgia. *Am. J. Surg. 24:*447–455.

Fox, J.L. (1971). Intractable facial pain relieved by percutaneous trigeminal tractotomy. *JAMA* 218:1940–1941.

Friedman, A.H., B.S. Nashold, Jr., and J. Ovelmen-Levitt (1984). Dorsal root entry zone lesions for treatment of post-herpetic neuralgia. *J. Neurosurg.* 60:1258–1262.

Furlow, L.T. (1942). Tic douloureux of the nervus intermedius (so-called idiopathic geniculate neuralgia). *JAMA* 119:255–259.

Gardner, W.J. (1962). Concerning the mechanism of trigeminal neuralgia and hemifacial spasm. *J. Neurosurg.* 19:947–958.

Gardner, W.J. and M.V. Miklos (1959). Response of trigeminal neuralgia to "decompression" of sensory root: Discussion of cause of trigeminal neuralgia. *JAMA* 170:1773–1776.

Grantham, E.G. and L.D. Segerberg (1952). An evaluation of palliative surgical procedures in trigeminal neuralgia *J. Neurosurg.* 9:390–394.

Hakanson, S. (1981). Trigeminal neuralgia treated by the injection of glycerol into the trigeminal cistern. *Neurosurgery* 9:638–646.

Hitchcock, E. (1970). Stereotactic trigeminal tractotomy. *Ann. Clin. Res.* 2:131–135.

Hosobuchi Y. (1980). The current status of analgesic brain stimulation. *Acta Neurochir.* 30(Suppl.):219–227.

Hosobuchi, Y., J.E. Adams, and H.L. Fields (1974). Chronic thalamic and internal capsular stimulation for the control of facial anesthesia dolorosa and dysesthesia of thalamic syndrome. *Adv. Neurol.* 4:783–787.

Hosobuchi, Y. and B. Rutkin (1971). Descending trigeminal tractotomy: Neurophysiological approach. *Arch. Neurol.* 25:115–125.

Hunt, J.R. (1907). On herpetic inflammations of the geniculate ganglion: A new syndrome and its complications. *J. Ner. Ment. Dis.* 34:73–96.

Jaeger, R. (1957). Permanent relief of tic douloureux by gasserian injection of hot water. *Arch. Neurol. Psychiatry* 77:1–7.

Jannetta, P.J. (1985). Trigeminal neuralgia: Treatment by microvascular compression. I *Neurosurgery* (R.H. Wilkins and S.S. Rengachary, eds.), pp. 2357–2363. McGraw-Hill, New York.

Kirschner, M. (1932). Zur elektrokoagulation des ganglion gasseri. *Zentralbl. Chir.* 47:2841–2843.

Leavens, M.E., C.S. Hill, D.A. Cech et al. (1982). Intrathecal and intraventricular morphine for pain in cancer patients: Initial study. *J. Neurosurg.* 56:241–245.

Lunsford, L.D. (1985). Trigeminal neuralgia. Treatment by glycerol rhizotomy. In *Neurosurgery* (R.W. Wilkins, and S.S. Rengachary, eds.), pp. 2351–2356. McGraw-Hill, New York.

Mazar, G.J., L. Merienne, and C. Cioloca (1979) Comparative study of electrical stimulation of posterior thalamic nuclei, periaqueductal gray, and other midline mesencephalic structures in man. *Adv. Pain Res.* 3:541–552.

McKenzie, K.G. (1954). Trigeminal tractotomy. *Clin. Neurosurg.* 2:50–70.

Meyerson, B.A., J. Boethius, and A.M. Carlsson (1979). Alleviation of malignant pain by electrical stimulation in the periventricular-periaqueductal region: Pain relief as related to stimulation sites. *Adv. Pain Res.* 3:525–529.

Mundinger, F. and H. Neumuller (1982). Programmed stimulation for control of chronic pain and motor diseases. *Appl. Neurophysiol.* 45:102–111.

Nashold, B.S., Jr. (1972). Extensive cephalic and oral pain relieved by midbrain tractotomy. *Conf. Neurol.* 34:382.

Nashold, B.S., Jr. (1986). "Trigeminal DREZ for craniofacial pain." In *Surgery in and around the Brainstem* (M. Samii, ed.) pp. 53–58. Springer-Vertog, Heidelburg.

Nugent, G.R. (1985). Trigeminal neuralgia: Treatment by percutaneous electrocoagulation. In

Neurosurgery (R.W. Wilkins, and S.S. Rengachary, eds.), pp. 2345–2350. McGraw-Hill, New York.

Nugent, G.R. and B. Berry (1974). Trigeminal neuralgia treated by differential percutaneous radiofrequency coagulation of the gasserian ganglion. *J. Neurosurg.* 40:517–523.

Onofrio, B.M. (1975). Radiofrequency percutaneous gasserian ganglion lesions. Results in 140 patients with trigeminal pain. *J. Neurosurg.* 42:132–139.

Onofrio, B.M., T.L. Yaksh, and T.G. Arnold (1981). Continuous low-dose intrathecal morphine administration in the treatment of chronic pain of malignant origin. *Mayo Clin. Proc.* 56:516–520.

Pennybacker, J. (1961). Some observations on trigeminal neuralgia. In *Scientific Aspects of Neurology* (H. Garland, ed.), p. 153, Livingstone, Edinburgh.

Pulec, J.L. (1976). Geniculate neuralgia: Diagnosis and surgical management. *Laryngoscope* 86:955–964.

Putnam, T.J. and A.O. Hampton (1936). A technique of injection into the gasserian ganglion under roentgenographic control. *Arch. Neurol. Psychiatry* 35:92–98.

Quinn, J.H. (1965). Repetitive peripheral neurectomies for neuralgia of second and third division of trigeminal nerve. *J. Oral Surg.* 23:600–608.

Richardson, D.E. and Akil, H (1977). Pain reduction by electrical brain stimulation in man. Part I. Acute administration in periaqueductal and periventricular sites. *J. Neurosurg.* 47:178–183.

Schvarcz, J.R. (1980). Chronic self-stimulation of the medial posterior inferior thalamus for the alleviation of deafferentation pain. *Acta Neurocir.* 30(Suppl.):295–301.

Sicard, J.A. and V. Robineau (1920). Algievelopharyngie essentielle: Traitment chirurgical. *Rev. Neurol.* 36:256–277.

Sjoquist, O. (1938). Studies on pain conduction in the trigeminal nerve. *Acta Psychiatr. Scand.* 17(Suppl.):1–139.

Stookey, B. and J. Ransohoff (1959). *Trigeminal Neuralgia: Its History and Treatment.* Charles C. Thomas, Springfield, Ill.

Sweet, W.H. and J.C. Wepsic (1974). Controlled thermocoagulation of trigeminal ganglion and rootlets for differential destruction of pain fibers: Pt. 1. Trigeminal neuralgia. *J. Neurosurg.* 40:143–156.

Sweet, W.H., C.E. Poletti, and J.B. Macon (1981). Treatment of trigeminal neuralgia and other facial pains by retrogasserian injection of glycerol. *Neurosurgery* 9:647–653.

Tenicela, R., Lovasik, D., and Eaglstein, W. (1985) Treatment of herpes zoster with sympathetic blocks. *Clin. J. Pain* 1:63–68.

Tew, J.M. (1979). Treatment of trigeminal neuralgia. *Neurosurgery* 4:93–94.

Tew, J.M., Jr. (1982) Treatment of pain of glossopharyngeal and vagus nerves by percutaneous rhizotomy. I *Neurological Surgery,* 2nd ed. (J.R. Youmans, ed.), pp. 3609–3612. W.B. Saunders, Philadelphia.

Turnbull, I.M. (1984). Brain stimulation. In *Textbook of Pain* (P.D. Wall, R. Melzack, eds), pp. 706–714. Churchill-Livingstone.

Walker, A.E. (1942). Relief of pain by mesencephalic tractotomy. *Arch. Neurol. Psychiatry* 48:865–883.

Weisenburg, F.M. (1910). Cerebellopontine tumor diagnosed for six years as tic douloureux. The symptoms of irritation of the ninth and tenth cranial nerves. *JAMA* 59:1600–1604.

White, J.C. and W.H. Sweet (1969). *Pain and the Neurosurgeon, a Forty Year Experience.* Charles C Thomas, Springfield, Ill.

Wilkins, R.H. (1985). Trigeminal neuralgia: Introduction. I *Neurosurgery* (R.H. Wilkins, S.S. Rengachary, eds.), pp. 2337–2344, McGraw-Hill, New York.

22

Life Stress, Personality Factors, and Reactions to Headache

RUSSELL C. PACKARD

Headache is a symptom that occurs in a variety of contexts and has a diverse etiology, nearly always multifactorial. The intertwining factors of life stress, personality traits, and reaction to headache affect virtually all headache patients. The difficulty comes in determining the degree of involvement for each individual patient, who may or may not be reacting to certain life stresses, who has a personality that may or may not influence the headache pattern, and who may react to a headache along a continuum from simply taking two aspirin and ignoring it to fearing the worst and being totally incapacitated both physically and socially. The headache complaint always involves a dynamic balance for each individual patient between cause, sensation, and reaction (Packard, 1979a).

Life is a constant, dynamic process of responding to stimuli, pressures, and demands that may originate internally or externally. What often complicates an accurate evaluation of stress or personality factors in a headache patient is that most patients experience a changing susceptibility to these and other stimuli as they age and adapt, so that these factors may exert an inconsistent and variable influence on headache attacks. For instance, a patient who is perfectionistic and suppresses feelings of anger at age 20 might suffer from periodic migraine (and/or muscle contraction headache), but at age 30 he may have relaxed his perfectionistic ways and become more expressive of his feelings. These adaptive changes (or others) could improve his headache problems (Saper, 1983). This variability and inconsistency makes it difficult to isolate the numerous emotional (and biological) stressors involved in headache evaluation. Most specialists agree, however, that careful attention to these influences is important in evaluating and managing patients with headache.

LIFE STRESS AND HEADACHE

Physicians have long been aware that emotionally stressful factors could trigger head-aches. In the late 1880s, Breuer and Freud (1955) noticed that patients' complaints of headache often disappeared after they reached an improved emotional equilibrium. Wolff (1963), in his investigations of psychiatric factors in headache, wrote that "since the human animal prides himself on 'using his head,' it is perhaps not without meaning that his head should be the source of so much discomfort . . . or that the vast majority of discomforts and pains of the head . . . are accompaniments of resentments and dissatisfactions." The first five groups of the American Medical Association Ad Hoc Committee on Classification of Headache (1962) encompassed those headaches that, in the committee's words, "May be the principal manifestation of temporary or sustained difficulties in life adjustment." These groups are vascular headache of migraine type, muscle contraction headache, combined headache—vas-cular and muscle contraction—headache of nasal vasomotor reaction, and headaches of delusional, conversion, or hypochondriacal states. "Temporary or sustained diffi-culties in life adjustment" could easily be termed, "life stress."

Stress has been variously defined. Rose and Gawel (1979) commented that "stress is one of the most misused words in the English language and its precise meaning is often forgotten." They define it from the shorter Oxford English Dictionary as sim-ply "a demand upon energy." They feel this is a difficult concept to apply to the human body and not a factor that can easily be measured. Selye (1976) defined stress as "the non-specific response of the body to any demand made upon it." Schafer (1983) modified this definition slightly by defining stress as "an arousal of mind and body in response to demands made upon it."

A common thread in these definitions is the word "demand." It seems clear that we cannot go through life without certain demands being placed on our energy, body, and mind. Stress and the arousal it produces are a universal part of life. Response to stress involves virtually every set of organs and tissues in the body, and thoughts and feelings are clearly intertwined with physiologic processes.

When the level of arousal becomes too high (or too low), either temporarily or chronically, then stress can become distress (Schafer, 1983). This may lead to symp-toms such as trembling hands, churning stomach, tight shoulders, edginess, or poor concentration. If a person ignores or "doesn't listen to" these early warning symp-toms, they may become chronic and develop into one of several stress-related ill-nesses, such as migraine, muscle contraction headache, peptic ulcer, irritable colon, or high blood pressure. It is important to bear in mind that reactions to stress are a function of perception, personality, age, status, life stage, unrealized expectations, prior experiences, social support systems, and one's capacity to respond adequately or adapt (Christensen, 1981).

The psychophysiologic mechanisms whereby migraine and muscle contraction headache may develop are discussed more fully in the chapters dealing with these specific headache types. It is still unclear how stress provokes migraine and, in fact, why some attacks occur after a period of prolonged stress and not during the period of stress (Saper, 1983). Simply stated, stress can contribute to headache development in three ways: (1) by imposing long-term wear and tear on the body and mind, reducing resistance, (2) by directly precipitating sustained muscular contraction or changing vascular reactivity in migraine, or (3) by aggravating an already existing headache.

The line between psychological distress symptoms and psychiatric illness is often not distinct. Symptoms tend to shade gradually into more serious states of anxiety or depression. Psychologic distress symptoms frequently accompany physical illness or headache because of the intricate interplay of mind and body. This area will be discussed further in the last section on reactions to headache.

Evaluation of Stress

Because emotionally stressful factors appear in such a high proportion of patients with headache, it is important to evaluate these areas in depth. Unfortunately, patients often cloud over stressful issues, present them in a vague manner or conceal them. Although patients are sometimes truly unaware of stressful events, often they are aware of stress but believe the physician will not be interested or does not have time, or they themselves see their complaint as embarrassing or a sign of weakness (Brodsky, 1984). Some physicians, in fact, want to avoid this type of evaluation because it does take time, involvement with the patient, and some awareness of life stress factors and issues (Packard, 1983). Lance (1981) also feels that careful attention must be given to the patient as a person and to his or her work and home environments to prevent unnecessary fluctuations in stress or emotional tone. For proper evaluation, the physician must be aware of some common and high-risk stressors, because patients are frequently unaware of these factors and their role in symptom formation.

Change

One of the major factors to consider is unpredictability and change (Brett, 1980). This may involve social change, referring to the environment in which the patient lives and works, or personal change in an individual's life such as moving, changing jobs, getting older, retiring, or becoming more assertive (Schafer, 1983). Toffler (1971), in his book *Future Shock,* discusses the accelerating pace of social change in our current age, with its faster pace, increased population growth and crowding, rapid technological growth, and new knowledge. In such a rapidly changing world, more frequent and faster adjustments are needed and more stress can set in.

Even though human beings have an excellent capacity to adjust and adapt to change, this capacity is variable depending on the individual (Schafer, 1978). We also can easily delude ourselves into believing we are adapting simply because we feel "comfortable" with a highly demanding job, the fast pace of our life, or a bad marriage. This apparent adjustment is really not successful adaptation. In time, our bodies give way in one way or another. Selye (1976) maintains that our deep adaptive reserves are limited and can be used up. It is important to note how frequently a "change" in one's headache pattern may reflect a change in one's circumstances or life situation.

Life Pace

It is important to get some concept of the patient's pace of life. Patients are often overloaded, cramming more into an hour, a day, a week. A good example is the so-called Type A personality, who is driven to accomplish as much as possible in the shortest possible time (Dembrosky et al., 1978). These people are often chronically impatient with "wasted time" as well as the slow pace of others. Friedman and Rosenman (1974) point out that American culture places a high value on speed, number, and accomplishment. It is not unusual for these patients to outwardly present as "free of stress" because they have deluded themselves into believing they are race horses. However, a fast pace of life without pause for rest can be a significant source of tension, stress, and distress that may lead to headache symptoms or a change in headache pattern. Some headache patients will report having two jobs, a divorce, family responsibilities, church duties, community activities, and no awareness of stress. Interestingly, although these patients are seeking explanation and relief from headache, they frequently will not have time for appointments with the doctor, biofeedback, or biofeedback practice.

Transitions

Another type of experience that frequently causes distress is transition from one set of habits to another. This is similar to and actually represents a form of change. But every change requires a transition, and transition requires adjustment. These factors have even been quantitated to some extent by the Holmes–Rahe social readjustment rating scale (1967). For instance, moving geographically, even though the move may be to a better job or a nicer neighborhood, represents a change from the familiar to the unfamiliar. A promotion involves a role transition in our current society. Marriage, divorce, and remarriage are common stressful transitional factors in life. Also, becoming a parent or a student can bring about major changes in one's life-style. A serious loss can be a very traumatic occurrence, especially the loss of a spouse or one's home. Even retirement represents a type of loss. Whatever the loss, people pass through remarkably similar steps of mourning (Horowitz, 1976).

Many studies have documented the contribution of individual life changes to physical and psychological distress (Rahe, 1979). Another common pattern, however, among highly stressed patients involves too much change in too short a time. A growing number of studies have shown that the greater the clustering of life events, the greater the chance of developing symptoms or becoming ill (Rahe, 1968; Garrity et al., 1977). Again, patients with headache often present with a "laundry list" of recent changes, transitions, and events, all clustered together, and they have little awareness of the role these may be playing in their headache symptom formation.

Work Stress, Role Conflicts, and Expectations

A recent comprehensive review by Brodsky (1984) thoroughly discussed work stress and its role as a stressor in 2000 patients over an 18-year period. An exploration of the patients' feelings about their job situations and roles in life is very important. A role is the cluster of expectations associated with a social or work position such as teacher, student, husband, or neighbor. When a person's own desires conflict with what others expect or want, a role conflict may result. Probably the most common situation is a job problem in which one is unable or unwilling to do what others expect because one wants something different or one's skills do not fit the situation. Conflicting expectations almost always create stress.

The expectations of a patient with headache are equally important to clarify, especially if the patient is expecting or hoping for "total relief." This expectation is rarely expressed verbally but frequently expressed on a patient history form (Packard, 1985). Patients with headache may also expect or want something from the doctor other than what the doctor expects, such as an explanation for the cause of the headache, rather than pain relief (Packard, 1979b). These are important issues to clarify.

The physical environment is often taken for granted, but noise has been noted to be perhaps the most troublesome and common of all stressors in the physical environment. Girdano and Everly (1979) point out that noise can produce a stress response in three ways: (1) by causing physiologic reactions from stimulation of the sympathetic nervous system, (2) by being annoying and subjectively displeasing, and (3) by disrupting ongoing activities. Another distressing stressor in the physical environment is improper lighting (Ivancevich & Matteson, 1980). The increased amount of time many individuals spend in front of a computer screen can also be quite irritating and can aggravate or even precipitate some headaches. Extreme temperatures can also have direct and indirect effects on stress.

Other

Other important areas of stress are understimulation (Schafer, 1983), social isolation or loneliness (Berkman & Syne, 1976), financial uncertainty or unemployment, and a number of minor but irritating "daily hassles." These "daily hassles," according to Lazarus (1981), may do the most damage of all. Most frequently, these involve concern about weight, health of a family member, rising prices, home maintenance, and too many things to do. Neurotic life-styles can also lead to chronic or intermittent stressful situations, such as when a person's fear of failure, fear of success, or perception of what one thinks one should be is in conflict with what one actually is. Patients who are rigid and perfectionistic have their own set of problems and difficulties; these will be discussed more in the next section under personality factors.

When Patients Deny Stress

Many patients with headache initially deny having any emotional difficulties or stress in their lives. This should not discourage the examiner from a careful evaluation of the patient's situation preceding or accompanying the onset of headache. The factors noted above should be listened for carefully. The coincidence of a major change or an acute emotional state with the appearance of headache is quite suggestive, even if the connection between the psychological event and the symptom is unrecognized by the patient (Packard, 1980). At times a relative or close friend may clarify many confusing areas, whereas further direct questioning of the patient will probably be of little benefit. The patient must essentially be allowed to tell his or her own story at his own or her own rate. It is often helpful to have the patient begin keeping a headache diary to report events preceding and during a headache, as well as to grade the headaches' intensity. This technique may enable the patient to develop an awareness of feelings or situations previously ignored or denied, and it can be useful for evaluating treatment.

The examiner should be alert for clues concerning psychological stresses that may be related to the patient's difficulties. An angry rejection or denial of possible psychological factors involved in a headache situation is in itself a measure of the degree of underlying emotional conflict. Some people simply are not in touch with their inner needs and feelings, however, and find it difficult to verbalize them.

Indirect questioning may help bring the psychological factors to light. Ask the patient what he or she does for fun. It is surprising how many patients who describe a wonderful and problem-free life with their job and spouse cannot think of a single thing that is fun. This realization will often open an important doorway to emotional issues. Also, inquire about whether the patient has ever known anyone with a similar type of headache problem. The answer may reveal unconscious attitudes about the patient's own situation and clues concerning the origin. Ask what the headache keeps the patient from doing. The answer here will often provide material concerning the psychodynamic significance of the symptoms as well as the secondary gain. Equally important is to find out the reactions of key relatives or the spouse to a patient's headache. Often one of two patterns may emerge: a spouse who is the perfectly understanding and sympathetic caretaker, or just the opposite, one who totally lacks sympathy and understanding. It may also be helpful to ask if the patient is concerned about a brain tumor. This is a common fear that is seldom spontaneously expressed.

PERSONALITY FACTORS IN HEADACHE

Personality factors in migraine have been more intensively studied over the years than those in other forms of headache, probably because migraine is a fairly well-defined syndrome. The thinking about personality factors in migraine has gone through an interesting evolutionary process over the years. Early studies in the 1930s and 1940s were heavily psychoanalytic, then as the varied and interesting vascular and biochemical discoveries came to light, migraine became "psychosomatic" (Pearce, 1977) and the physiologic aspects seemed to become more central. Recently, there seems to be a tendency to either dismiss personality factors, as evidenced in a book on *Advances in Migraine Research and Therapy* (Rose, 1982), which does not contain a single page dedicated to personality factors, or consider these factors separately, as in a recent book dedicated entirely to the psychiatric aspects of headache (Adler et al., 1987).

It is clear that personality factors are important to consider in patients with migraine and other headache types as well. As noted in other parts of this chapter, every headache is a multifactorial symptom occurring in a person with a unique personality. The headache is not an abstraction existing in a pool of chemicals or blood vessels outside a person. Even if headaches are caused primarily by hereditary and physiologic factors, treatment must still be directed, for the most part, to the person suffering from the headache (Lance, 1981; Packard, 1979a). This section reviews personality factors and their role in headache.

Early Studies

In 1743, Junkerius wrote that the primary cause of migraine is anger, especially when it is tacit and suppressed (Jonckheere, 1971). This theme echoes regularly through the early case studies of migraine patients. In an early study, Touraine and Draper (1934) suggested that it may be possible to identify a "constitutional" personality susceptible to migraine, with retarded emotional development but superior intelligence, frequent exaggerated dependence on the mother, and rather unsatisfactory sexual adjustment.

Knopf (1935), in a detailed study of 30 cases of migraine, described them as being "dignified," very ambitious, reserved, repressed, sensitive, domineering, resentful of authority, and, perhaps the most serious defect, possessing very little sense of humor. Fromm-Reichman (1937), in describing a series of eight patients treated by psychoanalysis, related the etiology of migraine to envious hostile impulses, often followed by guilt and turned back against the self.

Wolff (1937), in a paper on personality features and reactions of subjects with migraine, emphasized a number of characteristics described in these persons as compulsive, perfectionistic, rigid, ambitious, competitive, unable to delegate responsibility, and commonly in a state of chronic resentfulness.

Selinsky (1939) described migraine as particularly frequent in women with high intellectual abilities and inhibited behavior, who commonly led the life of a harried housewife. Trowbridge et al. (1943) felt the patient with migraine was deliberate, often to the point of displaying hesitation that rendered decisions difficult. It was difficult for these patients to face new situations, and they frequently had an exaggerated feeling of personal insecurity. Marcussen (1949) and Alexander (1950) related the occurrence of migraine to suppressed resentment and anger or a state of repressed rage.

In the 1950s, although several studies continued to describe the personality pattern in patients with migraine as inflexible, perfectionistic, rigid, resentful, and ambitious (Weiss & English, 1957), Friedman and Brenner (1950) commented that the relationship to suppressed anger was not entirely specific and that on occasion other conflicts might precipitate a migraine attack. Further, Friedman (1958) stated that he believed the personality manifestations were extremely variable in migraine patients and could include a variety of emotional factors, mostly unconscious. These factors include hostility, identification with a family figure, the wish to remain in a position of dependency as a means to gain love, affection, or attention. Conflicts most frequently seem to concern hostile impulses associated with feelings of guilt. There was little evidence of specificity of the precipitating or psychodynamic factors. Friedman concluded that not all patients with migraine were compulsive, perfectionistic, or rigid.

Kolb (1963) thought that the majority of patients with migraine who went to psychiatrists showed a rigid form of behavior in which they denied the expression of direct or verbal aggression. These patients often came from families who took great pride in attainment. In a dynamic formulation, the consequence of the arousal of conflict with associated anxiety over inevitably emerging hostility (while trying to maintain the family standards as a means of continuing the desired relationships) formed the interpersonal matrix that triggered the headache. Boag (1968) reviewed these early studies in detail and summarized that a wide range of personality characteristics could be described in patients suffering from migraine. There seemed to be general agreement that repressed anger was a major common factor. However, Boag believed that considerable evidence showed this does not hold in all cases; other emotional states, particularly anxiety in a setting of tense control or depression, may be equally important in an undefined proportion of cases.

Recent Studies

Jonckheere (1971) noted that 11 of 16 typical patients with migraine headaches were obsessional, aggressive, or both and that their aggression, along with their headaches, had a tendency to disappear when psychotherapy permitted its expression.

Using detailed histories and psychometric tests in a controlled study of 100 patients with migraine, Henryk-Gutt and Rees (1973) found that emotional stress was important, in that more than half of their subjects suffered their first migraine attacks during a period of emotional stress. However, there was no objective evidence that the subjects experienced greater stress than the controls. They concluded that migraine subjects were predisposed by constitutional factors (and not by environmental factors), to experience a greater than average reaction to a given quantity of stress. They were unable to confirm that migraine subjects were especially obsessional or ambitious and suggested that previous studies were insufficiently comprehensive because the groups studied were self-selected and not fully representative of migraine subjects in general.

In a review study, Phillips (1976) concluded that there was only minimal support for the view that migraine sufferers were more neurotic than age-matched normals. In a random sample of 1500 patients in a general practice, he found 39 migraine patients, 24 tension headache patients, and 5 patients with migraine and tension headaches. No significant group differences were found in neuroticism, extroversion, or psychotic behavior. These cases, collected without reference to a headache complaint, cannot be distinguished from normal subjects.

In a review of four Minnesota Multiphasic Personality Inventory (MMPI) studies (Steinhilber et al., 1960; Martin et al., 1967; Martin, 1972; and Rogado et al., 1974), 325 subjects with various types of headache complaints showed a common profile characterized by a "conversion V." This suggested that the patients' anxiety was being held in check by compulsive defenses and expressed by somatic complaints. Although psychological factors may be a cause of or a predisposition to headache, it should be noted that the neuroticism observed in headache patients may be a consequence of the risks of sudden intense pain or of adaptation to being a patient.

A recent trend has been for studies to indicate an absence of a discreet border between migraine and tension headache (Cohen, 1978). In a controlled study of personality in headache type by Passchier et al. (1984), very little difference was found in personality factors among migraine and tension headache patients. Achievement motivation was found to be elevated in both headache groups. The tension headache patients also exhibited greater rigidity than the migraine headache group and the controls, a finding not previously reported in earlier studies. Both headache groups showed raised achievement motivation and rigidity with more fear of failure than controls. No evidence was found for higher prevalence of neuroticism or obsessive–compulsive behavior in the headache groups. Adler, Adler, and Packard (1987) review personality factors in detail elsewhere.

In summary, it is difficult to derive a concise statement regarding personality factors in migraine. In broad terms, migraine seems to represent a vascular mechanism for coping with life situations that are stressful to the individual. It is probable that many stresses—social, economic, and psychological—may activate this unique vascular response. Some of the factors described may be very important in some patients with migraine and less important or even unimportant in others. If these personality factors are identified, they can be useful in the evaluation and management of these patients. As an example, a structured individual who only has migraine attacks on Saturday mornings can often be helped simply by rising a bit earlier or planning some weekend activity in advance. Other patients may be able to deal with accumulating tension and repressed or suppressed hostility up to a certain point, but beyond this they cannot continue and a headache may ensue that forces them to a halt.

It is clear that awareness of personality characteristics and the stresses that provoke or aggravate the migraine response is essential to effective treatment of these patients. The physician has a unique opportunity to assist the patient in modifying responses to the external factors he or she considers stressful, and more important, to change the patient's reaction to any unrealistically rigid internal demands that may be present.

Personality Factors and Other Headache Types

Muscle Contraction Headache

Muscle contraction is a common cause of headache. Chronic muscle contraction headaches are usually related to tension, anxiety, depression, repressed hostility, unresolved dependency needs, or psychosexual conflicts (Saper, 1983). One can see that many of the personality factors discussed in the previous sections on life stress and migraine can also lead to sustained contraction of skeletal muscle and development of muscle contraction headache, although the actual mechanisms are still unclear (Lance, 1981). These may be the most common headaches seen in medical practice and are often demonstrably associated with emotional stress or tension (Packard, 1979a; 1983). Friedman (1950) found emotional factors to be present in 100% of the patients with tension (muscle contraction) headaches.

One of the difficulties in delineating personality factors in cases of muscle contraction headache has been the vague and ambiguous terminology applied. Terms such as psychogenic, nervous, and tension have been used in different senses by different authors (Blumenthal, 1968). At least one study showed the term psychogenic headache to be variously defined and neither precise nor diagnostic (Packard, 1976). There always seems to be some doubt as to whether tension implies emotional tension or muscle tension.

Graham (1964) believes that a deep-seated reflex, apparently little altered by evolution, underlies muscle contraction headache. He compares the turtle shrugging back his head and the ape pulling his head down between his shoulders in the face of fear or danger to what the human being now does before the "slings and arrows of outrageous fortune." This type of headache may occur in occupational settings or in attempts to reduce the pain of a vascular headache or painful disorders of the neck, but most often it is part of a total reaction against psychological pressures. Although it seems clear that these headaches are often clearly related to environmental stress, anxiety, or strongly repressed or suppressed anger, there does not seem to be any clear personality type or profile associated. Adler, Adler, and Packard (1987) have made a thorough review.

Cluster Headache

Cluster headaches seem to occur more often in men who drink more alcohol and smoke more than the average male population without cluster headaches (Kudrow, 1979). Psychological tests and MMPI studies on a series of cluster headache patients demonstrated high scores on traits such as conscientiousness, perseverence, responsibility, self-sufficiency, precision, and resourcefulness; the patients were also found to be tense, frustrated, driven, and overwrought (Kudrow, 1979). MMPI results from patients with migraine and cluster headaches are noted to be almost indistinguishable (Kudrow, 1983).

A more detailed study of a small number of cluster headache patients demonstrated obsessive–compulsive behavior traits in aggressive, hard-driving, goal-oriented men. These men seemed to push themselves until they faltered because of the symptoms or until they reached their set goals, at which time they often collapsed with a seige of headache. Many times it was noted that a cluster seemed to begin during or just after stressful events in the person's life (Graham, 1969). Graham (1969) also described facial characteristics shared by many cluster headache patients as leonine in appearance. Observations also suggested that the presence of sustained stress and rage may provoke a bout of episodic cluster, and disturbance of sleep and mood may also occur before the onset of the headaches (Kudrow, 1980).

Some feel the cluster headache patient displays the most deep-seated emotional difficulties of all (Adler et al., Adler, 1982) Cluster patients will not acknowledge these difficulties, invariably denying them. The typical cluster patient is often an "iron clad man." Often severe and overwhelming early losses, frequently of a parent, have been experienced. What is remarkable is that in describing these occurrences, the cluster headache patient shows little feeling. He seems to have shut off the most upsetting emotional experience of his life behind a steel door. He does not betray intense emotion because he does not consciously feel intense emotion, but when the cluster headache begins, then there is tearing and thrashing and overwhelming agitation, depression, aggression, and sometimes even suicide. These problems are so well repressed and the affect is so isolated from awareness that they may be undetectable on the MMPI. These patients are often extremely resistant to traditional forms of psychotherapy but may very much need a less confrontational type of treatment, along with medical treatment.

REACTIONS TO HEADACHE

Headaches or any physical symptoms or illnesses have the capacity to initiate strong regressive tendencies in any individual (MacKinnon & Michels, 1971). Depending on basic character structure, one patient may submit to these tendencies by lapsing into a helpless and dependent state, whereas another may deny and/or try and hide symptoms and insist on maintaining usual activity. If headaches become long-lasting, chronic, or severely disabling, they may provoke a variety of psychological reactions in the patient and his or her family. This section considers some common patterns of reaction among patients with headache. An awareness by the physician of some of these factors can lead to improved treatment planning and management of patients with headache problems.

Personality and Emotional Reactions to Headache

Any major change in an individual's body functioning and way of living requires adaptation. Headache often represents a change that is unplanned, unscheduled, and unwanted, as well as producing pain and possibly other symptoms that may make adaptation difficult. The individual's reaction to this type of problem often depends on several factors, but especially important is one's own basic personality and the degree to which one has responded successfully to previous life stresses. Basic personality structure has become an important element in the psychological management of any patient who is physically ill, even when the patient is psychologically a normal, well-functioning person (Kahana & Bibring, 1964). Naturally, if there is marked accentuation of character traits, neurotic or psychotic symptoms, a limited capacity for work, or impaired ability for social relationships, then treatment becomes more difficult.

The basic nature and severity of the headache is also important, including its actual meaning and symbolic significance to the patient. Many laypersons still consider the head and brain as synonymous (Kolb, 1959). The family dynamics for coping play an important role, as do situational demands from the patient's environment, such as his or her level of responsibility and work. Expectations of both the patient and the physician are also important, especially if the patient is hoping for or expecting total relief (Packard, 1985).

Fortunately, most headaches are minor, short-lived, and self-limiting symptoms that impose little or no actual disability, but headache can become disabling, both physically and emotionally. It can drain an individual's energy, cause lost time at work, disrupt the family, and lead to medication overuse or abuse (Mathew, 1985). Anxiety generated by more significant headache or poor ability to cope may even sufficiently interfere with the patients adaptive capacity that he or she will be unable to participate effectively in managing the headache problem and its care (Horenstein,

1983). Simple anxiety in headache patients usually responds well to reassurance, a good physician–patient relationship, and a period of well-being or stability of the underlying headache symptom (Graham, 1985). The more a patient's life has changed, however, the more overwhelming the emotional response is likely to be, and certain types of reaction can often be defined. The most common of these are denial, depression, hostility, anger, and the development of dependency (Horenstein, 1983).

Denial

Some form of denial is not uncommon as a reaction to headaches or other physical symptoms or illnesses (Weinstein & Kahn, 1955). Denying the extent of one's symptoms by withdrawal may temporarily relieve the attendant anxiety. Denial may also protect the patient from painful reality by delaying necessary steps in diagnosis and treatment. For instance, many headache patients continue to work while feeling ill with a headache, continue a hectic pace that may aggravate their symptoms, or do not take time to see their doctor or take their medication. This type of reaction may actually be part of the underlying process that causes or precipitates some headaches. In a sense, it is "easier" for the patient to get a headache or have one get worse than to deal with the underlying fears, concerns, guilt, or harsh expectations. A patient may also delay treatment by seeking other medical advice, trying fads, or rejecting advice or medication.

Denial may also be coupled with projection; the patient may externalize the cause for his or her discomfort by blaming family members or even the physician. By this mechanism the patient may deny his or her own role in an auto or industrial accident that produced a post-traumatic headache. It may serve as a barrier to the patient's acceptance of his diagnosis, assumption of responsibility for participation in his or her own care, and involvement in long-term planning. These difficulties frequently arise with headache patients who present searching for a cure or total relief, despite explanations and the definition of realistic goals. Patients may even nod in understanding, only to call back in 2 days, reporting, "the headache isn't gone." Another common difficulty is the patient who is continually searching for "the cause," despite adequate evaluation, testing, and reassurance.

For the most part, denial tends to disappear with time and requires little special treatment other than careful explanation and understanding on the part of the physician. When one is confronted with a patient who is actively in a period of denial, it is often fruitless and frustrating to demand the patient's involvement in planning or participation in headache management. Prolonged or severe degrees of explicit denial may require psychotherapeutic intervention, which the patient may also balk at or reject. These situations may occur with hypochondriasis, in which the patient has a poor sense of self-worth and turns to the physician to provide what is not solidly established by the spouse or family (Adler, 1981). These patients will often be demanding, searching, complaining, and unresponsive to explanations and treatment measures.

Similarly, a patient presenting with a continuous or chronic headache and denial of any emotional and interpersonal difficulties, idealization of family relationships, excessive activity prior to the onset of the headache, and excessive passivity after its onset would fit a profile of "pain-prone disorder," as described by Blumer and Heilbronn (1981). These pain-prone patients are often not candidates for psychotherapy and are best managed in a pain or headache clinic where a treatment team consistently deemphasizes pain from headache, encourages activity, and slowly eliminates treatment with analgesics (Blumer, 1985). Denial also represents a key feature in conversion headache, in which the patient may complain bitterly about headache but seem affectually indifferent (Packard, 1980).

Depression

Depression is a common reaction to chronic headache, but both depression and headache are prevalent clinical problems that often coincide (Diamond, 1987). Either may antedate the other or they may appear simultaneously. Depression may occur in a "realistic sense" when the patient is aware of his or her limitations with a headache and its direct effect on his or her life, or it may be enhanced by the many symbolic meanings that the patient may attach to this problem. These reactions vary considerably from one patient to another and vary with each individual's situation. For instance, a minor vascular headache with a 5-minute visual aura may provoke considerable anxiety and depression in an airline pilot who anticipates occupational disability and dependency. This type of situation in a laborer would most likely be trivial. The symbolic meaning of headache invariably plays some part in the patient's reaction to illness.

The underrecognition of pain and depression has been highlighted by the effectiveness of antidepressants in treating pain with or without accompanying depression. It is an increasing practice of pain centers or headache clinics to focus on the diagnosis of depression and to treat the condition with antidepressant medication. It is not clear whether depression is simply a psychologic consequence of the pain or headache experience or represents part of a reverberating circuit between pain and depression or is an aspect of a fundamental psychobiologic disorder (Lindsay & Wyckoff, 1981). Whatever the precise mechanisms involved, mounting evidence suggests that it is best viewed as a single entity rather than as a condition in which each aspect is merely a symptom of the other. Further aspects of depression in headache and the biochemistry of affective disorders in headache can be found elsewhere in this book.

Hostility, Anger, and Dependency

Hostility and anger may dominate one's reaction to headache. As noted in the section on personality factors, many patients with headache have difficulty expressing angry or hostile feelings. Frequently these feelings emerge as a reaction to a headache— that is, the patient is angry because he or she has a headache or angry because there is no cure. In this situation the patient's family and/or physician may be the object of this displaced anger. If the patient has difficulty expressing his feelings, his or her behavior may become passive–aggressive, he or she may become depressed, and the headache may become worse.

An underlying quality of anger is common when the headache is associated with or has resulted from an industrial accident or personal injury (Massey & Scherokman, 1983). Under these circumstances, the patient may blame others entirely for his difficulty, thereby denying his own responsibility or even his own negligence. He may try to punish those responsible for his difficulty through law suits. Search for gain or compensation may become a predominant element in his reaction to post-traumatic headache. Although this is not a problem in all post-traumatic headache patients (Speed, 1985), it seems to be a general fact that as long as these issues remain unresolved, the patient is likely to remain symptomatic, respond poorly to management, and develop new symptoms, especially in response to treatment.

Dealing with a patient's anger requires more patience and thoughtfulness than many physicians can muster (Groves, 1978). In treatment, the psychological issues should be defined as clearly as possible, appropriate investigations should be conducted, and a therapeutic contract established with the patient in which therapeutic goals are mutually defined and pursued. In post-traumatic cases, usually little or no progress will be made until outstanding medical and legal issues have been settled, and settlement should be a condition of treatment (Horenstein, 1983). Any other therapeutic approach without prospect of medical-legal settlement is likely to fail and confirm the patient's symptoms. More details on post-traumatic headache can be found in the chapter devoted to that topic.

The development of dependency and the abandonment of efforts at independence frequently complicates long-term headache problems. Dependency reactions can often be anticipated to occur in patients with a past history of passivity and immaturity. Once established, these reactions are difficult to manage. The patient who reacted initially with depression may also become quite dependent.

A hostile patient often elicits a reciprocal feeling of anger in the physician that may lead to distancing from or rejection of the patient (Gorlin & Zucker, 1983). Such behavior only intensifies the patient's reaction. A coping strategy would be simply to acknowledge and analyze the patient's anger, use behavioral approaches, and not attempt to like the unlikable patient. If the situation is intolerable, the patient is best transferred to another physician.

The management of emotional reactions to headache is based on a good patient–physician relationship. It may be helpful for the physician to realize that the patient's reaction is not conscious or voluntary. Also, to some degree the family and others in the environment participate in the development and management of the emotional disorder. As effective treatment is instituted and physical improvement ensues, the emotional reactions tend to become less severe. For those patients with persistent denial, depression, hostility, or dependency, a psychiatric evaluation or psychotherapy should be considered as part of the treatment.

SUMMARY

- The intertwining factors of life stress, personality factors, and reaction to headache affect essentially all headache patients to some degree. An accurate evaluation of these factors is often difficult because most patients experience a changing susceptibility to these and other stimuli as they change, grow, and adapt, so that these factors may exert an inconsistent and variable influence on headache attacks. However, careful attention to these factors is important for effective evaluation and management of patients with headache.
- Because emotionally stressful factors appear in such a high proportion of pa-

tients with headache, it is important to evaluate these areas in depth. For proper evaluation, the physician must be aware that these areas are often clouded over or denied by patients. Also, some awareness of life stresses and their role in symptom formation are reviewed, such as change, life pace, transitions, work stress, role conflict, and expectations of both patients and physicians.

- Personality factors in migraine have been studied intensively for many years. Earlier studies focused on psychodynamic aspects of repressed anger, compulsiveness, rigidity, and perfectionism in pathogenesis. Recent studies have shown less specificity for these personality factors in migraine (although they are still present in many patients) and very similar dynamics in other types of headache. It is probable that many different stresses or personality factors may activate the unique vascular and/or muscle contraction mechanisms in headache. It is clear that awareness of personality features and characteristics in patients with headache can be useful in both diagnosis and treatment.
- Headaches are often unplanned, unscheduled, and unwanted and may provoke a variety of reactions, depending to a considerable degree on a patient's basic personality. The most common reactions noted in headache patient's are denial, depression, hostility, anger, and the development of dependency. These reactions are usually not conscious or voluntary and will improve with a good patient–physician relationship and/or resolution of symptoms. If they persist, a psychiatric evaluation or psychotherapy may be required.

REFERENCES

Ad Hoc Committee on Classification of Headache; special report (1962). *JAMA 179:*717–718.

Adler, G. (1981). The physician and the hypochondriacal patient. *N. Engl. J. Med. 304:*1394–1396.

Adler, C.L., S.M. Adler, (1982). Psychodynamics of cluster headache *Panminerva Medica 24:*167–172.

Alexander, F. (1950). *Psychosomatic Medicine.* W.W. Norton & Co., New York.

Berkman, L.F. and S.L. Syne (1976). Social class, susceptibility and sickness. *Am. J. Epidemiol. 104:*1–8.

Blumenthal, L.S. (1968). Tension headache. In *Handbook of Clinical Neurology,* Vol. 5 (P.J. Vinken and G.W. Bruyn, eds.), pp. 157–171. North Holland Publishing, Amsterdam.

Blumer, D. (1987). Chronic muscle contraction headache and the pain prone disorder. In *Psychiatric Aspects of Headache* (C.L. Adler, S.M. Adler, and R.C. Packard, eds.). Williams & Wilkins, Baltimore. In press.

Blumer, D. and M. Heilbronn (1981). The pain prone disorder: A clinical and psychological profile. *Psychosomatics 22:*395–402.

Boag, T.F. (1968) Psychogenic headache. In *Handbook of Clinical Neurology,* Vol. 5. (P.J. Vinken and G.W. Bruyn, eds.) pp. 247–257. North Holland Publishing, Amsterdam.

Brett, J.M. (1980). The effect of job transfer on employees and their families. In *Current Concepts in Occupational Stress* (C.L. Cooper and R. Payne, eds.), pp. 99–136. John Wiley & Sons, New York.

Breuer, J. and S. Freud (1955). Case histories. In *The Complete Psychological Works of*

Sigmund Freud, Studies on Hysteria, Vol. 2. (J. Strachey, ed.), p. 23. The Hogarth Press, London.

Brodsky, C.M. (1984). Long-term work stress. *Psychosomatics 25:*361–368.

Christensen, J.F. (1981). Assessments of stress: Environmental intrapersonal, and outcome issues. In *Advances in Psychological Assessment,* Vol. 5. (P. McReynolds, ed.), pp. 62–123. Jossey-Bass, San Francisco.

Cohen, M.J. (1978). Psychophysiological studies of headache: Is there similarity between migraine and muscle contraction headaches? *Headache 18:*189–196.

Dembrosky, T.M., M. Feinleib, S.E. Haynes et al. (1978). *Coronary Prone Behavior.* Springer, New York.

Diamond, S. (1987). Depression and headache. In *Psychiatric Aspects of Headache* (C.L. Adler, S.M. Adler, and R.C. Packard, eds.). Williams & Wilkins, Baltimore. In Press.

Friedman, A.P. (1958). The mechanism and treatment of migraine and tension headache. *Miss. V. Med. J. 80:*141–146.

Friedman, A.P. and C. Brenner (1950). Psychological mechanisms in chronic headache. *Assoc. Res. Nerv. Dis. Proc. 29:*605–608.

Friedman, M. and R.H. Rosenman (1974). *Type A Behavior and Your Heart,* Chapter 13. Fawcett Crest, New York.

Friedman, A.P., J.C. VonStorch, and H.H. Merritt (1954). Migraine and tension headache; A clinical study of two thousand cases. *Neurology 4:*773–774.

Fromm-Reichmann, F. (1937). Contribution to the psychogenesis of migraine. *Psychoanal. Rev. 24:*26–33.

Garrity, T.F., M.D. Marx, and G. Somes (1977). Personality factors in resistance to illness after recent life changes. *J. Psychosom. Res. 21:*23–32.

Girdano, D.A. and G.S. Everly (1979). *Controlling Stress and Tension,* pp. 100–101. Prentice-Hall, Englewood Cliffs, N.J.

Gorlin, R. and H.D. Zucker (1983). Physician's reactions to patients. *N. Engl. J. Med. 308:*1059–1063.

Graham, J.R. (1964). *Treatment of Muscle Contraction Headache, Modern Treatment,* Vol. 1, pp. 1399–1403. Harper & Row, New York.

Graham, J.R. (Oct. 1969). Cluster headache. Presented at the International Symposium on Headache. Chicago, Ill.

Graham, J.R. (1987). The headache patient and the doctor. In *Psychiatric Aspects of Headache* (C.S. Adler, S.M. Adler, and R.C. Packard, eds.). Williams & Wilkins, Baltimore. In press.

Groves, J.E. (1978). Taking care of the hateful patient. *N. Engl. J. Med. 298:*883–887.

Henryk-Gutt, R. and W.L. Rees (1973). Psychological aspects of migraine. *J. Psychosom. Res. 17:*141–153.

Holmes, T.H. and R.N. Rahe (1967). The social readjustment rating scale. *J. Psychosom. Res. 11:* 213–218.

Horenstein, S. (1983). Emotional aspects of neurologic disease. In *Clinical Neurology,* Vol. 4 (A.B. Baker and L.H. Baker, eds.), Chapter 64, pp. 1–3. Harper & Row, Philadelphia.

Horowitz, M.J. (1976). *Stress Response Syndrome,* p. 56. Jason Aronson, Inc., New York.

Ivancevich, J.M. and M.T. Matteson (1980). *Stress and Work,* p. 113. Scott, Foresman and Company, Glenview, Ill.

Jonckheere, P. (1971). The chronic headache patient. *Psychother. Psychosom. 19:*53–61.

Kahana, R.J. and G.L. Bibring (1964). Personality types in medical management. In *Psychiatry and Medical Practice in the General Hospital* (N.E. Zinberg, ed.), pp. 108–123. International University Press, New York.

Knopf, O. (1935). Preliminary report on personality studies in thirty migraine patients. *J. Nerv. Ment. Dis. 82:*270–285.

Kolb, L.C. (1959). Psychiatric and psychogenic factors in headache. In *Headache, Diagnosis and Treatment* (A.P. Friedman and H.H. Merritt, eds.) pp. 259–298. F.A. Davis, Philadelphia.

Kolb, L.C. (1963). Psychiatric aspects of the treatment of headache. *Neurology 13:*34–37.

Kudrow, L. (1979). MMPI pattern specificity in primary headache disorders. *Headache, 19:*18–24.

Kudrow, L. (1980). *Cluster Headache: Mechanisms and Management.* Oxford University Press, London.

Kudrow, L. (1983). Cluster headache; New concepts. In *Neurologic Clinics: Symposium on Headache.* Vol. 1 (R.C. Packard, ed.), pp. 369–383. W.B. Saunders, Philadelphia.

Lance, J.W. (1981). Headache. *Ann. Neurol.* 10:1–10.

Lazarus, R.S. (1981). Little hassles can be dangerous to health. *Psychology Today (July):*58–62.

Lindsay, P.G. and M. Wyckoff (1981). The depression-pain syndrome and its response to antidepressants. *Psychosomatics 2:*571–577.

MacKinnon, R.A. and R. Michels (1971). The psychosomatic patient. In *The Psychiatric Interview in Clinical Practice,* p. 365. W.B. Saunders, Philadelphia.

Marcussen, R.M. (1949). Vascular headache experimentally induced by presentation of pertinent life experiences: Modification of course of vascular headache by alternations of situations and reactions. *Assoc. Res. Nerv. Ment. Dis. Proc. 29:*609–614.

Martin, M.J. (1972). Muscle contraction headache. *Psychosomatics 13:*16–19.

Martin, M.J., H.P. Rome, and W.M. Swenson (1967). Muscle contraction headache; A psychiatric review. *Res. Clin. Stud. Headache 1:*184–204.

Massey, W. and B. Scherokman (1983). Post-traumatic headaches. In *Neurologic Clinics: Symposium on Headache,* Vol. 1 (R.C. Packard, ed.), pp. 457–464. W.B. Saunders, Philadelphia.

Mathew, N. (1987). Headache patients and drug abuse. *In Psychiatric Aspects of Headache* (C.L. Adler, S.W. Adler, and R.C. Packard, eds.). Williams & Wilkins, Baltimore. In Press.

Packard, R.C. (1976). What is psychogenic headache? *Headache 16:*20–23.

Packard, R.C. (1979a). Psychiatric aspects of headache. *Headache 19:*168–172.

Packard, R.C. (1979b). What does the headache patient want? *Headache 19:*370–374.

Packard, R.C. (1980). Conversion headache. *Headache 20:*266–268.

Packard, R.C. (1983). Emotional aspects of headache. In *Neurologic Clinics: Symposium on Headache,* Vol. 1 (R.C. Packard, ed.), pp. 445–456. W.B. Saunders, Philadelphia.

Packard, R.C. (1987). Expectations of patients with headache and their physician. In *Psychiatric Aspects of Headache.* Williams & Wilkins, Baltimore. In press.

Passchier, J., H. VanderHelm-Hylkema, and J.F. Orlebeke (1984). Personality and headache type: A controlled study. *Headache 24:*140–146.

Pearce, J. (1977). Migraine: A psychosomatic disorder. *Headache 17:*125–128.

Phillips, C. (1976). Headache and personality. *J. Psychosom. Res. 20:*535–542.

Rahe, R.A. (1968). Life change measurement as a predictor of illness. *Proc. Roy. Soc. Med. 61:*1124–1126.

Rahe, R.A. (1979). Life change events and mental illness: An overview. *J. Human Stress 5:*2–10.

Rogado, A.Z., R.H. Harrison, and J.R. Graham (1974). Personality profiles in cluster headache, migraine, and normal controls. *Arch. Neurobiol.* 37 (Suppl.):227–241.

Rose, C.L., ed. (1982). *Advances in Migraine Research and Therapy.* Raven Press, New York.

Rose, C.L. and M. Gawel (1979). What brings on a migraine attack? In *Migraine: The Facts,* p. 42. Oxford University Press, London.

Saper, J.R. (1983). Migraine: Precipitating factors. In *Headache Disorders: Current Concepts and Treatment Strategies,* p. 34. Wright-PSG Publishers, Mass.

Schafer, W. (1978). *Stress, Distress and Growth.* International Dialogue Press, Davis, Calif.

Schafer, W. (1983). *Wellness Through Stress Management,* pp. 24–26.

Selinsky, H. (1939). Psychologic study of the migrainous syndrome. *Bull. N.Y. Acad. Med. 15:*757–763.

Selye, H. (1976). *The Stress of Life,* p. 412. McGraw-Hill, New York.

Speed, W.G. (1987). Psychiatric aspects of post-traumatic headache. In *Psychiatric Aspects of Headache* (C.S. Adler, S.M. Adler, and R.C. Packard, eds.). Williams & Wilkins, Baltimore. In Press.

Steinhilber, R.M., J.S. Pearson, and J.G. Rushton (1960). Some psychological considerations of histamic neuralgia. *Proc. Staff Meetings Mayo Clin. 35:*691–699.

Toffler, A. (1971). *Future Shock.* Bantam Books, New York.

Touraine, G.A. and G. Draper (1934). The migrainous patient; A constitutional study. *J. Nerv. Ment. Dis. 80:*1–23.

Trowbridge, L.S., O. Cushman, M.G. Gray, et al. (1943). Notes on the personality of patients with migraine. *J. Nerv. Ment. Dis. 97:*509–517.

Weatherhead, D.L. and R.C. Packard (1987). Conversion headache. In *Psychiatric Aspects of Headache.* Williams & Wilkins, Baltimore. In press.

Weinstein, E.A. and R.L. Kahn (1955). *Denial of Illness.* Charles C Thomas, Springfield, Ill.

Weiss, F. and O.S. English (1957). *Psychosomatic Medicine.* W.B. Saunders, Philadelphia.

Wolff, H.G. (1937). Personality features and reactions of subjects with migraine. *Arch. Neurol. Psychiat. 37:*895–921.

Wolff, H.G. (1963). Cranial pain sensitive structures. In *Headache and Other Head Pain,* 2nd ed., pp. 59–97. Oxford University Press, New York.

23

Behavioral Therapies and Headache

RICHARD A. STERNBACH

BEHAVIORAL ANALYSIS OF PAIN

Because there is no purely objective measure of pain, behavioral signs are very important. Pain may be thought of as a symptom of an underlying disease, as is fever, and thus a nonspecific symptom. But whereas a thermometer can give accurate and repeated readings of the fever, there is nothing comparable in conscious or unconscious animals and humans for measuring pain. We depend on behavior to assess pain.

If a patient says, smilingly, that he or she is in pain, we are not overly impressed with its severity. If a patient, restless and perspiring, tells us the pain is not severe, we are more likely to believe our eyes than our ears. Thus, there are three major kinds of pain behaviors we attend to: verbal, motor, and physiologic, especially autonomic. All three kinds are easily susceptible to conditioning or learning procedures, and so neither words, motor behavior, nor autonomic patterns will bear a perfect relationship to "real" pain, because all reflect sociocultural influences as well as "pure" neurologic activity (Lang et al., 1972).

Fordyce (1976) has pointed out that pain behaviors of all three kinds may be thought of as either respondent or operant. Respondents are elicited by antecedent noxious stimuli, and thus are usually reflexive: the sudden withdrawal, vocalization, and increased pupillary diameter and pulse rate, for example. Such respondents are conditioned in the classic or Pavlovian manner; any stimulus regularly paired with the noxious stimulus will itself acquire the ability to elicit similar responses—the dentist's office, or a parent's angry voice, for example.

In contrast, operants are emitted behaviors governed by the reinforcers that follow them: moaning behavior, rewarded by attention from the family; taking analgesics, rewarded by a decrease in pain; being bedridden, rewarded by respite from unpleasant work but punished by a decline in income. These operations are conditioned in the Skinnerian manner; any behavior followed by a favorable consequence (positive reinforcer) is more likely to recur—it will increase in frequency. Any behavior followed by an aversive consequence (negative reinforcer, punishment) or no positive consequences will be likely to recur. It should be noted that a decrease of pain is usually a positive reinforcer, and whatever diminishes pain is likely to be repeated (or sought).

In practice, one usually encounters chronic pain patients who show a mixture of respondent and operant behaviors. This is usually reflexive behavior to antecedent pathogenic stimulation, and operant behavior maintained by contingent environmental consequences. The analysis of any patient's pain may not be advanced by questions as to "psychogenic" versus "somatogenic," but it may be furthered a great deal by attention to both reflexive respondents and contingent-controlled operants.

Such an analysis of pain abandons the disease model for a learning model. The disease model views pain as a symptom of underlying pathology, and the appropriate treatment is therefore directed toward the presumed cause, which can be diagnosed by appropriate tests. The learning model, on the other hand, views the pain behavior itself as the pathology to be modified, and attention is directed specifically to the operants (Fordyce et al., 1968). Although this may seem to be missing the point, to those accustomed to the traditional approach, and merely a technique to teach a stoicism while leaving "underlying" pain untreated, in fact, measures of subjective pain show improvement in follow-up studies of operant treatment for chronic pain (Fordyce et al., 1973; Ignelzi et al., 1977).

Because much if not most treatment of headaches is empirical rather than directed at "pathology," it follows that a systematic operant conditioning approach should be compatible with such treatment. Certainly for many of the muscle contraction and vascular headaches, the pain *is* the disease, and its elimination constitutes an effective treatment.

OPERANT CONDITIONING

If a person has a site of tissue injury or similar source of noxious stimulation, then respondent pain behaviors are quite likely to be elicited. There is adequate stimulation and automatic responses. Respondents are thus controlled by antecedent stimuli. However, if there is little or inadequate noxious stimulation, it is still possible for pain behaviors to be emitted, because they are receiving effective reinforcement. They are now occurring because of the reinforcing conditions that follow them.

Operant pain behaviors such as moaning, limping, and the like occur as a direct and automatic response to noxious stimulation, as with respondents, but in addition the operants come under the control of environmental consequences. Operant pain behaviors are more likely to occur when followed by positive or reinforcing conditions, or when healthy behaviors are punished or not rewarded. Pain behaviors are less likely to occur when they are not followed by positive reinforcement, or when they are punished and healthy behaviors are rewarded.

Conditioning of behaviors is temporary and can be maintained only by periodic reinforcement. However, once a behavior is in a person's repertoire, the reinforcers need not be frequent. In fact, they may be quite intermittent, and some of the behaviors most resistant to change are those that receive relatively infrequent reinforcement, such as gambling behavior and payoffs, or polysurgical addiction and the desired surgery.

Conditioning effects are usually specific to the conditions under which they take place, but they may generalize. Being ill in bed may bring temporary respite from unpleasant drudgery, and thus be reinforced, but the behavior recurs only in the setting of such drudgery. However, if other needs are met simultaneously by other effects, such as attention from an otherwise negligent spouse, then the sick behavior may occur again when attention is needed, or when the spouse is present.

There is a variety of operant pain behaviors that are troublesome to the patients, their families, and the health care personnel involved. These include limitations of physical activities, work disability, irritability at home, withdrawal from social interactions, hypochondriacal preoccupations, doctor-shopping, polysurgical addiction, and polypharmacy and drug dependence. Most of these represent operants that are reinforced by the satisfaction of dependency needs, but the drug problem is an especially involved one that requires separate consideration.

ANALGESIC USE AND ABUSE

Experience suggests that analgesic overuse is a problem in at least 50% of chronic pain patients in general, and headache patients in particular. In addition to the well-recognized associated problems of addiction, habituation, and toxicity, there is the central problem that the pain can be drug dependent. Many patients' *constant* and daily muscle contraction or vascular headaches are drug dependent. Andersson (1975) has shown that vascular headaches can become ergotamine dependent.

It is a truism that even nonnarcotic analgesics are not entirely benign when used frequently in large amounts: aspirin causes bleeding, phenacetin causes renal damage, acetaminophen causes liver damage. When these agents are combined with narcotics, as they frequently are, significant physiologic as well as behavioral pathology may result.

Fordyce (1976) has shown, by an analysis of the usual medication regimen for pain, how respondent pain can become operant pain—that is, the headache, which may initially occur because of a somatic pain generator, may come under environmental control from the use of medications prescribed for the pain. The result is that the pain is maintained by the analgesic designed to relieve it.

Typically, analgesics are prescribed on an "as-needed" *(prn)* basis. This is particularly true for intermittent pain problems, such as recurrent headaches. The intent is to limit the amount of analgesic ingested in order to avoid the problems just noted. The effect, however, can be the opposite, because of the reinforcing properties of the analgesics on the behaviors they follow (pain, associated affect such as anxiety or depression, other pain behaviors).

All that is necessary for any medication to be a powerful positive reinforcer is that it make the patient feel better. One of the most obvious ways it can make him or her feel better is by reducing the pain. Anything that reduces pain is a positive reinforcer; it increases the likelihood that the immediately preceding behaviors (pain, taking medication) will be repeated. The contingency is established that a feeling of well-being can follow the experience of pain and the expression of pain behaviors.

The effect of the analgesic is not limited to pain relief, however; it may relieve anxiety, counter depression, or treat insomnia. This is particularly important when the patient finds it easier to tolerate physical pain than emotional pain. He or she is likely to interpret or perceive the distressing affect as pain.

In addition to reinforcing (and maintaining) pain, analgesic use also reinforces the physician's prescription writing. The patient in pain is a person who usually demands relief. He or she can be insistent and even obnoxious, challenging the physician's self-image as a competent healer. Inasmuch as it may be impossible to treat the (assumed) underlying pathology, the physician can prescribe the analgesic the patient demands and thus satisfy part of his or her self-concept ("to comfort always"). This is a positive reinforcement. At the same time the physician escapes the unpleasant interaction with the patient, which is another positive reinforcer. Thus, the physician is rewarded for writing the script, as the patient has been for requesting it, and the interaction is therefore more likely to be repeated.

Such doctor–patient transactions are relatively common and subtle; physician and patient frequently manipulate each other in a variety of ways without mutual awareness, playing "pain games" (Sternbach, 1974). These transactions have not been adequately studied, although a beginning has been made. Bond and Pilowsky (1966) found that in patients with advanced cancer, their subjective rating of the severity of their pain did not always generate a proportionate request for analgesics; requests, when made, did not consistently lead to the administration of analgesics; and the strength of the medication was not proportionate to the pain levels. In a follow-up study, Pilowsky and Bond (1969) performed a factor analysis on such interactional data. They found that nursing staffs tended to withhold the stronger drugs from patients who had greater self-concepts of invalidism; but when such patients were women, the nurses more frequently took the initiative and medicated them with stronger analgesics. Older patients were likely to be given weaker medications.

From such data as these, it is obvious that requests for pain relief are not determined solely by the severity of the pain, and the administration of analgesics is influenced by a number of perceptions and motivations.

MANAGING PAIN MEDICATIONS

The patient who overuses medications probably has operant pain, or medication-dependent pain. He or she is probably also physically dependent on the drug, would show withdrawal symptoms if the medication were abruptly discontinued, and has habituated to the effects of the drug (i.e., initial doses no longer suffice to reduce pain). In addition, there are probably obvious and subtle pain behaviors associated with the ingestion of analgesics. Such a patient needs to be withdrawn from the analgesics and any associated drugs of abuse, such as sedatives, hypnotics, and psychotropics. This process almost invariably requires inpatient status, with good nursing supervision.

THE WITHDRAWAL PROCESS

It is not enough merely to detoxify the patient. That could be done by withholding medications and monitoring withdrawal symptoms over a week or two, allowing the patient to go "cold turkey." Only part of the problem is solved this way; no lasting behavior change results. The process should be gradual and systematic, not merely for the patient's physical comfort, but to extinguish the pain behaviors that led to analgesic use and to permit the acquisition and reinforcement of pain-incompatible behaviors.

Experience has shown that, for the withdrawal process to proceed smoothly and to have good long-term effects, several principles must be followed, without exception:

1. There must be *no* injections of *any* distress-relieving medications—analgesics, hypnotics, sedatives, or tranquilizers. Patients develop a "fix on the needle," or psychological dependence on the injection process, probably because of the very rapid and marked effect of the drug administered this way, which is a potent reinforcer.

   A corollary of this principle is that all such medications must be given orally. Rarely, if nausea and vomiting make this impractical, as in some migraine episodes, the drug may be administered *per rectum*. The needle should never be used.

2. Drugs must be given on a fixed time schedule, and never prn. This breaks up the contingent relationship between the pain and the medication. It makes it unnecessary for the patient to have an increase in severity of pain to get the reinforcing substance. Furthermore, by strictly following a regular clock schedule, the pain is not permitted to increase to severe levels nor fluctuate widely in severity, as frequently happen on a prn schedule. Consequently, the patient is kept comfortable, while the reinforcement of pain increments by the analgesic is extinguished.

3. Multiple drug usage should be reduced to the minimum and combined into one "pain cocktail." Patients frequently have been taking several analgesics, such as codeine, propoxyphene, and occasional meperidine. They often are taking several sedatives as well, such as diazepam and phenobarbital. Such combinations are unnecessary and may be reduced to a single agent for each class, representing analgesics, sedatives, and hypnotics.

   Analgesics can be converted into an equivalent dosage of methadone, for example, 5 mg every 6 hours (not to exceed 40 mg), sedatives represented by a sedating antihistamine such as hydroxyzine, and so on (Halpern, 1974). These agents can be combined into a single mix masked by cherry syrup or orange drink with a total volume of 10 cc, given every 4 hours around the clock. As the amount of the active ingredients is decreased each day, the amount of the masking vehicle is increased proportionately, to keep the volume constant (Fordyce, 1976).

   If the patient is depressed, and has a sleep disturbance, an antidepressant with hypnotic qualities can be added to the nighttime mixture. Amitriptyline or doxepin, 75 mg, is an appropriate starting dose. If depression is not a problem but insomnia is, temazepam, 30 mg, can be added to this cocktail.

4. Starting levels and decrements should be set in a manner that keeps the patient comfortable. It is unreasonable to expect analgesics to eliminate pain completely, especially with chronic use, but they should at least "take the edge off." The initial dosage level for 24 hours should be equal to or slightly higher than the amount the patient has actually been taking in a 24-hour period previously, at fixed 3- or 4-hour intervals.

   Dosages should be reduced daily by a rate of 10% of the initial daily dose. Thus, if methadone is given the first day at an adequate total daily amount of 30 mg in six divided doses, it is reduced each day by 3 mg. This should be done by reducing every other divided dose by 1 mg on the second day, reducing the remaining doses to 4 mg on the third day, and so on.

   The purpose of this approach, in addition to keeping the patient comfortable, is to make the daily reductions in strengths small enough, and yet the interval and amounts reliable enough, that the patient need not be preoccupied with the medication issue or the withdrawal process, and can turn his or her attention to more useful matters. Although the patient knows that withdrawal is taking place, the masking vehicle and fixed volume prevent his or her knowledge of the rate; because the patient is not uncomfortable with the withdrawal, he or she is not alarmed.

5. The patient should be kept as busy as is practical, with activities that simulate usual daily activities as much as possible. Merely lounging about in bed or in the hospital room is not satisfactory, because it does not give much opportunity for the production of pain-incompatible behaviors that can be reinforced. Physical therapy, occupational therapy, even volunteering a few hours each day at a work station, permit the shaping of healthy behaviors.

   Patients' whose pain is activity-related learn how to pace themselves to take a rest break before the pain increases. Waiting for an increase in pain severity, then resting, tends to reinforce the pain just as taking analgesics does, because rest is also a positive reinforcer for most persons. Consequently, rest breaks should also be on a fixed time schedule, and the patient can use the time in the hospital to learn an appropriate schedule.

6. An explicit understanding as to what is being done, and why, is essential to success. The patient must agree to the goals and methods of the withdrawal process. If this agreement is not absolutely clear and explicitly stated, it is likely to be doomed to failure: the patient may sabotage the effort by not taking medications when they are delivered, because of absence of severe pain, then requesting the next dose early or simply by leaving the hospital, remaining in bed all the time, or using other similar behaviors.

Similar explicit understandings with the nursing staff are essential. Unless the staff understands the goal and methods of the program, they may sabotage it. They may do so by not delivering the pain cocktail on time or waiting for the patient to ask for it, as they do with prn orders. Or they may not awaken the patient at night. They reinforce pain behaviors by acting sympathetic to complaints of pain instead of praising active healthy behaviors, and so on. All of these problems can be prevented by writing clear and specific orders, and also by conferring frequently with the nursing staff on each shift.

BIOFEEDBACK TECHNIQUES

A particular form of operant conditioning is that which uses biofeedback. This technique consists of detecting, transducing, amplifying, and displaying one of the subject's physiologic functions immediately and continuously. This may be the pulse rate, skin temperature, muscle tone, peripheral blood flow, or electroencephalogram (EEG). A subject who is appropriately motivated or rewarded can learn to increase or decrease the rate or amplitude of the displayed function "at will."

Miller (1969) summarized many carefully controlled animal studies that demonstrate laboratory animals can learn visceral and glandular responses for appropriate reinforcements. Normal human subjects are reinforced in the laboratory by monetary rewards for, say, raising skin temperature above a resting baseline. Patients presumably find the procedure intrinsically rewarding when advised that acquiring such "voluntary" control over a function may enable them to avoid a headache or other symptom.

Clinical experience suggests that most headache patients can acquire the desired response relevant to their symptom in a dozen or so laboratory training sessions. Those who then practice the technique regularly have good long-term results, while those who fail to practice do not.

BIOFEEDBACK FOR MUSCLE CONTRACTION HEADACHES

Budzynski et al. (1973) assigned 18 muscle contraction headache patients to one of three groups: electromyogram (EMG) frontalis muscle biofeedback; a similar group that received false feedback; and a control (no training) group. Auditory feedback was used, and there were 16 sessions of training, each of 20 minutes' duration. The first group showed a significantly lower EMG tension level after 3-month follow-up than the second. Four of six patients in the first group experienced significant improvement in headaches, compared with one in the second group and none in the third. After 18 months, three of four patients contacted from the first group continued improved.

Wickramasekera (1973) gave five patients verbal relaxation training, resulting in a very modest improvement in frontalis muscle EMG activity and headache frequency and intensity. This was followed by EMG biofeedback, which resulted in dramatic decreases in EMG readings and headache activity, maintained in a 9-week follow-up.

McKenzie et al. (1974) reported a clinically significant reduction in headaches in eight patients given 10 training sessions in EEG alpha-biofeedback. They showed greater improvement than eight patients who only listened to relaxation tapes. Results were sustained 2 months later. In a larger study with longer follow-up, two of these authors (Montgomery & Ehrisman, 1976) show that 13 of 22 patients who completed alpha training responded to questionnaires 6 months to 3 years later. They continued to report a statistically significant reduction in frequency and severity of headache.

Warner and Lance (1975) used only relaxation training, one 20-minute training session per week for 4 weeks, and instructed patients to practice daily. Of 17 patients, 13 had daily headaches, and 4 had headaches almost every other day. At 6-month follow-up, four were free of headache, four had one headache per month, three had fewer than one headache per week, and three had headaches as frequently as before, but much less severe. There were similar significant reductions in medication usage.

Bakal (1975) has pointed out that, although such empirical studies may be promising, in fact there is little evidence to relate psychological tension and muscle contraction headaches. He notes that most of these studies have not specified the critical psychologic and physiologic changes underlying the reduction of the headaches.

BIOFEEDBACK FOR VASCULAR HEADACHES

Learned relaxation techniques have been applied to vascular headaches as well as muscle contraction headaches. The rationale, aside from purely empirical results, has been that pain responses and relaxation responses are incompatible and that the latter could prevent the former. Gannon and Sternbach (1971) showed that a patient with post-traumatic vascular headaches could prevent these by entering a learned high-alpha state, although he could not stop a headache already present by this method.

Strictly behavioral methods, without biofeedback methodology but similar effects, have been reported by Mitchell and Mitchell (1971). Seventeen migraineurs were assigned to a relaxation training group, a combined desensitization–relaxation–assertiveness group, or a no-treatment control group. The combined treatment group showed a reduction in frequency and duration of migraine episodes, whereas the other two groups did not. In a second study, 20 migraineurs were assigned to a desensitization–relaxation group, a combined desensitization–relaxation–assertiveness group, or a no-treatment control group. The combined desensitization group showed a significant reduction in frequency and duration of attacks, whereas the desensitization–relaxation group alone was no different from the control group. However, Warner and Lance (1975) reported that simple training in relaxation techniques enabled 8 of 12 patients to reduce migraine episodes more than 50%, and 9 of the patients were able to reduce their medication by more than 30%.

Sargent et al. (1972, 1973) have shown that using autogenic training combined with biofeedback for learning hand warming has resulted in improvement in approximately 75% of 62 migraineurs. Solbach and Sargent (1977) reported on a follow-up survey of 110 patients more than 3 years after treatment. Seventy-four patients completed 270 days of training and follow-up; 76% of this group could be contacted. Thirty-six patients failed to complete the program, and only 33% of this group could be contacted. Those who completed training showed a greater decrease in headache intensity and duration and use of medications.

The concept of using hand-warming techniques rests on the assumption that migraineurs have a vasomotor instability, such that the headache episode is associated with peripheral vasoconstriction and cephalic vasodilatation; by increasing the blood volume in the extremities, there should be a reduced flow and dilatation in the cephalic vasculature, and thus less or no headache.

Elliott et al. (1974) have shown that, in fact, there is impaired reflex vasodilatation in the extremities of migraineurs compared with controls, confirming an earlier report of Appenzeller et al. (1963). In addition, Rickles et al. (1977) used psychophysiologic techniques and multivariate statistical analysis on 13 migraine patients compared with matched controls, and demonstrated individual response stereotypy in the patients. This consisted of cardiovascular variables showing the greatest responses to stimuli, even during headache-free periods, which was different from the response of headache-free controls.

However, although patients may learn to voluntarily control blood flow, temperature biofeedback would not appear to be an efficient technique, because surface temperature is a sluggish response to vasomotor activity, and other variables such as pulse volume would permit faster learning. Actually Koppman et al. (1974) have shown that seven of nine patients rapidly learned to constrict or dilate the superficial temporal artery, using feedback of the pulse volume.

Another problem complicating the whole application of such treatment methods to those with vascular headaches is the assumption of a uniform pathophysiology. Not every one with such headaches is a true migraineur, and certainly not all have peripheral vasomotor changes before or during their attacks. Mixed patient groups may give mixed results with such biofeedback training. Mitch et al. (1976) used autogenic instructions and hand-warming biofeedback on 20 patients: they found that 65% improved on two or more of four measures, and 35% improved on one or none. Ten of the patients were contacted at 6-month follow-up and, in general, they had maintained their improvement; however, the authors observed that those with mixed vascular and muscle contraction headaches were not helped.

Similarly, Medina et al. (1976) did a 1-year follow-up study of 27 patients with migraine or mixed migraine and muscle contraction headache. Patients were trained in both EMG and skin temperature methods, and assessment was made of severity and frequency of headaches and medication usage. Thirteen patients (50%) showed a significant improvement.

CONTROLLED STUDIES AND CRITICAL REVIEWS

It should be noted that controlled experimental studies of biofeedback treatment of headache (and other pain) have generally shown biofeedback to be more effective than no-treatment controls but no better than relaxation or cognitive therapy techniques.

Andrasik and Holroyd (1980) compared three frontalis muscle training techniques in the treatment of tension headache: increasing electromyographic readings, decreasing them, and maintaining them. These were compared with a no-treatment control group. All three treatment groups showed significant and comparable improvement in headaches at 3-month follow-up, and all three were equally superior to the control group.

Kewman and Roberts (1980) obtained comparable results using hand temperature feedback as a treatment for migraine. With double-blind techniques they compared hand-warming and hand-cooling training with a self-monitoring control group. They found no difference in outcome among the groups, with the control and treatment groups showing equivalent improvement. They conclude that it is not the specific temperature training that is effective in clinical outcome studies, but the nonspecific effects of using clinical procedures.

Using anxious college students, not headache patients, Plotkin and Rice (1981) found that either facilitation or suppression of alpha-EEG was effective in reducing anxiety. The anxiety decreased in direct proportion to the students' perceived success and was independent of the direction, magnitude, or duration of EEG changes.

Reviews of such experimental and controlled outcome studies have not supported the claims of uncontrolled clinical trials of biofeedback. Jessup et al. (1979), Turner and Chapman (1982a), and Turner and Romano (1984) concluded that relaxation training is as effective as biofeedback for either muscle contraction or migraine headache.

HYPNOSIS

We have already described hypnoticlike training procedures associated with biofeedback: relaxation training, desensitization, autogenic suggestions, and assertiveness training all involve the giving of instructions or suggestions to patients to produce responses incompatible with pain responses. The same can also be said of hypnosis, which has a longer history.

Unfortunately, the clinical research literature in hypnosis is quite sparse, particularly with respect to headaches. This is surprising, considering how long hypnosis has been used, and the large number of good experimental studies with normal subjects. For some reason, most of the clinical papers on this subject fail to use controls, or objective data, and usually consist of general statements and anecdotal case examples (Blumenthal, 1963; Kroger, 1963). However, Hilgard and Hilgard (1975) have written an excellent review of both the clinical and experimental literature on hypnotic relief of pain. Their review shows that hypnosis may indeed be an effective treatment for headache.

Harding (1961, 1967) reported first on a group of 25 chemotherapy-resistant migraineurs treated by hypnosis. Five had complete relief on follow-up ½ to 2½ years later, and six had 25 to 75% reduction in severity or frequency. He described his method in detail (Harding, 1961). Later, he reported on 90 such patients, with ½- to 8-year follow-up. Thirty-four reported complete relief, and 29 reported 25 to 75% reduction in frequency, duration, or intensity (Harding, 1967). Later, he reported the same 70% success rate for 200 patients (Hilgard & Hilgard, 1975).

Anderson et al. (1975) reported on 47 patients, randomly assigned to hypnotherapy ($N = 23$) or to chemotherapy with prophylactic prochlorperazine ($N = 24$). Monthly evaluations were made for 1 year, using as measures the number of attacks per month, the number who had grade-4 attacks, and the number experiencing complete remission. For those receiving hypnotherapy, the number of attacks and the number of blinding attacks were significantly lower than those of the prochlorperazine group, which did not improve on these two measures. Ten of 23 patients on hypnotherapy obtained complete remission during the last 3 months of the trial, compared with only 3 of 24 on the drug.

Thus, a clinical series and a controlled clinical study show hypnosis to be effective in migraine. Is it merely suggestion, or relaxation that is effective? Stacher et al. (1975) used four subjects and four experimental conditions: (1) waking and hypnotic relaxation suggestions, (2) waking and hypnotic analgesic suggestions, (3) measuring pain threshold, (4) and measuring pain tolerance to electric shock. They found suggestion of analgesia more effective in raising threshold and tolerance than suggestion of relaxation, in both waking and hypnotic states; and suggestions of both relaxation and analgesia were more effective in raising threshold and tolerance in the hypnotic than in waking state. Thus, hypnotic analgesia can most effectively raise pain threshold and pain tolerance.

An interesting comparison was made in a study of the mechanisms of acupuncture analgesia (Mayer et al., 1976). Acupuncture raised pain thresholds to electric shock by 27%, on the average, and its analgesic effects were reversed by the narcotic antagonist naloxone; hypnotic analgesia raised pain thresholds an average of 85%, and its effects were not reversible by this means.

Although the effectiveness of hypnotic analgesia seems fairly certain, its mechanism of action is not clear and is still the subject of much debate. The technique of such hypnosis for migraine, however, is well described by a number of authors. Harding (1961) and Anderson et al. (1975) both suggest control over vasomotor activity. Barber (1977) uses an indirect suggestion of comfort for all pain problems, and Maher-Loughnan (1975) uses intensive, prolonged, and indirect hypnotherapy on resistant cases. It appears that, over the years, clinical hypnosis techniques have tended to become less authoritarian and more permissive, and less magical and more rational in explanations to the patients. This seems to lower patient resistance and increase the rate of success.

Although the number of good clinical studies of hypnosis for headaches is small, the results to date suggest that it may be a useful treatment. Like biofeedback, it should certainly be tried on those resistant to chemotherapy. And considering their benign nature, both hypnosis and biofeedback may well be thought of as the first line of treatment, rather than the last (Finer, 1974). However, it cannot be stressed enough that good controlled studies of hypnosis are woefully lacking (Turner & Chapman, 1982b).

SUMMARY

- Patients with chronic pain usually show a mixture of respondent and operant behaviors. Usually they exhibit reflexive behavior to antecedent pathogenic stimulation and operant behavior maintained by contingent environmental consequences.
- Operant pain behaviors are more likely to occur when followed by positive or reinforcing conditions, or when healthy behaviors are punished or not rewarded.

- Experience suggests that analgesic overuse is a problem in at least 50% of chronic pain patients in general and headache patients in particular.
- Managing pain medications should include withdrawal, avoidance of injections, provision of drugs on a fixed time schedule, when possible, reduction of multiple drug usage, and attempts to increase the patient's activity. The patient must agree to the goals and methods of the withdrawal process.
- A particular form of operant conditioning is that using biofeedback. Electromyographic feedback may be useful for muscle contraction headaches. Autogenic training with associated hand warming has been shown to improve patients with migraine.
- Hypnosis may also be an effective treatment for headache, but controlled clinical studies have not been done.

REFERENCES

Anderson, J.A.D., M.A. Basker, and R. Dalton (1975). Migraine and hypnotherapy. *Int. J. Clin. Exp. Hypn. 23:*48–58.

Andersson, P.G. (1975). Ergotamine headache. *Headache 15:*118–121.

Andrasik, F. and K.A. Holroyd (1980). A test of specific and nonspecific effects in the biofeedback treatment of tension headache. *J. Consult. Clin. Psychol. 48:*575–586.

Appenzeller, O., K. Davison, and J. Marshall (1963). Reflex vasomotor abnormalities in the hands of migrainous subjects. *J. Neurol. Neurosurg. Psychiatry 26:*447–450.

Bakal, D.A. (1975). Headache: A biopsychological perspective. *Psych. Bull 82:*369–382.

Barber, J. (1977). Rapid induction analgesia: A clinical report. *Am. J. Clin. Hypn. 19:*138–147.

Blumenthal, L.S. (1963). Hypnotherapy of headache. *Headache 2:*197–122.

Bond, M.R. and I. Pilowsky (1966). Subjective assessment of pain and its relationship to the administration of analgesics in patients with advanced cancer. *J. Psychosom. Res. 10:*203–208.

Budzynski, T.H., J.M. Stoyva, C.S. Adler, and D.J. Mullaney (1973). EMG biofeedback and tension headache: A controlled outcome study. *Psychosom. Med. 35:*484–496.

Elliott, K., D.B. Frewin, and J.A. Downey (1974). Reflex vasomotor responses in the hands of patients suffering from migraine. *Headache 13:*188–196.

Finer, B. (1974). Clinical use of hypnosis in pain management. In *Advances in Neurology,* Vol. 4 (J. Bonica, ed.), pp. 573–579. Raven Press, New York.

Fordyce, W.E. (1976). *Behavioral Methods for Chronic Pain and Illness.* C.V. Mosby, St. Louis.

Fordyce, W.E., R.S. Fowler, Jr., J.F. Lehmann, and B.J. DeLateur (1968). Some implications of learning in problems of chronic pain. *J. Chronic Dis. 21:*179–190.

Fordyce, W.E., R.S. Fowler, Jr., J.F. Lehmann et al. (1973). Operant conditioning in the treatment of chronic pain. *Arch. Phys. Med. Rehabil. 54:*399–408.

Gannon, L. and R.A. Sternbach (1971). Alpha enhancement as a treatment for pain: A case study. *J. Behav. Ther. Exp. Psychiatry 2:*209–213.

Halpern, L.M. (1974). Psychotropic drugs and the management of chronic pain. In *Advances in Neurology,* Vol. 4 (J. Bonica, ed.), pp. 539–546. Raven Press, New York.

Harding, H.C. (1961). Hypnosis and migraine or vice versa. *Northwest Med. 60:*168–172.

Harding, C.H. (1967). Hypnosis in the treatment of migraine. In *Hypnosis and Psychosomatic Medicine* (J. Lassner, ed.), pp. 131–134. Springer-Verlag, New York.

Hilgard, E.R. and J.R. Hilgard (1975). *Hypnosis in the Relief of Pain.* Kaufmann, Los Altos, Calif.

Ignelzi, R.J., R.A. Sternback, and G. Timmermans (1977). The pain ward follow-up analyses. *Pain 3:*277–280.

Jessup, B.A., R.W.J. Neufeld, and H. Merskey (1979). Biofeedback therapy for headache and other pain: An evaluative review. *Pain 7:*225–270.

Kewman, D.G. and A.H. Roberts (1980). Skin temperature biofeedback and migraine headaches, a double blind study. *Biofeedback Self Regul. 5:*327–345.

Koppman, J.W., R.D. McDonald, and M.G. Kunzel (1974). Voluntary regulation of temporal artery diameter by migraine patients. *Headache 14:*133–138.

Kroger, W.S. (1963). Hypnotherapeutic management of headache. *Headache 3:*50–62.

Lang, P.J., D.G. Rice, and R.A. Sternbach (1972). The psychophysiology of emotion. In *Handbook of Psychophysiology* (N.S. Greenfield and R.A. Sternbach, eds.), pp. 623–643. Holt, Rinehart and Winston, New York.

Maher-Loughnan, G.P. (1975). Intensive hypnoautohypnosis in resistant psychosomatic disorders. *J. Psychosom. Res. 19:*361–365.

Mayer, D.J., D.D. Price, J. Barber, and A. Rafii (1976). Acupuncture analgesia: Evidence for activation of pain inhibitory system as a mechanism of action. In *Advances in Pain Research and Therapy,* Vol. I. (J. Bonica and D. Albe-Fessard, eds.), pp. 751–754. Raven Press, New York.

McKenzie, R.E., W.J. Ehrisman, P.S. Montgomery, and R.H. Barnes (1974). The treatment of headache by means of electroencephalographic biofeedback. *Headache 13:*164–172.

Medina, J.L., S. Diamond, and M.A. Franklin (1976). Biofeedback therapy for migraine. *Headache 16:*115–118.

Miller, N.E. (1969). Learning of visceral and glandular responses. *Science 163:*434–445.

Mitch, P.S., A. McGrady, and A. Iannone (1976). Autogenic feedback training in migraine: A treatment report. *Headache 15:*267–270.

Mitchell, K.R. and D.M. Mitchell (1971). Migraine: An exploratory treatment application of programmed behavior therapy techniques. *J. Psychosom. Res. 15:*137–157.

Montgomery, P.S. and W.J. Ehrisman (1976). Biofeedback alleviated headaches: A follow-up. *Headache 16:*64–65.

Pilowsky, I. and M.R. Bond (1969). Pain and its management in malignant disease: Elucidation of staff-patient transactions. *Psychsom. Med. 31:*400–404.

Plotkin, W.R. and K.M. Rice (1981). Biofeedback as a placebo: Anxiety reduction facilitated by training in either suppression or enhancement of alpha brainwaves. *J. Consult. Clin. Psychol. 49:*590–596.

Rickles, W.H., M.J. Cohen, and D.L. McArthur (1977). A psychophysiology study of ANS response patterns in migraine headache patients and their headache free friends. Paper presented at 19th annual meeting of the American Association for the Study of Headache, San Francisco.

Sargent, J.D., E.E. Green, and E.D. Walters (1972). The use of autogenic feedback training in a pilot study of migraine and tension headaches. *Headache 12:*120–124.

Sargent, J.D., E.D. Walters, and E.E. Green (1973). Psychosomatic self-regulation of migraine headaches. *Semin. Psychiatry 5:*415–428.

Solbach, P. and J.D. Sargent (1977). A follow-up evaluation of the Menninger pilot migraine study using thermal training. Paper presented at 19th annual meeting of the American Association for the Study of Headache, San Francisco.

Stacher, G., P. Schuster, P. Bauer et al. (1975). Effects of suggestion of relaxation or analgesia on pain threshold and pain tolerance in the waking and in the hypnotic state. *J. Psychosom. Res. 19:*259–265.

Sternbach, R.A. (1974). *Pain Patients: Traits and Treatment.* Academic Press, New York.

Turner, J.A. and C.R. Chapman (1982a). Psychological interventions for chronic pain: A critical review. I. Relaxation training and biofeedback. *Pain 12*:1–21.

Turner, J.A. and C.R. Chapman (1982b). Psychological interventions for chronic pain: A critical review. II. Operant conditioning, hypnosis, and cognitive-behavioral therapy. *Pain 12*:23–46.

Turner, J.A. and J.M. Romano (1984). Evaluating psychological interventions for chronic pain: Issues and recent developments. In *Advances in Pain Research and Therapy*, Vol. 7 (C. Benedetti, C.R. Chapman, and G. Moricca, eds.), pp. 257–296. Raven Press, New York.

Warner, G. and J.W. Lance (1975). Relaxation therapy in migraine and chronic tension headache. *Med. J. Aust. 1*:298–301.

Wickramasekera, I. (1973). The application of verbal instructions and EMG feedback training to the management of tension headache—preliminary observations. *Headache 13*:74–76.

24

Cervicogenic Headache

OTTAR SJAASTAD

It is generally believed in the West that although headache may originate in the cervical spine, this is indeed a rare phenomenon. There is also a general confusion about how headache originating from the neck materializes clinically. Our own studies of chronic paroxysmal hemicrania (CPH), a strictly unilateral headache, led us to believe that headache might be closely associated with disorders in the neck (Sjaastad et al., 1982). More than four years ago, we started recognizing a group of patients with a strictly unilateral headache, but a temporal pattern quite different from those of cluster headache and CPH. We have come to believe that this headache does originate in the neck and is a *cervicogenic headache* (Sjaastad et al., 1984). We have by now seen more than 30 patients who form a rather homogeneous picture: mostly female, relatively young patients (the mean age of onset around 30), who can provoke attacks by certain head and neck movements, as can patients with CPH.

In cervicogenic headache, the pain is a head pain and not just a neck and facial pain, it's *main* manifestation usually in the temporal, frontal, and ocular areas (Sjaastad et al., 1983). When particularly severe, the pain is occasionally felt on the opposite side as well. Attacks usually last hours to days. Some ipsilateral phenomena are frequently associated with the attack: slight lacrimation, conjunctival injection, nasal secretion/stenosis, tinnitus, moderate facial flush and in a few cases, we have observed lid edema, particularly of the lower lid. Ipsilaterally reduced vision is also noted fairly frequently. During severe attacks, migrainous phenomena, such as nausea, loss of appetite, vomiting, and phono- and photophobia, may occur. Dizziness is sometimes a symptom, and swallowing may be hindered. Ipsilateral, diffuse shoulder and arm pain is experienced by a number of patients. *Overt* Horner's syndrome has not been observed. There may be crepitation, and neck movements may be painful and restricted. Most patients are able to provoke attacks apparently identical to the spontaneously occurring ones by certain acts, such as moving the neck, coughing, sneezing, and bowel movements. Keeping the head in a locked position for a prolonged period may be a sufficient stimulus to provoke an attack. Awkward nocturnal positioning of the head may give rise to morning headache. Just like in CPH, even longlasting attacks may be precipitated by firm digital pressure on certain tender spots on the symptomatic side of the neck. These spots are located over the C_2 root, over the great occipital nerve, and over the transverse processes of C_4/C_5.

WHY IS THIS HEADACHE PROBABLY OF CERVICAL ORIGIN?

There are several pieces of evidence pointing to a cause and effect relationship between cervical disorders and cervicogenic headache: neck movements or pressure against certain trigger points precipitate attacks; stiffness and pain occur in the neck, with crepitation on movements; there is reduced motility of the neck; there is vague, annoying homolateral shoulder-, arm-, and hand-pain. Jointly these findings indicate the presence of a unilateral cervical disorder. Furthermore, ipsilateral local anesthetic blocks of the C_2 (and at times also C_3) root during the symptomatic periods resulted in complete or partial relief in 9 of 11 patients in our studies (Sjaastad et al., 1983). The latter findings seem to correspond to those of Hunter & Mayfield (1949), who carried out local anaesthetic blocks of the second cervical root. This eliminated pain in patients with a traumatic background (8 cases), but only alleviated it in those with a nontraumatic background (3 cases). The second sensory cervical root was then cut intraspinally on the symptomatic side, after which the pain disappeared completely (for an unspecified time period)—in our estimation, a most relevant observation. Unfortunately, these findings seem to have been neglected. Their patients were similar to ours in most respects (i.e., recurring unilateral attacks of headache, always appearing on the same side, with pain spreading to the entire head during the most severe attacks; attacks of varying duration, but usually rather long-lasting; the pain starting in the suboccipital region and spreading forward to the vertex and eye area; occasional vomiting and giddiness; excessive tenderness in the occipital/suboccipital area and ipsilateral tinnitus, tearing, nasal stenosis, and flushing of the face), although age of onset, female preponderance, visual disturbances, swallowing difficulties were not mentioned.

Immediate and durable results by uncoforaminectomy have been obtained by Kehr et al. (1976), who found an 87% success rate in the cervicocephalic syndrome with a corresponding figure in cases of pure headache of 78%. Grønbæk (1982) and Pasztor (1978) have reported similar results in their cases. We have no information about similar results in ordinary migraine.

We do not know whether this type of headache invariably stems from primary disorders of the spine itself. Consequently, we have purposely not used the term *vertebragenic* for this type of headache, which would purport that the headache derives from a lesion in the vertebra as such. In our opinion the term cervicogenic headache is the correct one, at this stage at least, since it seems to be a *neutral* term. Cervicogenic indicates the *region* where the headache originates and does not pinpoint the structure primarily affected. The term *migraine cervicale* should be abandoned, since this implies that we are faced with a migraine. The term *cervical headache* is not an adequate one either because this may convey the impression that the headache pain is *sited* in the cervical area and *not* that the pain *originates* in the neck.

Cervicogenic headache is strictly unilateral. Probably bilateral cases exist, (i.e., cases exhibiting unilaterality on both sides) and maybe such cases are more frequent than presently believed. However, unilateral cases may be diagnosed with reasonable certainty at the present time, whereas the diagnostic error may be unacceptably high in bilateral cases. We have a strong feeling that if we were to include bilateral cases

Table 24-1 Cervicogenic headache: Differential diagnostic aspects versus cluster headache and chronic paroxysmal hemicrania (CPH)

	Cluster headache	CPH	Cervicogenic headache
Sex	90% males	Female preponderance (approx 90% ?)	2/3 females (?)
Attack duration	+ +	+	+ + +
Frequency of attacks	1–3/day	>15/day (?)	1–3 (?)/week
Severity of pain	+ + +	+ + +	+(+)
Mechanical precipitation	−	+ +	+ + +
Overt Horner's syndrome	+(−)	−	−
Effect of indomethacin	−	+ + +	(+)
Effect of lithium	+ + +	− *	−
Ergotamine effect	+ +	−	−
Corneal indentation pulse (CIP) amplitude and intraocular pressure increase during attack	+	+	−

*CPH patients even deteriorate on lithium.

in scientific approaches in this field, we might once more bring discredit on the whole field. Bilateral cases should, therefore, be kept apart from unilateral cases for the time being.

DIFFERENTIAL DIAGNOSIS AND PATHOGENESIS

As for the diagnosis of cervicogenic headache, it must be differentiated from other unilateral headaches. Cervicogenic headache differs clearly from cluster headache and CPH in attack duration, attack frequency, and attack severity (Table 24-1). Supplementary test findings and drug effects also differ greatly from those in the two other groups. In groups of patients, there is thus a rather clear difference between these diagnostic categories; in the individual, however, differential diagnostic difficulties may arise. Particularly in the chronic cluster headache patient, such as when the characteristic cluster phenomenon is lacking, the differential diagnostic problems may be considerable. As a matter of fact, Hunter & Mayfield's cases (1949) have been misinterpreted as being cluster headache cases.

The differential diagnosis versus the ordinary, common migraine may also be intricate. In the diagnosis of cervicogenic headache, its strict unilaterality and ipsilateral associated phenomena (the tinnitus, rhinorrhea, conjunctival injection, lacrimation, the vague arm pains, etc.) are of importance. Emphasis should also be placed on symptoms and signs pertaining to the cervical spine. The visual disturbances in migraine proper are frequently bilateral and homonymous. The visual disturbances in cervicogenic headache are monocular and ipsilateral. Scintillating scotomata, as in classic migraine, have not been described in cervicogenic headache. One old migraine criterion that has been forgotten more or less in recent years, that the headache should alternate sides from one attack to the other (Graham, 1968) ought to be re-adopted. In ordinary migraine, attacks usually are not "sidelocked," although there probably are exceptions to this. We have probably also seen such cases, although rarely.

Thus we are probably faced with a distinct group of patients that differs in important respects from migraine patients. This group should be separated from migraine as far as categorization is concerned. It also differs from the other universally accepted headache groups, as listed in the National Institute of Neurological Disease and Blindness ad hoc committee's classification system (1962). Employing our criteria, this headache does not appear to be a rare one, contrary to the prevailing view in Western countries.

Etiology and pathogenesis in the cervicogenic headache are only very vaguely understood at present. It may well be that the uncovertebral joints (Krogdahl & Torgersen, 1940) play a fundamental role in the pathogenesis of this headache, although the pathogenesis in some cases may be somewhat more intricate and sophisticated (Hildebrandt & Jansen, 1984; Jansen & Spoerri, 1984). As far as the nosological status of this headache is concerned we are inclined to believe that groups like Barré's *syndrome sympathique cervical posterieur* (1926) and Bärtschi-Rochaix' *migraine cervicale* (1968) are rather similar. We do not feel convinced, however, that their cases represent distinct, homogeneous groups of patients. Headache of cervical origin, cervicogenic headache, is a controversical issue, and the time has come to sort out the controversies pertaining to this headache.

REFERENCES

Barré, M. (1926). Sur un syndrome sympathique cervical posterieur et sa cause frequente: 1. arthrite cervicale. *Rev. Neurol.* (Paris) *33*:1246–1248.

Bärtschi-Rochaix, W. (1968). Headache of cervical origin. In *Handbook of clinical neurology, Vol 5. Headache and cranial neuralgias* (Vinken, P.J. and G.W. Bruyn, eds.), pp. 192–203. North Holland Publishing Co., Amsterdam.

Graham, J.R. (1968). Migraine. Clinical aspects. In *Handbook of clinical neurology, vol V. Headache and cranial neuralgias* (Vinken P.J. and G.W. Bruyn, eds.), pp. 45–58. Amsterdam: North-Holland Publishing Co.

Grønbæk, E. (1982). Traumatic cervical pain generators. Abstract from scientific exhibition: *Scand. Neurosurgical Society 34 annual meeting, Trondheim, Norway.*

Hildebrandt, J. and J. Jansen (1984). Vascular compression of the C_2 root—yet another cause of intermittent hemicrania. *Cephalalgia 2*:167–170.

Hunter, C.R. and F.H. Mayfield (1949). Role of the upper cervical roots in the production of pain in the head. *Am J. Surg 48*:743–751.

Jansen, J. and O. Spoerri (1984). Atypical fronto-orbital pain and headache—due to compression of upper cervical roots. In *Proceedings of the 1. International Headache Congress Munich Sept. 1983*. (V. Pfaffenrath, P.O. Lundberg, and O. Sjaastad, eds.), pp. 14–16. Springer, Berlin.

National Institute of Neurological Disease and Blinness Ad hoc committee on classification of headache. (1962). *JAMA 179*:717–718.

Kehr, P., G. Lang, and F.M. Jung (1976). Uncusektomie und Uncoforaminektomie nach Jung. *Langenbecks Arch. Chir. 341*:111–125.

Krogdahl, T. and O. Torgensen (1940). Die "Unco-Vertebralgelenke" und die "Arthroses deformans uncovertebralis." *Acta Radiol. (Stockh). 21*:231–262.

Pasztor, E. (1978). Decompression of vertebral artery in cases of cervical spondylosis. *Surg. Neurol. 9*:371–377.

Sjaastad, O., D. Russell, C. Saunte, and I. Hørven (1982). Chronic paroxysmal hemicrania. VI. Precipitation of attacks. Further studies on the precipitation mechanisms. *Cephalalgia 2*:211–214.

Sjaastad, O., C. Saunte, and H. Breivik (1984). Chronisch-paroxysmale Hemikranie. Eine Sonderform des Zervikogenen (vertebragenen) Kopfschmerzes? In *Primäre Kopfschmerzen. Pathogenese, Diagnostic und Therapie* (V. Pfaffenrath, A. Schrader, and I.S. Neu, eds.), pp. 9–16. MMV Medizin Verlag, München.

Sjaastad, O., C. Saunte, H. Hovdal, H. Breivik, E. Grønbæk (1983). "Cervicogenic" headache. An hypothesis. *Cephalalgia 3*:249–256.

25

Clinical Observations on Headache

DONALD J. DALESSIO

INCIDENCE

The most common headaches are those associated with mood disorders, particularly depression, anxiety, and emotional tension. Next most commonly encountered are vascular headaches of the migraine type and associated variants including cluster headache. The headaches provoked by fever and septicemia probably rank next in frequency, and then come those due to nasal and paranasal, ear, tooth, and eye disease. The headaches of meningitis, intracranial aneurysm, brain tumor, and brain abscess, though very important and singularly dramatic, are less common.

INTENSITY

The most intense headaches are those due to ruptured intracranial aneurysm, meningitis, fever, migraine, and those associated with arterial hypertension. The subarachnoid hemorrhage resulting usually from ruptured intracranial aneurysm produces a headache that is sudden in onset, reaches great intensity in a very short time, and may be associated with feelings of faintness or with unconsciousness. The onset of pain is soon followed by the development of a stiff neck and the presence of blood in the lumbar spinal fluid. The intense headache of meningitis is accompanied by a very stiff neck, which prevents passive flexion of the head on the chest. The spasm of the muscles of the neck associated with the intense headaches of migraine may also inhibit flexion of the neck.

The intensity of the headaches associated with brain tumors, brain abscesses, sinus disease, and tooth and eye disease is usually only moderately severe. Hemorrhage into the parenchyma of the brain may not cause headaches unless the hemorrhage breaks through into the ventricular or subarachnoid spaces; then intense headache may result. Also, hemorrhage into a brain tumor causing additional and serious displacement of the brain may result in severe headache.

QUALITY OF HEADACHE

The headaches of fever, migraine, and hemangiomatous tumors, and those associated with arterial hypertension are characteristically throbbing or pulsating in quality. Headache associated with emotional tension or resulting from secondary muscle contraction from eye or sinus disease has the quality of tightness or external pressure or may be bandlike, caplike, or viselike. The headache of brain tumor and of meningitis, though occasionally pulsating, is usually of a steady aching quality.

SITE

Vascular headaches of the migraine type may occur anywhere in the head and face. The most common site of migraine headache is the temple. Migraine headache at times involves both right and left sides, although any one attack may be strictly unilateral. The headache of tooth, sinus, or eye disease is usually in the front of the head shortly after its onset, roughly in the region near the site of stimulation; subsequently, the pain may be predominantly in the back of the head and neck as a result of secondary muscle contraction. Headaches associated with pituitary adenomas and parasellar tumors are often bitemporal.

The headaches of posterior fossa tumors, early in the development of the tumor and before the beginning of general brain displacement, are usually over the occiput or behind the ear. Headaches from supratentorial tumors, before serious brain displacement occurs, are usually in the front or on top of the head. Occasionally, if the tumor involves the dura and the bone, the headache may be near or over the site of the lesion. Early in the course of the tumor or before general displacement of the brain has occurred, the headache is usually on the same side as the tumor.

Subdural hematoma produces a headache of considerable intensity, usually localized over or near the site of the lesion, most commonly over the frontoparietal areas. The headache may be intermittent but is usually present for some time each day, over a period of weeks, months, or longer. A history of almost continuous headache from the date of injury is characteristic.

The headaches associated with tumors of the cerebellopontine angle and acoustic neurinoma are often localized in the postauricular region. Like other brain tumor headaches, they are intermittent and of moderate intensity. They are associated with hyperalgesia of the postauricular region on the same side as the tumor. Headache is one of the earliest manifestations of acoustic neurinoma; it is a later manifestation of cerebellopontine angle tumors.

The headache or pressure sensations associated with emotional tension are usually first evident and most intense in the neck, shoulders, and occiput, but later spread to include the frontal region. They may be unilateral or bilateral.

Disease involving the dome of the diaphragm or the phrenic nerve causes pain high in the shoulder and neck. Similarly, in rare instances coronary occlusion and myocardial insufficiency cause pain in the lower jaw, high in the neck, and in the occiput. Disease and dysfunction of structures below the diaphragm induce headache only indirectly through fever, sepsis, or bacteremia.

TENDERNESS

Tenderness in the region of the dilated cranial arteries on the outside of the head and sometimes diffusely over the slightly edematous and aching side of the head may be conspicuous during vascular headache of the migraine type and for some hours thereafter. Also, there may be tenderness of the skin of the face as a result of inflammation of the nasal and paranasal spaces, of the teeth, and of the ear. Muscle in a state of sustained contraction, secondary to pain anywhere in the head, may become tender on palpation. Thus, brushing and combing the hair may be a painful experience during or after migraine headache. With myositis and myalgia there may be tender areas in the muscles of the head and neck. Because of the hyperalgesia, percussion of the head may cause pain over or near an underlying brain tumor.

Periostitis secondary to frontal, ethmoid, or sphenoid sinus disease or mastoiditis produces a pain of moderate to severe intensity associated with local tenderness at the site of disease. If the pain is sufficiently severe and continuous, it may become generalized. The tenderness or hyperalgesia associated with mastoid disease with periostitis is far greater than the hyperalgesia associated with posterior fossa brain tumor.

Tenderness at the site of a head injury, and often that associated with a scar, may persist for many years. Also, in post-traumatic headache tender muscles or nodules often occur in parts of the head remote from the site of injury. Headache of the vascular type akin to migraine with tenderness over the arteries may be initiated by head injury.

EFFECTS OF MANUAL PRESSURE

Pressure on the temporal, frontal, supraorbital, postauricular, occipital, and common carotid arteries often reduces the intensity of migraine headache and that associated with arterial hypertension. Support of the head makes any patient with headache feel more comfortable. The pain of chronic muscle contraction headache may be intensified by firm manipulation of tender muscles or regions of tenderness. Conversely, gentle massage and simple measures of physical therapy including heat and hot packs not infrequently produce muscular relaxation and relieve this form of headache.

EFFECTS OF POSITION AND BODY MOVEMENT

In many instances vascular headache of the migraine type is made worse by assuming a horizontal position and is relieved by an erect position. It is often made worse by ascending stairs, by moving about rapidly, or by lifting objects. Sitting quietly in an upright position often proves to be most comfortable. The lying-down position may at first intensify the headache associated with nasal and paranasal disease, but subsequently the headache subsides. A sudden change in position—usually from lying down to sitting up, and less frequently from sitting up to lying down—may make the headache of brain tumor more intense. Unlike the migraine headache, the headache of brain tumor is often worse when the patient is in the upright position. The head-down position aggravates most headaches, except those due to spinal drainage and occasionally those associated with brain tumor. Muscle tension headache is usually reduced in intensity by movements of the head and neck, which extend the contracted muscles.

Straining at stool and coughing increase all but muscle contraction headaches and those due to spinal drainage. Sharp flexion or extension of the head often reduces the intensity of postpuncture headache, whereas jugular compression increases the headache.

A major criterion that can be used in the diagnosis of cluster headache is the behavior of the patient during the attack. Pacing, walking, sitting, and rocking during the attack are considered pathognomonic of this disorder. Frantic activity may occur. There is no other primary headache disorder in which such behavior is an associated feature.

THE EFFECT OF HEAD JOLT

Headaches known to arise primarily from dilatation of pain-sensitive intracranial vessels, particularly arteries (i.e., the headache that follows the intravenous administration of histamine, that induced by hypoglycemia, and the headaches of fever, systemic infection, "hangover," postpuncture reaction, and the early postconcussion state), are easily aggravated by even mild head jolting. Patients with headaches known to arise primarily from inflammation of pain-sensitive intracranial arteries and veins and their adjacent structures (i.e., the headaches accompanying meningitis and those following ventriculography or pneumoencephalography) are particularly sensitive to head jolting. The threshold of jolt headache during these states may be depressed 2.0 to 3.0 g or more. In patients with intracranial masses (i.e., subdural hematoma or brain tumor), the threshold of jolt headache is usually depressed and the location of the headache induced by jolting may indicate the side of the lesion. The threshold of jolt headache may be lowered in relatively infrequent instances of vascular headaches of the migraine type that have a portion of their origin within the cranial cavity.

On the other hand, headaches arising from structures on the outside of the head (i.e., muscle tension headache, most migraine headaches, and the headache induced by the injection of hypertonic saline into the temporal muscle) are not significantly intensified by head jolting, and the threshold of jolt headache is not lowered.

CHRONOLOGICAL FEATURES

Vascular headaches may be as brief as 20 or 30 minutes, or may last for days or, rarely, for weeks. The usual headache is terminated within 24 hours. A striking feature of migraine is the freedom from headache between prostrating attacks. The headaches of brain tumor are intermittent but usually occur during part of every day, varying in intensity from time to time. Headache associated with chronic sinus disease is intermittent, but quite predictable; it may occur during the working hours of each day for weeks or even months. Muscle contraction headache or pressure sensations associated with sustained tension and anxiety may persist for days, weeks, or even years.

Headaches associated with hypertension and migraine most commonly have their onset in the early hours of the morning so that the patient awakens with the pain. Such migraine headaches characteristically diminish in intensity in the evening. Headaches of the cluster type very commonly occur during the sleeping hours from 12 to 2 A.M. The headache of brain tumor, if it is connected in any way with the time of day, is more severe in the early part of the day, though not in the early hours of the morning. The headache associated with nasal and paranasal disease usually begins and is worse in the morning and improves toward the late afternoon or when the patient retires. Headache associated with eye disease usually begins in the latter part of the day or evening. Muscle contraction headache or pressure sensations are usually worse at the end of the working day.

Vascular headaches of the migraine type are common during weekends, during the first period of vacation holidays, and immediately after vacation. They are very common just before the onset of menstruation. Patients with migraine-type headache often have fixed days of the week when their headaches occur.

Headache associated with nasal and paranasal disease is usually more common during periods when upper respiratory infections prevail, namely, the darker months of the year. Migraine headache occurs during periods of increased conflict, tension, or stress for the individual—for example, during early fall for the schoolteacher, during rush or holiday seasons for the merchant, during very hot or humid weather for those who feel ineffective and prostrated during such climatic states. Exacerbations of tic douloureux are common in the spring and fall, notably in March and October. The same may be true for cluster headaches.

Headaches that begin in childhood or at puberty and recur especially with menstruation and at certain fixed intervals over many years are, in all likelihood, of the migraine variety. The migraine variety of headache often stops at menopause. On the other hand, they occasionally begin at this time.

SUSTAINED CONTRACTION OF MUSCLE

Contractions of the muscles of the head and neck occur with all headaches. If the contractions are of sufficient duration, they themselves become a cause of headache. Headache and a very stiff neck accompanied by Kernig's sign are associated with widespread meningitis. Kernig's sign may be absent even late in the course of a carcinomatous invasion of the meninges at the base of the brain. Headache and stiff neck are common with tumors of the posterior fossa, but the stiff neck may be overcome by persuasion and the passive movements of the head by the examining physician.

Contraction of the muscles of the neck, head, and back may become so great with meningitis that the muscles cannot be relaxed and the patient assumes the position of opisthotonus. With posterior fossa tumors muscle spasm may cause tilting of the head or lifting of the shoulder. The muscle contraction headache associated with prolonged anxiety and tension may cause backward tilting of the head and half closing of the eyes. Muscle contraction is often an accompaniment of migraine headache and is one explanation of the slow relief afforded by ergotamine tartrate to some patients in whom this is a major component.

MUCOUS MEMBRANE INJECTION

Redness and swelling of the mucous membranes of the nose with or without nose-bleeds may occur with migraine. Also injection of the conjunctiva may be seen. The mucous membrane injection and engorgement may be conspicuous and give rise to headache in those with allergic sensitivities to inhaled dusts and pollens and in those in whom the nasal mucous membranes are involved during periods of major adaptive difficulties. With the rare exception of headache resulting from neoplastic invasion of paranasal structures and antral infection via the dental route, no headache associated with disease of the nasal and paranasal sinuses occurs without obvious congestion of the turbinates and nasal mucous membranes.

GASTROINTESTINAL DISTURBANCES

Anorexia, nausea, and vomiting, though most commonly associated with vascular headache of the migraine type, may be associated with any headache, and the more intense the headache the more likely these symptoms are to occur. Vomiting without nausea may occur with brain tumors, especially those of the posterior fossa. Nausea and vomiting with little or no headache may occur in persons with migraine. The headache associated with sinus or eye disease is seldom associated with vomiting. Constipation is commonly associated with migraine, although diarrhea also occurs. Distention and flatulence are common in migraine and tension headaches but are seldom associated with other headaches.

POLYURIA

Polyuria is commonly associated with migraine headache attacks and seldom occurs with other headaches. Tension states with headaches may be linked with frequency of urination.

VISUAL DISTURBANCES

Both scintillating scotomata and visual field defects, such as unilateral or homony-mous hemianopia, may occur with migraine headaches. Such defects in vision may occur with brain tumor headaches when the tumor is due to a lesion of the occipital lobes or is adjacent to the visual pathways. The visual disturbances of migraine, with the exception of blurred vision and diplopia, seldom occur with the headache but usually precede it. They are usually short-lived, that is, under 1 hour. Enlarged pupils and lacrimation may cause faulty vision during a migraine headache, but when defects in visual acuity or in the fields of vision outlast the headache attack, it is likely that a cerebral vascular accident or brain tumor is the cause. Defects in color vision and colored rings about lights may occur with headache associated with glaucoma. Ptosis of the eyelid may be an accompaniment of the headache of brain tumor or of a berry aneurysm of the circle of Willis, especially in the latter case when linked with a fixed and dilated pupil. Ptosis also occurs with ophthalmoplegic migraine, a symptom complex involving paresis of the muscles supplied by the third cranial nerve, and occasionally also of those supplied by the fourth and sixth cranial nerves. It usually has its onset late in the headache attack, persists for days or weeks, and is due to edema of tissue near or about the affected cranial nerves. Partial closure of the eyes due to edematous lids or to muscle contraction may lead to the complaint of faulty vision.

Horner's syndrome may appear as a manifestation of cluster headache. Photophobia is associated with any headache experienced chiefly in the front or top of the head. It is commonly noted in patients with meningitis, migraine, nasal and paranasal disease, eye disease, brain tumor, and muscle contraction headache. Injection of the sclera and conjunctiva may accompany such photophobia. If the intensity of the pain is very great, photophobia, lacrimation, and sweating of the homolateral forehead and side of the face also occur.

When headache is linked with papilledema, it is usually due to an expanding intracranial mass. However, in patients with brain tumor, headache often occurs without papilledema, and papilledema without headache. In the advanced phase of hypertensive encephalopathy, headache and papilledema are usual. Ruptured aneurysm and subdural hematoma may cause intense headache without papilledema. Ruptured intracranial aneurysms are sometimes accompanied by retinal hemorrhages, which when unilateral usually occur on the same side as the rupture. Meningitis does not affect the eye grounds except possibly to induce slight suffusion. During migraine headache, unilateral arterial and venous dilation in eye grounds may occur.

VERTIGO AND OTHER SENSORY DISTURBANCES

Vertigo may be a forerunner of a migraine headache attack. Vertigo is sometimes associated with the headaches of brain tumors, although feelings of unsteadiness are more common. Fleeting vertigo with sudden movement or rotation of the head often accompanies the post-traumatic headache and muscle tension headache.

Meniere's or the labyrinthine syndrome is occasionally associated with headache. Other sensory disturbances such as paresthesias of the hands and face may occur as a forerunner of the migraine headache. However, paresthesias that persist during or outlast the headache attack are more common in patients with brain tumors and in those with epilepsy.

MOOD

The wish to retire from people and responsibilities, a dejected, depressed, irritable, or negativistic mental state bordering on prostration or stupor is a dominant aspect of the migraine attack and may in some instances be more disturbing than the pain in the head. Apathy, listlessness, or even euphoria may be associated with brain tumor headache.

The headache associated with muscle tension may occur in a tense, irritable person, but the patient is usually more willing to accept attention, massage, or medication than the patient with a migraine headache attack, who commonly expresses the wish to be left alone. Exaltation or feelings of special well-being are rare sequels to the migraine headache attack. The suffering experienced with the headache of fever, meningitis, or ruptured aneurysm may be very great, but the mental state is that of reaction to severe pain.

SLEEP

Vascular headaches of the migraine type, even of the most severe type, do not disrupt sleep entirely, except for short periods. Those of brain tumor, sinus disease, and muscle contraction permit sleep. Therefore, when an individual complains of long periods of sleep loss because of headache, it is well to consider anxiety or depression as the dominant aspect of the illness. The headache of meningitis usually interrupts sleep. Migraine headaches of the vascular type may also occur after periods of excessively prolonged or very deep sleep.

Cluster headache often occurs during REM sleep.

FAMILY HISTORY

The headache of migraine and that associated with arterial hypertension are the only familial headaches.

CLINICAL PATHOLOGIC ABNORMALITIES AND HEADACHE

Slight elevations in body temperature are common during migraine headache attacks. Fever may be associated with the headache of carcinomatous meningitis and brain tumor.

Any fever, especially that during the onset of an infection, may be associated with headache. Unusually intense during this phase are the headaches of typhoid and typhus fever and "grippe." Headache may be the earliest manifestation of an infection.

The combination of headache, fever, and a very stiff neck is common with meningitis, meningismus, and blood in the subarachnoid space.

Chilly sensations and hot flashes without change in body temperature are common in patients with migraine attacks and the headache associated with muscle contraction. The headache of brain abscess is commonly accompanied by periodic elevations of temperature.

SOME OLD CLINICAL SAWS THAT NEED COMMENT

Unilaterality

If headache is always on the same side, should one suspect an aneurysm? What does it mean to have a persistent focal headache? Does a unilateral headache suggest aneurysm? Should the patient be studied? Are angiograms indicated?

The patient's history must be taken seriously, but is the patient providing the diagnosis, or is the history confusing both patient and physician? Focal headaches imply focal disease. The clinician should be alert for local infection such as sinusitis or inflammation (cranial arteritis) or diseases of the facial organs including the eyes and nose. He or she should also be concerned about endocrine and metabolic diseases, especially diabetes.

But if the headache is typically migrainous, or suggests cluster headache, then it should be accepted as such. Aneurysms are, by and large, nonpainful entities. Angiomas do not often produce pain. Angiomas may rupture, bleed, clot, calcify, provoke seizures, and eventually inhibit learning, but they do not usually hurt.

Many patients with migraine always have their headache on the same side, and there is no requirement that the headache must shift from side to side. This first maxim, then, has produced many unnecessary studies and evoked much needless worry among clinicians. If focal disease is not present, the clinician should accept the persistent repetition of unilateral throbbing head pain as compatible with vascular headache of several types, including migraine and cluster headaches.

Association of Vascular Lesions and Migraine

Are aneurysms common in patients with migraine? Migraine is a common disease; aneurysms are uncommon. It is reasonable to assume that the two entities may occasionally appear in the same patient, but there is little evidence that the two syndromes are related. Asymptomatic aneurysms are asymptomatic. If an aneurysm begins to expand rapidly, it will produce a particularly severe localized pain that is not likely to be mistaken for recurrent vascular headache.

Those aneurysms that do rupture evoke catastrophic headache, with associated neurologic signs and symptoms, related to a sterile inflammatory reaction produced by the presence of blood in the subarachnoid space.

Is migraine a common feature of cerebral arteriovenous anastomoses? It is true that angiomas may leak briefly and repeatedly. Because the source of the bleeding is usually from anomalous, often venous blood vessels, and not an artery, the headache is not as intense as in subarachnoid bleeding. If sufficient blood is liberated into the subarachnoid space, signs of meningeal irrigation also occur, indistinguishable from those associated with subarachnoid bleeding produced by the rupture of a typical berry aneurysm.

Hemispheric angiomas may produce almost any neurologic sign or symptom related to bleeding, calcification, and the production of seizures. Large angiomas may also produce headache.

Is headache therapy straightforward and easy, once the diagnosis is made? Successful treatment of a patient with headache may not be accomplished easily. The care and sympathy with which the physician relates to his patients is indispensable to effective management of each individual headache problem. Cures should not be promised. It is enough to advise the patient that attempts will be made to reduce the intensity and frequency of his or her headaches. The art of medical practice may be more important than scientific pharmacology. Patience and perseverance on the part of both physician and patient may be necessary. The physician may find his or her therapeutic suggestions have not brought forth the desired result. It is important, then, not to become angry at the patient. Sometimes simple structuring of the environment will help the patient modify some of his or her life goals. At times the patient will demand a type of practical office psychotherapy, an informal program directed toward guidance and reeducation of emotional responses. With careful attention to the whole patient, some resolution of the problem can be achieved in the majority of headache complaints. If the physician suspects a serious thought disorder, psychiatric consultation is mandatory.

Allergy

Is migraine frequently caused by allergy? It has not been possible to demonstrate that migraine results from any significant or specific antigen–antibody reaction, whether the antigen be an inhaled pollen, an injected material, or food. There is no specific correlation between positive skin tests for various allergens and the appearance of migraine.

Dietary migraine may be related to the ingestion of vasoactive substances in a person predisposed to overactivity of vasomotor responses. Thus, long trials of hyposensitization to presumed allergens are not indicated in the chronic treatment of migraine. Hives, allergic rhinitis, etopic eczema, bronchial asthma, and other manifestations of true allergic reactions cannot be equated with the migraine episode.

Brain Tumor

Is severe headache a common sign of brain tumor? Headache is certainly one of the cardinal signs of brain tumor, particularly of rapidly expanding tumors producing traction on the pain-sensitive structures of the head. This is especially the case if the ventricular system is compromised by obstruction of absorption or flow of cerebrospinal fluid, causing traction hydrocephalus. Headache is sometimes a prominent finding with increased intracranial pressure. But with more slowly growing tumors, headache may be transitory, mild, or easily relieved by common analgesics, and the patient's description of the head pain in this situation may be desultory. The worst head pains are not usually related to tumor but to vascular headaches or the major neuralgias. Some generalizations concerning headache and the localization of brain tumor seem justified, nonetheless:

1. Although the headache of brain tumor may be referred from a distant intracranial source, it approximately overlies the tumor in about one third of all patients.
2. If the tumor is above tentorium, the pain is frequently at the vertex, or in the frontal regions.
3. If the tumor is below the tentorium, the pain is occipital, and cervical muscle spasm may be present.
4. Headache is almost always present with posterior fossa tumor.
5. If the tumor is midline, it may be increased with cough or straining or sudden head movement. (This also occurs with migraine.)
6. If the tumor is hemispheric, the pain is usually appreciated on the same side of the head.
7. If the tumor is chiasmal, at the sella, the pain may be referred to the vertex.

How important are these clinical observations? Perhaps they are of modest value. The history of headache in patients with brain tumor is helpful most often when there is no previous history of headache; sudden appearance of headache in an adult should suggest an organic lesion of the brain. If the clinician feels that some pathologic process is producing headache, then the workup should be parsimonious and should search out suspected causes of headache in a logical fashion. The use of CT techniques for the examination of the cranial contents is suggested. More aggressive and potentially damaging studies such as arteriograms should not be done for the complaint of headache alone.

Is headache characteristic of chronic hydrocephalus (normal pressure hydrocephalus)? The clinical picture in occult hydrocephalus or the hydrocephalic syndromes includes disturbances of gait, mentation, and micturition. Almost all patients with this problem have a disturbance in gait, varying from slight disability to total inability to walk. When these patients are tested carefully by an experienced psychometrist, almost all of them will demonstrate significant mentational difficulties, particularly impairment of memory, distractibility, and inability to maintain attention and concentration span. Later, incontinence of sphincters occurs. It is not usually appreciated as urgency but almost always represents the incontinence of dementia, in which concern for incontinence is lacking or reduced or micturition may be performed in front of others, much as a child would. Problems with bowel incontinence are considerably less common, though flatus is often expelled without concern for social niceties. It should be emphasized that sphincter incontinence is almost always a late sign and is rarely seen early in the course of this disease.

Other symptoms of the hydrocephalic syndrome include dizziness, lightheadedness, faintness or weakness, falling spells, and brief episodes of unconsciousness. Complaints of headache, which is often the primary symptom of acute hydrocephalus, are absent.

MIGRAINE EQUIVALENTS

Migraine may express itself in forms other than hemicranial pain, and these different modes of expression are known as migraine equivalents. The equivalents are paroxysmal, recurrent symptom complexes characterized by the following:

1. No demonstrable organic lesion.
2. Previous history of typical migraine headache.
3. Replacement of headaches by the equivalent syndrome.
4. Absence of symptoms between attacks.
5. Family history of migraine.
6. Relief from the equivalent syndrome using appropriate drugs.

Migraine equivalents may take many forms, including abdominal, ophthalmic, and psychic.

Abdominal migraine is characterized by recurrent episodes of vomiting and/or abdominal pain in association with symptoms of the migraine attack. It is the most common visceral manifestation of migraine. Although it has been reported in patients from infancy to old age, it is most common between the ages of 2 and 11 years, and males are most often affected. Abdominal migraine is often characterized by a prodromal period of yawning, listlessness, drowsiness, or the typical aura of the migraine attack. The episode usually starts suddenly and is precipitated by a specific or stressful experience. The pain may be situated anywhere in the abdomen, but is usually epigastric or periumbilical. The individual bout of pain varies in severity, usually lasts 1 to 6 hours, and is frequently characterized by severe nausea and vomiting. There may also be associated a typical headache, constipation or diarrhea, lethargy, stuporous sleep, or irritability. Electroencephalography performed during the attack may show a mild generalized dysrhythmia.

Ophthalmic migraine is also a reasonably well-recognized syndrome, characterized by temporary scotomas, amblyopias, or hemianopsias that mark the height of the migraine attack instead of acting as a prodrome to the unilateral headache. Many of these patients are men. Some may develop ophthalmic migraine without the subsequent headache.

Psychic migraine is probably more common than realized and is characterized by transient mood disorders or psychotic states that replace a typical unilateral headache. Often there is a short prodromal period of lethargy or vigor, followed by a mood disorder lasting from a few hours to days. Many patients experience similar symptoms prior to a typical migraine attack, but in psychic migraine no headache occurs.

Various autonomic dysfunctions are common in patients with migraine. These include Raynaud's phenomenon, flushing, and even on occasion hemorrhage into the skin. Recurrent febrile episodes as a migraine equivalent have been reported. Recently three young women were seen who had reasonably typical migraine, and in addition, a not clearly defined form of connective tissue disease, perhaps a mixed connective tissue disease or Sjogren's syndrome.

Some migraine equivalents may be associated with intracranial vasoconstriction. For example, visual cortical ischemia almost certainly produces ophthalmic migraine, although the retinal artery may be involved as well. Cortical, subcortical, thalamic, or hypothalamic ischemia could evoke transient mood disorders. Ischemia in the thermal regulatory center could cause the febrile equivalent. Sensory or motor strip ischemia causes minor hemiplegic equivalents, with subsequent local cerebral edema causing the major hemiplegias. Ischemia in autonomic diencephalic centers would be capable of causing abdominal migraine.

GENERAL REMARKS ON THERAPY

Counseling

There are three basic approaches to migraine therapy: the symptomatic approach using medications to abort the acute attack; a preventive approach using methods of prophylaxis; and, finally, prevention by encouraging adjustments in the patient's behavior to avoid situations or substances known to precipitate migraine.

Once the diagnosis is established, it is good practice to educate the patient about his or her disorder, with a detailed description of suspected mechanisms and common precipitating factors. Contributing psychological factors should also be noted with encouragement for the patient to communicate personal feelings about what has been presented. Patients are often relieved to find out that their head pain is neither secondary to an organic disease nor "merely" psychogenic.

Abortive versus Prophylactic Therapies

The frequency and duration of migraine attacks are the principal criteria for deciding between the abortive and the prophylactic approach. If the migraine attacks occur two or more times a month, each attack lasting a day or more, then it is appropriate to consider prophylaxis.

It is important to provide the patient with treatment alternatives that cover all of the potential types of head pain identified in the history. Migraine patients often suffer from muscle contraction headaches, either as an independent syndrome or as a consequence of muscle tension remaining after the migraine attack. Also, some patients on prophylactic medications experience "breakthrough" migraine attacks. Abortive medications can be used in this contingency; one should also identify under what circumstances the patient should contact the physician during an attack for further treatment.

All medications in the proposed treatment regimen should be discussed in relation to latency periods, side effects, and complications. With patients on supplemental or replacement estrogen therapy, some adjustments in dose and scheduling may be desirable. Also, patients with a history of chronic head pain often develop a strong overreliance on analgesics. It is always important to consider the possibility of an established pattern of drug abuse and to provide specific guidance about the use or avoidance of pain medications other than those prescribed.

Continuing Care

A headache calendar is a useful tool for refinement of the therapeutic approach. When the treatment regimen is prescribed, the patient can be shown how to maintain this record of pain episodes, using codes to indicate headache characteristics and associated factors, such as menses, diet, and physical or psychological states. This record helps the physician analyze the effectiveness of the prescribed regimen and ascertain what additional steps might be constructive.

Since migraine is a recurrent disorder, medical management is required on a periodic basis. A typical pattern of continuing care would be a follow-up visit 1 month after prescription of the initial treatment regimen, again in 6 weeks, and every 2 weeks to 3 months thereafter. At each visit, the patient's vital signs can be obtained, the effects of the medication reviewed, and the headache calendar examined.

SPECIFICS ON MEDICATION

Abortive Treatment of the Acute Attack

Analgesics

If taken during the early states of a migraine attack, aspirin and other nonnarcotic analgesics such as acetaminophen and propoxyphene may raise the pain thresholds of some patients enough to give relief. If nausea and tension are associated problems, analgesics can be combined with sedatives or antiemetics.

If the patient gets more than one or two migraines a month, analgesics are not likely to provide satisfactory control of migraine pain. However, because many migraine patients have muscle contraction headaches in addition to, or as an aftermath of, their migraine attacks, it is likely that they will continue to use analgesics for head pain relief. For that reason, it is important for the physician to inquire circumspectly about a migraine patient's use of analgesics, to advise the patient about the consequences of overuse, and to encourage use of alternative coping strategies.

Ergot Alkaloids

If migraine attacks occur less than twice a month with relatively short durations, then ergotamine tartrate is the drug of choice for abortive therapy. Ergotamine is an alpha-adrenergic blocking agent with a direct stimulating effect on the smooth muscle of peripheral and cranial blood vessels, and produces depression of central vasomotor centers in the brain. It is also a serotonin antagonist. Some preparations combine ergotamine with additives: caffeine to increase the rate of absorption and to aid vasoconstriction; and sedatives to control anxiety.

To effectively abort a migraine attack, ergotamine must be taken soon after onset and in adequate dosage. Patients should be advised to carry the drug with them for immediate availability.

Side Effects of Ergotamine

Frequent use may cause ergotamine-bound headaches, adding to the pain problems that already exist. Other side effects reported by patients who abuse ergotamine include worsening headaches, drowsiness, anorexia, and cold extremities. Long-term, uninterrupted use may cause severe vasoconstriction and endarteritis. In very rare instances this may result in gangrene of the extremities.

Ergotamine tartrate is contraindicated in patients with hypertension, occlusive vascular disease, renal or hepatic disease, severe pruritus, sepsis, hypersensitivity to ergot alkaloids, and pregnancy.

Isometheptene

A combination product containing primarily isometheptene (Midrin), which produces vasoconstriction through indirect adrenergic stimulation, is also effective in migraine, especially for those patients who cannot take ergot products.

Prophylactic Treatment of Migraine

If the patient has two or more migraine attacks a month, or only one migraine that lasts for several days, abortive therapies will have inherent limits. First, even if the abortive medications are effective, the patient still suffers some unavoidable disability during the initial hours of the attack. Second, the frequent use of ergot alkaloids may produce adverse side effects. Finally, some patients do not tolerate ergotamine very well, and for others ergotamine is contraindicated. For these patients, prophylaxis should be considered.

Methysergide

Methysergide—prescribed as a 2-mg tablet used two to four times daily—is the oldest medication specifically indicated for migraine prophylaxis. It acts as a serotonin antagonist by a mechanism that is still unclear. An important disadvantage of methysergide therapy is that it must be interrupted for a period of 3 to 4 weeks after each 6-month course of treatment to avoid the rare but dangerous side effect of retroperitoneal and pleuropulmonary fibrosis. Less dangerous side effects such as nausea, dizziness, abdominal pain, drowsiness, and leg pain may also limit its usage in some patients.

Beta-Blockers

Mode of Action

Beta-adrenergic blocking agents are widely used in antihypertensive therapy and prophylaxis of angina pectoris, and are indicated for the prophylaxis of common migraine.

Their prophylactic effect against migraine occurs because of a nonselective blocking action that alters neural stimulation, not only of the beta-1 receptors, found primarily in the heart, but also of the beta-2 receptors, found primarily in the arterioles. If the beta-2 receptors were stimulated, they would cause the smooth muscle to relax, which contributes to vasodilation. When these beta-2 receptors are blocked by propranolol, alpha-receptor activity in the smooth muscle is unopposed and the result is increased vascular tonus.

Contraindications

Beta-adrenergic blockers are contraindicated in (1) bronchial asthma, (2) allergic rhinitis during the pollen season, (3) sinus bradycardia and greater-than-first-degree block, (4) cardiogenic shock, (5) right ventricular failure secondary to pulmonary hypertension, (6) congestive heart failure, and (7) patients on adrenergic-augmenting psychotropic drugs (including MAO inhibitors), and during the 2-week withdrawal period from such drugs.

Dosage Schedule for Propranolol Hydrochloride in Migraine

Dosage must be individualized often beginning with an initial dose of 80 mg of propranolol daily, in divided doses. The usual effective dose is between 80 and 160 mg. The dosage may be increased gradually to achieve optimum migraine prophylaxis.

If a satisfactory response is not obtained within 4 to 6 weeks, or after reaching a maximum dose of 240 mg per day, then propranolol therapy should be discontinued. It may be advisable to withdraw the drug gradually over a period of several weeks.

Nadolol is also effective in migraine prophylaxis, in dosages of 80 to 160 mg per day, as is Timolol in dosages of 30 mg per day.

Calcium-Channel Antagonists

The calcium-channel antagonists (CCA) affect the influx of calcium into vascular smooth muscle, and so alter the ability of vessels to constrict. Although they may therefore be perceived as vasodilators, their ability to alter excessive vasomotor reactivity at least provides a theoretical basis for their use in the prophylaxis of migraine. Some CCAs are selective for intracerebral as opposed to peripheral blood vessels.

Preliminary studies have established that several of these compounds, including nimodipine, nifedipine, verapamil, flunarizine, and cinnarizine, are effective in headache prophylaxis. In addition, other drugs known to be useful in headache prophylaxis, including cyproheptadine and amitriptyline, have been shown to have significant calcium antagonistic properties and can be considered as nonspecific calcium-channel antagonists.

The exact role of the CCA in the treatment of migraine (and cluster headache) remains to be determined. It seems likely, however, that this novel class of vasoactive compounds will prove useful in the prophylaxis of several types of vascular headache.

INDEX